Amputation Rehabilitation

Editors

ALEX DONAGHY
ALBERTO MIRANDA

PHYSICAL MEDICINE AND REHABILITATION CLINICS OF NORTH AMERICA

www.pmr.theclinics.com

Consulting Editor
BLESSEN C. EAPEN

November 2024 • Volume 35 • Number 4

ELSEVIER

1600 John F. Kennedy Boulevard • Suite 1800 • Philadelphia, Pennsylvania, 19103-2899

http://www.theclinics.com

PHYSICAL MEDICINE AND REHABILITATION CLINICS OF NORTH AMERICA Volume 35, Number 4
November 2024 ISSN 1047-9651, 978-0-443-29690-1

Editor: Megan Ashdown
Developmental Editor: Nitesh Barthwal

Reprints. For copies of 100 or more of articles in this publication, please contact the Commercial Reprints Department, Elsevier Inc., 360 Park Avenue South, New York, NY 10010-1710. Tel.: 212-633-3874; Fax: 212-633-3820; E-mail: reprints@elsevier.com.

Physical Medicine and Rehabilitation Clinics of North America (ISSN 1047-9651) is published quarterly by Elsevier Inc., 360 Park Avenue South, New York, NY 10010-1710. Months of issue are February, May, August, and November. Business and Editorial Offices: 1600 John F. Kennedy Blvd., Suite 1800, Philadelphia, PA 19103-2899. Customer Service Office: 3251 Riverport Lane, Maryland Heights, MO 63043. Periodicals postage paid at New York, NY and additional mailing offices. Subscription price per year is $352.00 (US individuals), $100.00 (US students), $400.00 (Canadian individuals), $100.00 (Canadian students), $506.00 (foreign individuals), and $210.00 (foreign students). For institutional access pricing please contact Customer Service via the contact information below. Foreign air speed delivery is included in all *Clinics* subscription prices. All prices are subject to change without notice. Orders, claims, and journal inquiries: Please visit our Support Hub page https://service.elsevier.com for assistance.

Physical Medicine and Rehabilitation Clinics of North America is indexed in *Excerpta Medica, MEDLINE/ PubMed (Index Medicus), Cinahl,* and *Cumulative Index to Nursing and Allied Health Literature.*

Contributors

CONSULTING EDITOR

BLESSEN C. EAPEN, MD
Division of Physical Medicine and Rehabilitation, David Geffen School of Medicine at UCLA, VA Greater Los Angeles Health Care System, Los Angeles, California

EDITORS

ALEX DONAGHY, MD
Clinical Assistant Professor, Physician, Department of Physical Medicine and Rehabilitation, University of Michigan, Ann Arbor, Michigan

ALBERTO MIRANDA, MD
Health Sciences Associate Clinical Professor, Department of Medicine, David Geffen School of Medicine at UCLA, Department of Physical Medicine and Rehabilitation, Greater Los Angeles VA Healthcare System, Los Angeles, California

AUTHORS

SHALIZ AFLATOONI, BS
Morsani College of Medicine, University of South Florida, Tampa, Florida

MATTHEW N.M. BARTELS, MD, MPH
Professor and Chair, Department of Rehabilitation Medicine, Montefiore Medical Center, Albert Einstein College of Medicine, Bronx, New York

THOMAS M. BEACHKOFSKY, MD, FAAD
Dermatologist, Dermatology Department, James A. Haley Veterans' Hospital; US Department of Veterans Affairs, Tampa, Florida

KATE BEEKMAN, BS
Morsani College of Medicine, University of South Florida, Tampa, Florida

WAYNE T. BIGGS, BS, CPO
Regional Clinical Director, Regional Amputation Center, Rehabilitation Care Services, VA Puget Sound Health Care System, Seattle, Washington

CHRISTOPHER A. BONILLA, MD, MS
Department of Physical Medicine and Rehabilitation, Veterans Affairs Puget Sound Health Care System, Seattle, Washington

ERIC BRUNK, DO
PM&R Resident Physician, Department of Physical Medicine and Rehabilitation, Johns Hopkins University School of Medicine, Baltimore, Maryland

MERIDETH BYL, DO, MBA
PM&R Resident, Department of Physical Medicine and Rehabilitation, Greater Los Angeles Veteran Affairs HealthCare System, Division of PM&R, Department of Medicine, UCLA Health, Los Angeles, California

MARY E. CALDWELL, DO, FAAPMR, CAQSM
Assistant Professor, Department of Physical Medicine and Rehabilitation, Residency Assistant Program Director, VCU Physical Medicine and Rehabilitation, Virginia Commonwealth School of Medicine, Medical Director of Sportable, Richmond, Virginia

NICOLETTE CARNAHAN, PhD
Assistant Professor, Department of Physical Medicine and Rehabilitation, Johns Hopkins University School of Medicine, Baltimore, Maryland

JUAN CAVE II, MSPO, CPO
Advanced Research Prosthetist-Orthotist, Department of Rehabilitation Medicine, University of Minnesota, Minneapolis VA Health Care System, Minneapolis, Minnesota

PAUL S. CEDERNA, MD
Professor, Department of Biomedical Engineering, Robert Oneal Collegiate Professor of Plastic Surgery, Department of Surgery, University of Michigan Medical School, Ann Arbor, Michigan

ALEX DONAGHY, MD
Clinical Assistant Professor, Physician, Department of Physical Medicine and Rehabilitation, University of Michigan, Ann Arbor, Michigan

MICHAEL GALLAGHER, MD, MA
Department of Physical Medicine and Rehabilitation, Veterans Affairs Puget Sound Health Care System, Seattle, Washington

ANDREW GITKIND, MD
Associate Professor, Vice Chair, Department of Rehabilitation Medicine, Montefiore Medical Center, Albert Einstein College of Medicine, Bronx, New York

MARLÍS GONZÁLEZ-FERNÁNDEZ, MD, PhD
Associate Professor, Department of Physical Medicine and Rehabilitation, Johns Hopkins University School of Medicine, Baltimore, Maryland

MARLIS GONZÁLEZ-FERNÁNDEZ, MD, PhD
Associate Professor, Department of Physical Medicine and Rehabilitation, Johns Hopkins University School of Medicine, Baltimore, Maryland

AMNA HAIDER, DO
Physician, Department of Physical Medicine and Rehabilitation, Johns Hopkins University School of Medicine, Baltimore, Maryland

ELIZABETH G. HALSNE, PhD, CPO
Principal Investigator, Department of Rehabilitation Medicine, University of Washington, Seattle, Washington

JEFFREY T. HECKMAN, DO
Collaborative Associate Professor, Morsani College of Medicine, University of South Florida, Medical Director, James A. Haley Veterans' Hospital & Clinics, Tampa, Florida

ALISON W. HENDERSON, PhD
Research Scientist, VA Center for Limb Loss and Mobility (CLiMB), VA Puget Sound Health Care System, Seattle, Washington

KERRY HENNESSY, MD
Dermatologist, Department of Dermatology and Cutaneous Surgery, Morsani College of Medicine, University of South Florida, Tampa, Florida

MICHAEL JASON HIGHSMITH, PhD, DPT, CP, FAAOP
Orthotic, Prosthetic & Pedorthic Clinical Services (OPPCS) Program Office (12RPS4), Rehabilitation and Prosthetic Services, US Department of Veterans Affairs, Washington, DC; School of Physical Therapy and Rehabilitation Sciences, Morsani College of Medicine, University of South Florida, Tampa, Florida

CHAD M. HIVNOR, MD, FAAD
Dermatologist, Dermatology Department, US Department of Veterans Affairs, South Texas Veterans Health Care System, San Antonio, Texas

LINDSEY HOLBROOK, PhD
Neuropsychology Fellow, Department of Physical Medicine and Rehabilitation, Johns Hopkins University School of Medicine, Baltimore, Maryland

RACHEL C. HOOPER, MD
Clinical Assistant Professor, Section of Plastic Surgery, Department of Surgery, University of Michigan Medical School, Ann Arbor, Michigan

BRANDON KALASHO, DO
PM&R Resident, Department of Physical Medicine and Rehabilitation, Greater Los Angeles Veteran Affairs HealthCare System, Division of PM&R, Department of Medicine, UCLA Health, Los Angeles, California

BRIAN KELLY, DO
Professor, Division of Orthotics and Prosthetics, Department of Physical Medicine and Rehabilitation, University of Michigan Medical School, Ann Arbor, Michigan

MARY S. KESZLER, MD
Physiatrist, Department of Physical Medicine and Rehabilitation, Johns Hopkins University School of Medicine, Baltimore, Maryland

ERIC M. LAMBERG, EdD, PT, CPed
Associate Dean, School of Health Professions-Dean's Suite, Professor, Department of Physical Therapy, Stony Brook University, President, American Amputee Soccer Association, Stony Brook, New York

MARY E. MATSUMOTO, MD
Medical Director, Department of Physical Medicine and Rehabilitation, Regional Amputation Center, Minneapolis VA Health Care System, Minneapolis, Minnesota

DAVID C. MORGENROTH, MD
Assistant Professor, VA Center for Limb Loss and Mobility (CLiMB), VA Puget Sound Health Care System, Seattle, Washington

DANIEL C. NORVELL, PhD
Investigator, VA Center for Limb Loss and Mobility (CLiMB), VA Puget Sound Health Care System, Seattle, Washington

SANJOG PANGARKAR, MD
Professor, Department of Physical Medicine and Rehabilitation, David Geffen School of Medicine at UCLA, Greater Los Angeles Veterans Affairs Healthcare System, Los Angeles, California

QUYNH GIAO PHAM, MD
Professor, Department of Physical Medicine and Rehabilitation, David Geffen School of Medicine at UCLA, Greater Los Angeles Veterans Affairs Healthcare System, Los Angeles, California

STEPHANIE RAND, DO
Residency Program Director, Assistant Professor, Department of Rehabilitation Medicine, Montefiore Medical Center, Albert Einstein College of Medicine, Bronx, New York

JOHN SHAFFER, CPO
Prosthetist, Department of Rehabilitation Medicine, University of Minnesota, Minneapolis VA Health Care System, Minneapolis, Minnesota

AMAAN SHEIKH, DO
PM&R Resident, Department of Physical Medicine and Rehabilitation, Johns Hopkins University School of Medicine, Baltimore, Maryland

PETER R. SHUMAKER, MD
Dermatologist, Dermatology Department, US Department of Veterans Affairs, Veterans Administration San Diego Healthcare System, San Diego, California

GEOFFREY SIEGEL, MD
Associate Professor of Surgery, Division of Musculoskeletal Oncology, Department of Orthopedic Surgery, University of Michigan Medical School, Ann Arbor, Michigan

YUNNA L. SINSKEY, MD
Department of Physical Medicine and Rehabilitation, Mary Free Bed Rehabilitation Hospital, Grand Rapids, Michigan

REBECCA A. SPECKMAN, MD, PhD
Medical Director, Regional Amputation Center, Rehabilitation Care Services, VA Puget Sound Health Care System, Assistant Professor, Department of Rehabilitation Medicine, University of Washington, Seattle, Washington

MARY CATHERINE SPIRES, MD
Professor, Department of Physical Medicine and Rehabilitation, University of Michigan, Ann Arbor, Michigan

TUSHARA SURAPANENI, MD
Physician, Department of Rehabilitation Medicine, Albert Einstein College of Medicine, Bronx, New York

MELISSA J. TINNEY, MD, FAAPMR
Clinical Assistant Professor, Department of Physical Medicine and Rehabilitation, University of Michigan; Amputation Specialty Clinic and Adaptive Sports Program Director, Lieutenant Colonel Charles S. Kettles VA Medical Center, Ann Arbor, Michigan

JENNIFER TRAM, MD
PM&R Resident, Department of Physical Medicine and Rehabilitation, Greater Los Angeles Veteran Affairs HealthCare System, Division of PM&R, Department of Medicine, UCLA Health, Los Angeles, California

JENNIFER VIOLA, DO
PM&R Resident Physician, Department of Physical Medicine and Rehabilitation, Johns Hopkins University School of Medicine, Baltimore, Maryland

JENNY XU, MD
PM&R Resident, Department of Physical Medicine and Rehabilitation, Johns Hopkins University School of Medicine, Baltimore, Maryland

Contents

The main causes of limb loss include trauma, complications from diabetes and peripheral arterial disease, malignancy, and congenital limb deficiency. There are significant geographic variations in the incidence of upper and lower, and major and minor limb loss worldwide. Limb loss is costly for patients and the health care system. The availability of orthotic and prosthetic services, along with cost of services, represents barrier to care and contributes to morbidity and mortality. More research is needed, especially in low-income and middle-income countries to describe the extent of limb loss.

Limb-loss is a significant medical event with lifelong consequences, impacting various aspects of a patient's well-being. Care for these often-complex patients involves providers from many different specialties working toward a set of patient-centered goals. This article aims to highlight the important role of physiatrists in directing the interdisciplinary care for these patients. Through evidence-based concepts, the authors aim to lay a roadmap for comprehensive, longitudinal management of these patients from pre-amputation assessment through lifelong care.

Pediatric limb loss or limb deficiency is uncommon in the United Sates occurring 1 per 1943 live births per year, with a ratio of 2:1 upper to lower extremity.[1] Causes include congenital limb deficiency, and less frequently, limb loss secondary to trauma, cancer, or other illnesses. Vascular disruption, particularly as seen in amniotic band syndrome, stands as the leading suspect in the multifaceted and intricate causes of congenital limb loss. Children with limb difference and deficiency present unique medical and rehabilitation challenges. Physical Medicine and Rehabilitation (PM&R) physicians are uniquely equipped to navigate these complexities. Prosthetic prescription and fabrication for children require balancing scientific principles with individual needs. A "one-size-fits-all" approach is ineffective. Many diverse factors impact prosthetic prescription and fabrication, including amputation level, residual limb characteristics, cognitive/developmental age, family goals, financial resources, and medical literacy.

and physical factors (eg, pain and prostheses). While many patients experience posttraumatic growth and successfully reintegrate back into their lives, others have a more difficult adjustment. Interdisciplinary teams can best facilitate reintegration through early screening for barriers to reintegration such as depression, pain, body image, and inaccessible environments, to intervene early after amputation. With these barriers addressed, amputees may be able to return to driving and other valued activities more quickly, resulting in improved reintegration across life domains.

This article reviews emerging surgical techniques and prosthetic innovations related to amputation rehabilitation. Osseointegration is discussed from conception to modern implant designs. Motor and sensory reinnervation techniques are reviewed and compared. Prosthetic socket casting, interface, and design innovations are discussed, including direct molded sockets, water casting, adjustable sockets, and magnetic suspension. Advanced components with hydraulic and microprocessor control, power and crossover prosthetic feet are described.

Much of the burden of living with a disability is concentrated among those populations least financially able to bear the burden. As the price of 3 dimensional (3D) printing decreases, individual access to this technology increases. 3D-printed prostheses can be designed specifically for use in resource-poor settings, including developing countries, to minimize the cost of consumable parts while optimizing durability in harsh environmental conditions.

PHYSICAL MEDICINE AND REHABILITATION CLINICS OF NORTH AMERICA

SERIES OF RELATED INTEREST

Orthopedic Clinics
https://www.orthopedic.theclinics.com/
Neurologic Clinics
https://www.neurologic.theclinics.com/
Clinics in Sports Medicine
https://www.sportsmed.theclinics.com/

VISIT THE CLINICS ONLINE!
Access your subscription at:
www.theclinics.com

Foreword

Advances in Amputee Care, Recovery, and Rehabilitation

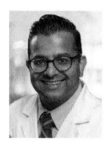

Blessen C. Eapen, MD
Consulting Editor

The management of amputee care has evolved remarkably over the last century due to advances in medical, surgical, and wound care management, along with *early* primary prevention measure. Despite these advancements, in the United States, over 2 million individuals are living with limb loss, and over 185,000 amputations occur annually. The majority of amputations are related to either vascular disease, trauma, or cancer, with hospital costs associated estimated to be over $8 billion dollars.

The integration of prosthetics, advancements in surgical techniques, and innovative rehabilitation strategies have transformed the landscape of limb loss, offering new possibilities for individuals facing limb loss that were not previously available. Amputee rehabilitation often involves an interdisciplinary team approach to provide a holistic approach to provide physical, emotional, and social engagement to maximize functional independence, overall well-being, and effective community reintegration.

This special issue provides a thorough exploration of current best practices, emerging research, and practical approaches to rehabilitation management by bridging the gaps in knowledge and practice. This issue provides a comprehensive overview of amputee care from preamputation care through life-long care. The team delves into *special* topics, including dermatologic conditions, pain management, health care disparities, community reintegration after amputation, adaptive sports, 3D printing, and adaptive sports.

We want to thank Drs Donaghy and Miranda and our esteemed academic, civilian, and Department of Veterans Affairs colleagues for leading this special issue and for

Phys Med Rehabil Clin N Am 35 (2024) xv–xvi
https://doi.org/10.1016/j.pmr.2024.08.007
1047-9651/24/© 2024 Published by Elsevier Inc.

sharing their valuable experience and expertise with the physical medicine and rehabilitation community!

Blessen C. Eapen, MD
Division of Physical Medicine
and Rehabilitation
David Geffen School of Medicine at UCLA
VA Greater Los Angeles Health Care System
11301 Wilshire Boulevard
Los Angeles, CA 90073, USA

E-mail addresses:
beapen@ucla.mednet.edu; blessen.eapen2@va.gov

Preface

Insights and Innovations in Amputation Rehabilitation

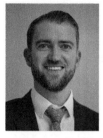 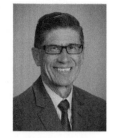

Alex Donaghy, MD   Alberto Miranda, MD
Editors

We are delighted to present this issue of *Physical Medicine and Rehabilitation Clinics of North America* focusing on the care of the person with limb loss. Several exciting advancements in the care of persons with limb loss have come about in the past several years. Although reviewing all such advancements and innovations for a topic as vast and complex as is the care of persons with limb loss would be out of reach of a single issue, our aim was to select topics that highlight some of these recent advancements. Topics were selected to allow the reader to explore current and new management practices ranging from the preamputation shared decision-making process, surgical planning and techniques, prosthetic restoration, health care disparities, and community reintegration.

As co-editors, we aimed to bring expertise from our combined experiences in working within well-supported interdisciplinary teams. These combined experiences include civilian, academic, and federal (VA) work, with a full spectrum of patients seen in urban, rural, and telehealth settings. This issue presents evidence-based reviews and clinical insights from a host of authors from various disciplines, including physiatry, epidemiology, pain management, surgery, dermatology, therapy, and prosthetics/orthotics. We certainly hope this mix of authors with various backgrounds and experiences can provide a well-rounded view of our role as health care providers for persons with limb loss and may help to foster better communication and collaboration in our readers' practices. This issue should be a helpful resource for any provider caring for the person with limb loss, regardless of discipline or practice setting.

We are extremely grateful to the esteemed authors that contributed their time and expertise to the development of this issue. Their commitment to advancing the care and quality of life for persons with limb loss is evident in their clinical and academic

Phys Med Rehabil Clin N Am 35 (2024) xvii–xviii
https://doi.org/10.1016/j.pmr.2024.08.006
1047-9651/24/© 2024 Published by Elsevier Inc.

works. We would also like to thank our mentors and teachers, who through their guidance have instilled in us a curiosity and desire to do the same.

DISCLOSURES

The authors have no conflicts of interest to disclose.

Alex Donaghy, MD
Department of Physical Medicine
and Rehabilitation
University of Michigan
325 East Eisenhower Parkway
Ann Arbor, MI 48108, USA

Alberto Miranda, MD
Department of Medicine
David Geffen School of
Medicine at UCLA
Los Angeles, CA, USA

Department of Physical Medicine
and Rehabilitation
Greater Los Angeles VA Healthcare System
11301 Wilshire Boulevard (117)
Los Angeles, CA 90073, USA

E-mail addresses:
Donaghya@gmail.com (A. Donaghy)
Alberto.Miranda@va.gov (A. Miranda)

Epidemiology and Impact of Limb Loss in the United States and Globally

Jenny Xu, MD, Amna Haider, DO, Amaan Sheikh, DO,
Marlis González-Fernández, MD, PhD*

KEYWORDS

• Limb loss • Epidemiology • Amputation • Global

KEY POINTS

- Limb loss is a major cause of morbidity and mortality, and an economic health burden worldwide.
- The main causes of limb loss include complications from diabetes mellitus and peripheral arterial disease, trauma, malignancy, and congenital limb deficiency.
- Significant geographic variations exist regarding the incidence of major and minor, as well as upper and lower extremity limb loss.

INTRODUCTION

Limb loss is a major cause of morbidity and mortality as well as an economic health burden worldwide.[1–4] The main causes of limb loss include peripheral vascular disease, diabetes mellitus, malignancy, trauma, and congenital limb deficiency.[5,6] Limb loss can be subdivided into major and minor limb loss. Major limb loss is defined as a transhumeral, transradial, transfemoral, or transtibial amputation while minor limb loss is defined as a hand, digit, toe, or midfoot level amputation.[7] Among countries where data are available, significant geographic variations have been noted regarding the incidence of major and minor, as well as upper and lower extremity limb loss.[8] A meta-analysis of observational studies in North America, Europe, Japan, Taiwan, Singapore, and Australia found a decreasing incidence of major amputations and increasing rate of minor amputations from 2010 to 2020.[9,10] Another study found a similar decreasing trend for major amputations, where major amputations occurred more frequently in countries with low health care expenditures and gross domestic product (GDP) per capita.[8] While established registries exist in countries such as

Department of Physical Medicine and Rehabilitation, Johns Hopkins University School of Medicine, North Wolfe Street, Phipps Building, Suite 160, Baltimore, MD 21287, USA
* Corresponding author. 600 North Wolfe Street, Phipps Building, Suite 160, Baltimore, MD 21287.
E-mail address: marlis@jhmi.edu

Phys Med Rehabil Clin N Am 35 (2024) 679–690
https://doi.org/10.1016/j.pmr.2024.05.003
pmr.theclinics.com

England, Scotland, Sweden, and Australia,[11] poor record keeping due to lack of human and physical resources in low-income and middle-income settings makes it difficult to quantify the extent of limb loss worldwide.[2]

Morbidity and Mortality

Factors such as accessibility and affordability of resources and services impact morbidity and mortality after limb loss. Globally, the demand for orthotist and prosthetist services, especially in low-income and lower-middle-income settings is expected to double by 2050.[12] Few countries have a national assistive technology policy or high public access to assistive technology.[13] For patients with limb loss, proper fitting, training, and follow-up of prosthesis fit with trained personnel are essential to prevent complications. However, travel, affordability, and fear of stigmatization are all barriers.[13,14] Without appropriate care and maintenance, there is an increased risk for injury, falls, and overuse.[15]

Economic Health Burden

Limb loss contributes to the economic health burden worldwide. In the United States, in 2013, the estimated annual indirect cost for limb loss was estimated to be $75,000 per person over 3years, and lifetime health care cost after lower extremity amputation was estimated at $649,953. Furthermore, 42% of people in the United States were estimated to be unable to work 7 years after a traumatic lower limb loss.[4] In France, Spain, Italy, Germany, and the United Kingdom, the direct cost of diabetes-related foot amputation was estimated to be $13,842 in 2001 and $83,728 from 2005 to 2009.[3] The estimated financial cost of major lower limb amputation to the National Health Service in England is between 10,000 and 15,000 pounds per procedure, approximating to between 50 and 75 million pounds annually.[16] In the South Africa province of KwaZulu-Natal, the national cost of diabetes-related lower limb loss was estimated to be at least 3 million USD.[17] In Mexico, from 2005 to 2015, the total direct cost of diabetes-related lower extremity amputations hospitalization was approximately 132.51 million USD.[18] This variation highlights how the economic burden experienced by the individual as well as a country's health system is not standardized but rather relative to region.

Upper Limb Loss

Upper limb loss can be classified as trans-phalangeal, trans-metacarpal, trans-carpal, wrist disarticulation, trans-radial, elbow disarticulation, trans-humeral, shoulder disarticulation, and forequarter amputation.[19] While upper limb loss occurs less frequently and in younger individuals than lower limb loss, it is difficult to have clear estimates due to lack of epidemiologic data.[20,21]

Lower Limb Loss

Lower limb loss can be classified as hemipelvectomy, hip disarticulation, transfemoral, knee disarticulation, transtibial, ankle disarticulation (Syme), partial foot, trans-metatarsal, and toe amputation.[22–24] Significant variation in reporting methods also makes it difficult to fully quantify the extent of lower limb loss.[9] One analysis estimated the highest rates of lower extremity limb loss were among Native-American men in the Navajo region of the United States, and the lowest rates were in Okayama, Japan.[6] The global variation in incidence can be associated with differences in ethnicity, socioeconomic determinants of health, as well as rates of trauma, diabetes, vascular disease, and malignancy.[9,24] Lower limb loss is associated with impaired functional mobility, physical, and mental health issues including phantom limb pain and depression.[25]

CAUSES OF LIMB LOSS—TRAUMA

In 2017, an estimated 57.7 million people worldwide were living with limb loss from trauma, with the most common causes being falls, followed by road injuries, other transportation injuries, and mechanical forces. The highest rates of traumatic amputations occurred in East and South Asia, followed by Western Europe, North Africa, the Middle East, North America, and Eastern Europe.[11]

North America

As of 2021, greater than 2.1 million people live with limb loss in the United States with an estimated 185,000 amputations yearly, of which lower limb amputations account for 65%.[26] The average age of amputation in the United States was 50 years and ranged from 18 to 84 years.[26] African Americans were 4 times more likely to have an amputation than white Americans and 3 times more likely when compared to other demographic groups.[26] Approximately 45% of amputations in the United States are due to trauma, whether from motor vehicle collisions, machinery accidents, or military injuries.[27] Since 2001, more than 1700 service members have lost limbs from wars in Afghanistan and Iraq.[26] In the pediatric population, children aged 15 to 18 years were the most common age group to have a traumatic upper extremity amputation, with 92.5% of amputations involving the digits.[28]

Latin America

In tropical Latin America, 6% of amputations were due to trauma, whereas in southern, central, and and ean Latin America 0.98%, 0.42%, and 0.39% of amputations, respectively, were from trauma.[11] For example, in Brazil, trauma contributed approximately 3% of the minor amputations and 2.8% of the major amputations from 2009 to 2020.[29] In Colombia, a study estimated 32.6% of the agricultural transtibial amputations were from farm accidents, 18.4% from anti-personnel landmines, and 16.3% from traffic accidents, with males experiencing 91.8% of the agricultural trans-tibial amputations. An estimated 70% of anti-personnel landmines and unexploded ordinances, of which 98% detonate in rural areas, resulted in amputation. The Colombian Association of Physical Medicine and Rehabilitation estimated the incidence of amputation to be 200 to 300 people per 100,000.[15]

Europe

In Europe, traumatic amputations vary within the continent by region. In 2017, between Central, Eastern, and Western Europe there were 2478, 2096, and 1294 traumatic amputations per 100,000 individuals (**Table 1**). In England, from 2003 to 2008, 13.9% of the patients undergoing major lower extremity amputation had a diagnosis of injury or trauma.[16]

Table 1
Traumatic amputations in Europe[11]

Region	Traumatic Amputations in 2017
Central Europe	2478 per 100,000 individuals
Eastern Europe	2096 per 100,000 individuals
Western Europe	1294 per 100,000 individuals

Middle East

In Iran, from 2003 to 2011, the most common cause of upper and lower limb amputations was trauma (45.2% of all cases),[30] with motor vehicle accidents as the number 1 cause, occurring more often in men. This may be due to the fact that tradition in the region favors a male predominant society where it is uncommon to have female drivers or female study participants.[31] While lower limb amputations were significantly more common than upper limb amputations, up to 75% of upper limb amputations were trauma related. Similarly, in Saudi Arabia, from 2013 to 2018, trauma was the leading cause of upper limb amputations in the region. Males under 40 years old had a significantly higher rate of traumatic amputations,[32] this likely related to younger males being involved in more dangerous endeavors.

Australia

Australia has around 8,000 yearly lower limb amputations, with trauma accounting for a smaller percentage at 8%.[33] Australia sees more vascular disease-related amputations than trauma. More research is needed to evaluate the demographics and causes of trauma-related amputations.

Africa

In Nigeria, from 2008 to 2014, trauma was the main cause for limb loss, with lower limb amputations being significantly more common and occurring more frequently in males. In Ethiopia, trauma was also the main cause for both upper and lower limb loss.[34] Trauma was previously the largest factor for both upper and lower limb amputations across Africa until recent trends saw an increase in vascular-related disease.

Asia

In South Korea, from 1970 to 1994 and from 2011 to 2010, the most common cause of amputation was trauma.[35,36] In 2019, workers compensation insurance data showed 38.3 amputations per 100,000 people, with finger amputation accounting for 93.7%.[36] From 2001 to 2010, in Kitakyushu City, Japan, the most common cause of limb loss was from trauma, and partial hand amputation was the most frequent upper limb loss.[37] In Kolkata, India, from 2008 to 2010, trauma was the most common cause of limb loss as well, occurring more often in younger individuals.[38]

CAUSES OF LIMB LOSS—COMPLICATIONS FROM DIABETES MELLITUS & VASCULAR DISEASE

In 2017, 425 million people worldwide (?) were estimated to have diabetes. This number is expected to increase to 629 million by 2045.[39] Diabetic foot disease is associated with foot infection, ulceration, and bony destruction, and is one of the most common as well as costly causes of hospital admissions.[40,41] Compared to people without diabetes, people with diabetes have a 7.4 to 41.3 times higher risk of lower extremity amputation.[42] From 2010 to 2020, the estimated global annual incidence of diabetes-related minor and major amputations was 139.97 and 94.82 cases/100,000 people, respectively, with a higher incidence in patients with type 1 diabetes and in men.[10]

Peripheral arterial disease (PAD) results from atherosclerotic narrowing of peripheral arterial vasculature, mainly in the lower limbs, and affects more than 230 million people worldwide. The most severe complication is critical limb ischemia, which can result in limb loss. In people with diabetes, PAD not only develops more easily, but also progresses more rapidly.[41] From 2010 to 2014, an analysis of 12 countries found the lowest rates of lower extremity amputation from PAD in New Zealand and the highest rates in Hungary.[8]

North America

Vascular disease secondary to diabetes and/or PAD is the most common cause of limb loss in the United States, accounting for an estimated 85% of new amputations and 54% of people with limb loss. Approximately 130,000 amputations per year are due to diabetes and nearly half of people with vascular limb loss die within 5 years.[43] In 2014, 69% of the amputations in the United States occurred in males, who were more likely to have diabetes-related lower extremity loss.[26]

In Canada, the average age-adjusted rate of lower extremity amputations from 2006 to 2011 was 22.9 per 100,000 individuals. From 2006 to 2011, the number of lower extremity amputations increased, with 65% of the cases attributed to diabetes. The average age for lower extremity amputations was 65.7 years[44] and for upper extremity amputations was 42 years.[45]

In Mexico, approximately 75 people are amputated per day. In 2013, the Mexican Social Security Institute estimated 187 major amputations and 166 minor amputations over the year in southern Mexico City.[46] From 2004 to 2005, hospital admissions in Mexico due to diabetic foot disease increased by 10% with a concomitant 4% increase in major amputations.[46] From 2005 to 2015, the average age of hospitalization for lower extremity amputation due to diabetes was 64.5 years.[18]

Latin America

In Brazil, PAD is the primary cause of lower extremity amputation, representing 47.65% of the major amputations from 2009 to 2020, followed by diabetes at 15.55%. In 2020, both diabetes and PAD contributed to approximately 35% of the minor amputations. Although minor amputation occurs more often than major amputations, rates of major lower extremity amputations are increasing in Brazil, where limb loss occurs more often in males. Until the age of 70, minor amputations were more frequent.[29]

Middle East

In the Middle East, Kuwait, Saudi Arabia, and Bahrain are among the top 10 countries with the highest prevalence of type 2 diabetes worldwide[47] and in these regions lower limb loss has become more common. One study conducted in Saudi Arabia between 2008 and 2019 showed 75% of the amputations were related to diabetic complications.[48] In Saudi Arabia, from 2013 to 2018, lower limb amputations were significantly more common, with vascular and diabetes-related complications as the leading cause of lower limb amputation.[32]

Europe

A report based on the European Society of Vascular Surgery Registry attributed 25.7% to 74.3% of the amputations to be due to diabetes.[42] Diabetes is the most prominent cause of both major and minor amputation and affects 1 in 3 amputees.[16] From 2003 to 2008, 39.4% of the patients undergoing major lower extremity amputation had a diagnosis of diabetes. In England, diabetes is a major cause of all major and minor amputations.[49] PAD accounted for the most leg and foot amputations, with 80% of patients having concurrent diabetes. Approximately 5,000 major amputations are performed yearly in individuals over 50 years of age, with over 90% attributed to complications of PAD.[45] In Germany, 50.7% of patients who underwent major amputations had peripheral arterial disease and 18.5% had diabetes.[45] In Italy, patients with diabetes had an amputation rate of 128.7 per 100,000 compared with only 8.6 per

100,000 for patients without diabetes.[50] In 2013, in Poland, major non-traumatic lower amputations in diabetic patients comprised 57.15% of the total lower limb amputations performed in 2013.[51] In Switzerland, from 1990 to 1999, the rate of amputation varied from 1.8 to 11.4 per 100,000 patients per year. The yearly incidence of amputation for people with diabetes in Switzerland is 19.9 per 100,000 per year and 1.8 per 100,000 for individuals without diabetes. During this time, PAD was the most common cause of amputation.[52]

Australia

Australia has around 8,000 yearly lower limb amputations,[33,53] with 53% of lower limb amputations attributed to type 2 diabetes mellitus (T2DM), followed by non-diabetic PAD at 18%.[54] A study from 2007 to 2012 shows that in general, older males with type 2 diabetes have an increased risk of lower limb amputation. However, this was not in the Northern Territory[55] where in 2020, Aboriginal females in the Northern Territory and Central Region had a higher rate of amputations.[33] Several studies show Aboriginal females have poorer health outcomes than non-Aboriginals and a shorter 14-year life expectancy.[56,57] This is possibly due to remote living situations and access to health care; however, more research needs to be done in this regard. Nonetheless, diabetes remains the number 1 cause of lower limb amputation across the country.

New Zealand

In New Zealand, diabetes is the number 1 cause of lower limb amputation. While major lower limb amputations vary by nearly 4-fold across the country, diabetes remains the leading cause.[58] In the region of Tairawhiti, Māori individuals with diabetes were 65% more likely to undergo major lower-limb amputation than individuals identifying as European/Other, even after adjusting for sex, age, deprivation, rurality, comorbidity, and prior amputation.[59] The reasons behind the increase within this specific population is most likely multifactorial with lack of access to adequate health care services, including high-quality foot care services playing a factor.

Africa

In South Africa, the most common indication for lower limb amputation currently is diabetes and PAD, with a study noting equal sex distribution among participants. Previous literature from sub-Saharan Africa reported trauma and tumors as predominant causes for lower limb amputations,[60–63] but this has seen a recent shift. In Ethiopia, diabetic foot ulcers were the second most common cause for upper and lower limb loss.[34] In Tanzania, from 2008 to 2010, diabetes complications resulted in 41.9% of all the amputations.[63] Overall, there is an increase in diabetic-related disease across the region, overtaking trauma and tumors as the predominant cause of amputations.

Pacific Islands Countries and Territories

In the Pacific Islands Countries and Territories, it is estimated up to 1 in 3 adults have T2DM.[64,65] In Fiji, the mean age for lower extremity limb loss in people with T2DM was 58 years, compared to 70 years for people with T2DM in developed countries. More people in indigenous communities with T2DM experienced lower limb loss compared to other ethnicities.[65] In Vanuatu, Nauru, and the Solomon Islands, delays in treatment were common prior to limb loss.[66]

Asia

In South Korea, from 1970 to 1994 and from 2011 to 2020, the second most common cause of limb loss was PAD.[35,36] Limb loss from vascular disease was 10 to 15 times higher in patients with diabetes compared to patients without diabetes.[36] In Kitakyushu City, Japan, from 2001 to 2005, transtibial followed by transfemoral limb loss were the most common sites of limb loss caused by diabetes and vascular disorders.[37] In China, diabetic foot was the leading cause of non-traumatic limb loss, with an up to 14.4% annual mortality rate.[67] In Singapore, major and toe/ray amputation rates, at 92.1% and 89.0%, respectively, were stable in people with diabetes from 2008 to 2017.[42]

CAUSES OF LIMB LOSS—MALIGNANCY

Bone sarcomas, which include osteosarcoma, chondrosarcoma, and Ewing sarcoma, are rare and associated with limb loss when limb salvage cannot occur.[68,69] Factors associated with limb loss included advanced stage, advanced age, greater comorbidities, large tumor size, and lower income.[69] In areas where limb salvage is not an option, amputation remains the most common surgery for malignant bone tumors.[70]

United States

Approximately 2% of the US population has had cancer-related limb loss, of which above knee amputations represented 75% of amputations. A study found that limb loss due to cancer occurred at an average of 30 years[26]; however, rates of amputation due to malignancies have been decreasing.[7]

Canada

In Canada, 34% of amputations were attributed to malignant neoplasms arising in connective and soft tissue of the lower limb and hip. Malignant neoplasms in the long bones of the lower limb resulted in 21% of oncological amputations, the skin of the lower limb including hip 10%, and the bone and bone marrow 10%.[71]

Europe

From 2004 to 2015, 587 of the 2442 patients registered in the National Cancer Database in Germany underwent amputation.[69] In Switzerland, from 1990 to 1999, the rate of amputation varied from 1.8 to 11.4 per 100,000 patients per year with only 5.7% of the amputations in this 10-year period due to causes including tumors, trauma, and non-arterial conditions.[52] In England, from 2003 to 2008, 2.2% of the patients undergoing major lower extremity amputation had a diagnosis of neoplasm.

CONGENITAL DIFFERENCES

Congenital limb differences include radial, ulnar, humeral, fibular, tibial, femoral, or multiple limb deficiency, and are associated with genetic variation, teratogen exposures, and gene environment interactions.[6,72] Limb deficiency can be classified as transverse, if limb elements are absent distal to a level across the long axis of a limb, or longitudinal, if there is aplasia or hypoplasia along the long axis. Transverse deficiencies are the most common and radial deficiencies are the most common transverse deficiency.[72] In a study looking at the prevalence of birth limb deficiency from 1964 to 1993, upper limb deficiency occurred 2 to 3 times more often than lower limb deficiency with a stable rate in congenital limb deficiency in the United States, Europe, and Canada.[6]

LIMITATIONS

While this review attempts to gather data distributed globally regarding limb loss and amputation, it is limited by research and data availability in each region. This highlights the importance of further delving into the epidemiology of regions less rich in these studies to provide greater awareness and stimulate the mobilization of appropriate care to people with limb loss.

SUMMARY

Globally, limb loss results from factors such as trauma, complications from diabetes and peripheral vascular disease, malignancy, and congenital limb deficiency.[1–4] There are significant geographic variations in the incidence of upper and lower, and major and minor limb loss.[8] With increasing global rates of diabetes and PAD, lower limb loss has become more common; however, trauma remains a common cause of both upper and lower extremity amputation.[10,11,42] The availability of orthotic and prosthetic services, along with cost of services, represents barrier to care and contributes to mortality rates after amputation.[13,14] Overall, understanding the epidemiology and impact of limb loss in the United States and globally can help identify how to prevent and decrease the morbidity, mortality, and economic burden of limb loss.

CLINICS CARE POINTS

- Lower extremity limb loss occurs more often than upper extremity limb loss and can be attributed to the rising rates of diabetes and vascular disease complications.

- Age, sex, and cultural factors play a significant role in causes of limb loss, including trauma, diabetes, vascular disease, malignancy, and congenital limb deficiency.

- Health care access, attitudes toward disabilities, and lifestyle choices can impact the incidence and management of limb loss across diverse populations.

- More studies are needed to fully comprehend the global scale of limb loss.

DISCLOSURE

The authors declare that they have no relevant or material financial interests that relate to the research described in this paper.

REFERENCES

1. Kadam D. Limb salvage surgery. Indian J Plast Surg 2013;46(2):265–74.
2. Okello TR, Magada SM, Atim P, et al. Major limb loss (MLL): an overview of etiology, outcomes, experiences and challenges faced by amputees and service providers in the post-conflict period in Northern Uganda. J Glob Health Rep 2019;3. https://doi.org/10.29392/joghr.3.e2019028.
3. Tchero H, Kangambega P, Lin L, et al. Cost of diabetic foot in France, Spain, Italy, Germany and United Kingdom: A systematic review. Ann Endocrinol (Paris) 2018; 79(2):67–74.
4. Ma VY, Chan L, Carruthers KJ. Incidence, prevalence, costs, and impact on disability of common conditions requiring rehabilitation in the United States: stroke, spinal cord injury, traumatic brain injury, multiple sclerosis, osteoarthritis, rheumatoid arthritis, limb loss, and back pain. Arch Phys Med Rehabil 2014; 95(5):986–95.e1.
5. Hughes W, Goodall R, Salciccioli JD, et al. Editor's Choice - Trends in Lower Extremity Amputation Incidence in European Union 15+ Countries 1990-2017. Eur J Vasc Endovasc Surg 2020;60(4):602–12.

6. Ephraim PL, Dillingham TR, Sector M, et al. Epidemiology of limb loss and congenital limb deficiency: a review of the literature. Arch Phys Med Rehabil 2003;84(5):747–61.

7. Varma P, Stineman MG, Dillingham TR. Epidemiology of limb loss. Phys Med Rehabil Clin N Am 2014;25(1):1–8.

8. Behrendt C, Sigvant B, Szeberin Z, et al. International variations in amputation practice: A VASCUNET report. Eur J Vasc Endovasc Surg 2018;56(3):391–9.

9. Moxey PW, Gogalniceanu P, Hinchliffe RJ, et al. Lower extremity amputations–a review of global variability in incidence. Diabet Med 2011;28(10):1144–53.

10. Ezzatvar Y, García-Hermoso A. Global estimates of diabetes-related amputations incidence in 2010-2020: A systematic review and meta-analysis. Diabetes Res Clin Pract 2023;195:110194.

11. McDonald CL, Westcott-McCoy S, Weaver MR, et al. Global prevalence of traumatic non-fatal limb amputation. Prosthet Orthot Int 2021;45(2):105–14.

12. Clarke L, Puli L, Ridgewell E, et al. Regulation of the global orthotist/prosthetist workforce, and what we might learn from allied health professions with international-level regulatory support: a narrative review. Hum Resour Health 2021;19(1):1–83.

13. World Health Organization. 2023. "Assistive technology." Web page. Available at: https://www.who.int/news-room/fact-sheets/detail/assistive-technology. Accessed August 20, 2023.

14. Mishra S, Laplante-Lévesque A, Barbareschi G, et al. Assistive technology needs, access and coverage, and related barriers and facilitators in the WHO European region: a scoping review. Disabil Rehabil Assist Technol 2022;19(2): 474–85.

15. Ortega Bedoya Y, Mejía Londoño V, Rendón Vélez E, et al. Mobility and postural limitations perceived by transtibial amputees undertaking agricultural activities: a qualitative study. Ann Med 2023;55(2):2258915.

16. Moxey PW, Hofman D, Hinchliffe RJ, et al. Epidemiological study of lower limb amputation in England between 2003 and 2008. Br J Surg 2010;97(9):1348–53.

17. Thompson AT, Bruce JL, Kong VY, et al. Counting the cost of preventable diabetes-related lower limb amputations at a single district hospital in KwaZulu-Natal: what does this mean, what can be done? J Endocrinol Metabol Diabetes S Afr 2020; 25(2):44–50.

18. Ascencio-Montiel IdJ. 10 years Analysis of Diabetes-related Major Lower Extremity Amputations in Mexico. Arch Med Res 2018;49(1):58–64.

19. Maduri P and Akhondi H. Upper limb amputation, In: *Upper limb amputation*, 2023, StatPearlsStatPearls Publishing. Available at: http://www.ncbi.nlm.nih.gov/books/NBK540962/. Accessed November 15, 2023.

20. Jiménez Cotes EA, López Rios AA, Vásquez Sañudo V, et al. Descriptive study of patients with upper limb amputation as possible candidates for a hand transplant in Medellín, Colombia. Cureus 2022;14(2):e22527.

21. Watve S, Dodd G, MacDonald R, et al. Upper limb prosthetic rehabilitation. Orthopaedics and Trauma 2011;25:135–42.

22. Gholizadeh H, Baddour N, Botros M, et al. Hip disarticulation and hemipelvectomy prostheses: A review of the literature. Prosthet Orthot Int 2021;45(5):434–9.

23. Meier RH3, Melton D. Ideal functional outcomes for amputation levels. Phys Med Rehabil Clin N Am 2014;25(1):199–212.

24. Molina CS and Faulk J. Lower Extremity Amputation, In: *Lower extremity amputation*, 2023, StatPearlsStatPearls Publishing, Available at: http://www.ncbi.nlm.nih.gov/books/NBK546594/. Accessed November 15, 2023.

25. Amtmann D, Morgan SJ, Kim J, et al. Health-related profiles of people with lower limb loss. Arch Phys Med Rehabil 2015;96(8):1474–83.

26. Cain JJ, Ignaszewski D, Blymire C. Living Well After Amputation: Lessons in Innovation, Peer Support, and Health Policy. Tech Orthop 2021;36(4):360.

27. Sheehan TP, Gondo GC. Impact of limb loss in the United States. Phys Med Rehabil Clin N Am 2014;25(1):9–28.

28. Vakhshori V, Bouz GJ, Mayfield CK, et al. Trends in pediatric traumatic upper extremity amputations. Hand (N Y) 2019;14(6):782–90.

29. Biagioni RB, Louzada ACS, Biagioni LC, et al. Cross-sectional analysis of 180,595 lower limb Amputations in the State of Sao Paulo Over 12 Years. World J Surg 2022;46(10):2498–506.

30. Mousavi AA, Saied AR, Heidari E. A survey on causes of amputation in a 9-year period in Iran. Arch Orthop Trauma Surg 2012;132(11):1555–9.

31. Killawi A, Khidir A, Elnashar M, et al. Procedures of recruiting, obtaining informed consent, and compensating research participants in Qatar: findings from a qualitative investigation. BMC Med Ethics 2014;15:9.

32. Alshehri FM, Ahmed SA, Ullah S, et al. The patterns of acquired upper and lower extremity amputation at a Tertiary Centre in Saudi Arabia. Cureus 2022;14(4): e24026.

33. Stuart L, Kimmel L, Jolly A. Incidence of lower limb amputation in Central Australia. Aust Health Rev 2021;45(3):361–7.

34. Sume BW, Geneti SA. Determinant Causes of Limb Amputation in Ethiopia: A Systematic Review and Meta-Analysis. Ethiopian journal of health sciences 2023; 33(5):891–902.

35. Kim YC, Park CI, Kim DY, et al. Statistical analysis of amputations and trends in Korea. Prosthet Orthot Int 1996;20(2):88–95.

36. Bok S, Song Y. Fact Sheet of Amputee 10-Year Trends in Korea: From 2011 to 2020. Ann Rehabil Med 2022;46(5):221–7.

37. Ohmine S, Kimura Y, Saeki S, et al. Community-based survey of amputation derived from the physically disabled person's certification in Kitakyushu City, Japan. Prosthet Orthot Int 2012;36(2):196–202.

38. Pooja GD, Sangeeta L. Prevalence and aetiology of amputation in Kolkata, India: A retrospective analysis. Hong Kong Physiother J 2013;31(1):36–40.

39. Forouhi NG, Wareham NJ. Epidemiology of diabetes. Medicine (Abingdon) 2014; 42(12):698–702.

40. Feldman EL, Callaghan BC, Pop-Busui R, et al. Diabetic neuropathy. Nat Rev Dis Primers 2019;5(1):42–9.

41. Mascarenhas JV, Albayati MA, Shearman CP, et al. Peripheral arterial disease. Endocrinol Metab Clin North Am 2014;43(1):149–66.

42. Riandini T, Pang D, Toh MPHS, et al. National rates of lower extremity amputation in people with and without diabetes in a multi-ethnic asian population: a ten year study in Singapore. Eur J Vasc Endovasc Surg 2022;63(1):147–55.

43. Robbins JM, Strauss G, Aron D, et al. Mortality rates and diabetic foot ulcers: is it time to communicate mortality risk to patients with diabetic foot ulceration? J Am Podiatr Med Assoc 2008;98(6):489–93.

44. Imam B, Miller WC, Finlayson HC, et al. Incidence of lower limb amputation in Canada. Can J Public Health 2017;108(4):e374–80.

45. Efanov JI, Tchiloemba B, Izadpanah A, et al. A review of utilities and costs of treating upper extremity amputations with vascularized composite allotransplantation versus myoelectric prostheses in Canada. JPRAS Open 2022;32:150–60.

46. Moya-Jiménez S, Morales-Ochoa Y, Serrano-Lozano J. Incidence of major ampu-tations secondary to diabetic foot prior and after endovascular revascularization. Rev Mex Angiol 2020;48(1):11–6.

47. Saeedi P, Petersohn I, Salpea P, et al. Global and regional diabetes prevalence estimates for 2019 and projections for 2030 and 2045: Results from the Interna-tional Diabetes Federation Diabetes Atlas, 9(th) edition. Diabetes Res Clin Pract 2019;157:107843.

48. AlMehman DA, Faden AS, Aldahlawi BM, et al. Post-amputation pain among lower limb amputees in a tertiary care hospital in Jeddah, Saudi Arabia: A retro-spective study. Saudi Med J 2022;43(2):187–96.

49. Ahmad N, Thomas GN, Gill P, et al. The prevalence of major lower limb amputa-tion in the diabetic and non-diabetic population of England 2003-2013. Diab Vasc Dis Res 2016;13(5):348–53.

50. Walter N, Alt V, Rupp M. Lower Limb Amputation Rates in Germany. Medicina (Kaunas) 2022;58(1):101.

51. Wierzba W, Krasnodębski P, Śliwczyński A, et al. Geographic variability of major non-traumatic lower limb amputations in diabetic and non-diabetic patients in Poland. Ann Agric Environ Med 2020;27(1):76–9.

52. Carmona GA, Hoffmeyer P, Herrmann FR, et al. Major lower limb amputations in the elderly observed over ten years: the role of diabetes and peripheral arterial disease. Diabetes Metab 2005;31(5):449–54.

53. Dillon MP, Kohler F, Peeva V. Incidence of lower limb amputation in Australian hos-pitals from 2000 to 2010. Prosthet Orthot Int 2014;38(2):122–32.

54. Lazzarini PA, O'Rourke SR, Russell AW, et al. What are the key conditions asso-ciated with lower limb amputations in a major Australian teaching hospital? J Foot Ankle Res 2012;5(1):12.

55. Dillon MP, Fortington LV, Akram M, et al. Geographic Variation of the Incidence Rate of Lower Limb Amputation in Australia from 2007-12. PLoS One 2017; 12(1):e0170705.

56. Care, Australian Government Department of Health and Aged, National women's health policy 2010, 2023, Australian Government Department of Health and Aged Care, Available at: https://www.health.gov.au/resources/publications/national-womens-health-policy-2010?language=en. Accessed November 15, 2023.

57. Australian Bureau of Statistics. (2015-2017). Life Tables for Aboriginal and Torres Strait Islander Australians methodology. ABS. Available at: https://www.abs.gov.au/methodologies/aboriginal-and-torres-strait-islander-life-expectancy-methodology/2015-2017. Accessed August 20, 2024.

58. Gurney JK, Stanley J, York S, et al. Regional variation in the risk of lower-limb amputation among patients with diabetes in New Zealand. ANZ J Surg 2019; 89(7–8):868–73.

59. Gurney JK, Stanley J, York S, et al. Risk of lower limb amputation in a national prevalent cohort of patients with diabetes. Diabetologia 2018;61(3):626–35.

60. Sarfo-Kantanka O, Sarfo FS, Kyei I, et al. Incidence and determinants of diabetes-related lower limb amputations in Ghana, 2010-2015- a retrospective cohort study. BMC Endocr Disord 2019;19(1):27–8.

61. Sarfo-Kantanka O, Kyei I, Mbanya JC, et al. Diabetes-related foot disorders among adult Ghanaians. Diabet Foot Ankle 2018;9(1):1511678.

62. Gebreslassie B, Gebreselassie K, Esayas R. Patterns and causes of amputation in ayder referral hospital, mekelle, ethiopia: a three-year experience. Ethiop J Health Sci 2018;28(1):31–6.

63. Chalya PL, Mabula JB, Dass RM, et al. Major limb amputations: a tertiary hospital experience in northwestern Tanzania. J Orthop Surg Res 2012;7:18.
64. Tin STW, Lee CMY, Colagiuri R. A profile of diabetes in Pacific Island Countries and Territories. Diabetes Res Clin Pract 2015;107(2):233–46.
65. Khan S, Mohammadnezhad M, Ratu A, et al. Patterns and risk factors associated with index Lower Extremity Amputations (LEA) among Type 2 Diabetes Mellitus (T2DM) patients in Fiji. Prim Care Diabetes 2021;15(6):1012–8.
66. Win Tin ST, Gadabu E, Iro G, et al. Diabetes related amputations in Pacific Islands countries: a root cause analysis of precipitating events. Diabetes Res Clin Pract 2013;100(2):230–4.
67. Zhao W, Xu Z, Wang A, Journal of Diabetes and Clinical Research Commentary. Epidemiological characteristics of diabetic foot and affecting factors for amputation in China. J Diabetes Clin Res 2021;3(3). Available at: https://www.scientificarchives.com/journal/journal-of-diabetes-and-clinical-research.
68. Nystrom LM, Morcuende JA. Expanding endoprosthesis for pediatric musculoskeletal malignancy: current concepts and results. Iowa Orthop J 2010;30:141–9.
69. Bläsius F, Delbrück H, Hildebrand F, et al. Surgical treatment of bone sarcoma. Cancers (Basel) 2022;14(11):2694.
70. Khan SA, Kumar VS, Poudel RR. Sarcoma: A multidisciplinary Approach to Treatment. Limb Salvage in India 2017;483–510.
71. Kayssi A, de Mestral C, Forbes TL, et al. A Canadian population-based description of the indications for lower-extremity amputations and outcomes. Can J Surg 2016;59(2):99–106.
72. Wilcox WR, Coulter CP, Schmitz ML. Congenital limb deficiency disorders. Clin Perinatol 2015;42(2):281–300, viii. https://doi.org/10.1016/j.clp.2015.02.004.

The Physiatrist's Approach to Limb Loss
Pre-amputation Through Lifelong Care

Alex Donaghy, MD[a,1,*], Mary S. Keszler, MD[b,2],
Christopher A. Bonilla, MD, MS[c,3]

KEYWORDS

- Amputation • Limb-deficiency • Physiatrist • Prosthetics • Rehabilitation

KEY POINTS

- Limb-loss management should incorporate a well-coordinated, interdisciplinary, long-term care approach led by a physiatrist.
- Physiatrists are ideally involved in all phases of limb-loss care: pre-amputation, post-operative, prosthetic restoration and rehabilitation, and lifelong care.
- Early physiatric involvement includes functional prognostication, patient education, and rehabilitation, while long-term follow-up involves prosthetic restoration and the management of any or all limb-loss sequelae.

INTRODUCTION

Amputation often represents a profound, life-altering event in one's life. Most proximally, a major amputation and its precipitating factors constitute a significant mortality risk, and more distally, trigger a shift in one's daily functioning, independence, and sense of self.[1,2] Physiatrists are well-suited to help patients navigate this shift, to guide and support patients through every phase of their amputation rehabilitation experience. Limb-loss prevalence is expected to double between 2005 and 2050[3] and resultant disability rates are high.[4–7] Moreover, persons with limb loss (PwLL) often have numerous comorbidities and downstream complications, making

[a] Department of Physical Medicine and Rehabilitation, University of Michigan, 325 East Eisenhower Parkway, Ann Arbor, MI 48108, USA; [b] Department of Physical Medicine and Rehabilitation, Johns Hopkins University School of Medicine, 600 North Wolfe Street, Suite 160, Baltimore, MD 21287, USA; [c] Department of Physical Medicine and Rehabilitation, VA Puget Sound Health Care System, 1660 South Columbian Way, Seattle, WA 98108, USA
[1] Present address: 325 E. Eisenhower Parkway, Ann Arbor, MI 48108
[2] Present address: 600 N. Wolfe Street, Suite 160, Baltimore, MD 21287
[3] Present Address: 1660 S Columbian Way, Seattle, WA 98108
* Corresponding author.
E-mail address: donaghya@umich.edu

Phys Med Rehabil Clin N Am 35 (2024) 691–705
https://doi.org/10.1016/j.pmr.2024.05.004
pmr.theclinics.com
1047-9651/24/© 2024 Elsevier Inc. All rights reserved, including those for text and data mining, AI training, and similar technologies.

specialized, long-term care necessary. In this sense, the physiatrist's role is essential, spanning pre-amputation assessments that shape decision-making, through the intricacies of post-amputation care, to the transformative phases of prosthetic adaptation, functional restoration, and psychosocial empowerment. A timeline of the phases of limb-loss rehabilitation and their associated goals can be found in **Fig. 1**. This article aims to highlight the multifaceted responsibilities undertaken by physiatrists in the comprehensive care of PwLL through an exploration of key concepts and evidence-based practice recommendations.

PRE-AMPUTATION

Amputation most commonly results from a few specific scenarios noted in decreasing order of incidence: complications from diabetes mellitus and/or vascular disease, trauma, and malignancy.[8,9] Trauma may result in acute amputation or elective amputation years later due to chronic complications including pain. In acute situations, the surgical team's primary goal is to prevent mortality by resecting compromised tissues in a timely manner and in a way that optimizes healing potential.[10] Regarding level-of-amputation, objective tests including vascular studies, epidemiologic data regarding

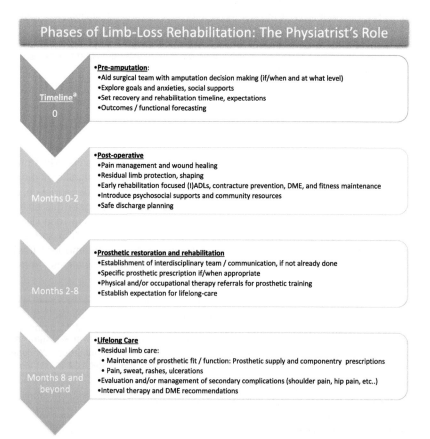

Fig. 1. Phases of limb-loss rehabilitation. [a]Representing typical post-lower extremity amputation time intervals, though may vary depending on various health and/or rehabilitative factors

revision rates, and surgical candidacy are essential tools for decision-making.[9,11] While surgical site healing and pain management are obvious short-term goals, optimizing functional outcomes remains a secondary, longer term objective, and is one that physiatrists may play an intangible consulting role.

Outside of the need for emergent amputation, there is often a requisite counseling and planning phase. In this stage, there are 2 important questions: 1. *Do we amputate?* And if so, 2. *At what level do we amputate?*

1. *Do we amputate*: This question excludes emergent or life-threatening scenarios including severe ischemia, sepsis, or malignancy. Many situations are more nuanced. In the setting of diabetic foot ulcerations (DFUs), one should first ensure patients have been evaluated by the proper team of specialists. Studies show that the incorporation of interdisciplinary teams for those with DFUs, which may include nurses, surgeons, registered dieticians, endocrinologists, and/or infectious disease specialists, may decrease amputations by 50% to 85%, lower costs, and lead to better quality of life outcomes.[12,13] Morbidity following ulceration is high, with recurrence rates of 65%, lifetime lower-extremity amputation risk of 20%, and 5-year mortality of 50% to 70%.[13] Amputation is often necessary and recommended in the setting of chronic, non-healing wounds. As alternatives to amputation, it is important to consider not only the possibility of definitive healing, but the possibility of treating non-healing wounds via careful monitoring and antibiotics when indicated. For patients with high perioperative risks or likelihood for significant functional decline post-amputation, this latter option may be considered. In a study, including 81 patients who underwent transtibial amputation (TTA) due to DFUs, quality of life measures improved in 75% but *worsened* in 25%[14]: might the latter group benefit instead from chronic wound care? A physiatrist is ideally suited to help predict functional capabilities in either scenario, and to counsel the patient and medical team regarding possible outcomes.

Patients with chronic pain and/or disability from prior limb trauma may seek elective amputation. While many of these patients have already undergone multiple limb-salvage surgeries and extensive rehabilitation, a thorough evaluation should be conducted by a physiatrist, exploring all therapeutic options before electing for amputation. Consulting physiatrists should carefully consider potential footwear solutions, orthoses, and durable medical equipment (DME). In a small study of injured active-duty military members, individuals with amputation compared to those with limb salvage who were provided a custom carbon fiber ankle-foot-orthosis (AFO) and intensive rehabilitation had similar performance outcomes.[15] In another study of service members with chronic limb injuries, participants were enrolled in a structured rehabilitation program utilizing a custom, dynamic AFO: patients' physical performance measures improved and 92% of the patients initially considering amputation subsequently favored limb salvage.[16] A careful medical history and physical examination should be performed to evaluate residual limb strength, range of motion, and functional weight-bearing capacity of the affected limb. In patients with Chronic Regional Pain Syndrome (CRPS), one should ensure appropriate multifaceted treatment approaches prior to consideration of amputation. Aman and colleagues proposed an algorithm for elective amputation combined with Target Muscle Reinnervation (TMR) to improve decision-making and outcomes for those with CRPS seeking amputation.[17] In a cross-sectional/longitudinal study of 47 patients who underwent amputation due to therapy-resistant CRPS, mobility and pain improved in 77% and 73%, respectively, but with self-reported recurrence of symptoms up to 51% (19% by Budapest criteria).[18] Patients should be counseled on the propensity for proximal recurrence of CRPS and phantom limb pain. A physiatrist is well qualified to provide the patient with guidance on functional expectations at the proposed level of amputation to help with informed decision-making.

2. *At what level do we amputate:* Preservation of residual limb length is a primary objective and is associated with improved functional outcomes.[19–22] Preservation of functional distal joints is nearly always preferable. At select levels of amputation, longer residual limbs provide more surface area for the prosthetic interface and result in longer "lever arms," allowing for greater force generation. However, there are important counterexamples to these principles. Gait efficiency is not superior following partial foot versus TTAs with prosthetic restoration.[22] TTAs may compare favorably to the more distal Syme's amputations as it allows for more prosthetic componentry options, results in lower rates of prosthetic failure, and is associated with similar functional outcomes.[23] In the case of TTAs, the ideal length is mid-shaft tibia, often cited between 12.5 and 17.5 cm measured from the medial joint line,[10] which allows for adequate distal soft tissue coverage and the use of higher energy returning prosthetic foot options. TTAs should be performed preferentially to through-knee or transfemoral amputations (TFAs) whenever medically feasible, as there are considerable differences in energy expenditure, prosthetic abandonment, and functional outcomes.[19,21] Through-knee amputations may result in improved "physical quality of life" and walking capabilities, though with more pain and lower rates of prosthetic usage compared to TFAs, and are associated with poor wound healing rates.[21,24] In rare cases, such as the patient who is non-ambulatory at baseline or is not expected to ambulate or transfer independently with amputation of any level, a TFA may be preferred to TTA due to improved healing times and lower frequency of surgical revisions.[25,26]

Beyond these 2 questions, it is important for physiatrists to meet with patient pre-amputation to address fears, make functional projections and disposition recommendations, and lay the groundwork for subsequent rehabilitation. Though a detailed discussion is beyond the scope of this article, there are various tools used to aid post-amputation functional predictions, including the AMPREDICT-Mobility model.[4]

POST-OPERATIVE

The same goals set during the pre-operative phase continue into the post-operative phase. These include communicating with the interdisciplinary team, optimizing the rehabilitation plan and recovery, and monitoring for adverse effects. Maintaining open communication with the surgical team during this phase is critical. In the case of dysvascular or complicated traumatic amputations, there is the potential for complications necessitating revision that can delay residual limb healing, hospital discharge, and ultimately prosthesis fitting. Additional surgeries can prolong periods of immobility, contributing to further deconditioning and contracture development, which may have an impact on the patient's functional prognostication.

During this phase, it is important to clarify the wound care and edema management plan, be it soft or rigid dressing, or an immediate post-operative prosthesis (IPOP). An IPOP requires a well-organized team involving a prosthetist to apply the cast in the immediate post-operative period and to re-apply as needed, along with therapists and nurses familiar with the post-operative activity protocols. While in theory an IPOP allows for earlier mobilization, some recent data suggest otherwise.[27] At most institutions, patients receive other forms of rigid dressings (such as traditional casts, removable casts, or prefabricated rigid removable dressings) or use soft dressing for compression. When available, rigid dressings are generally preferred as they provide compression, residual limb protection, and reduced risk of joint contractures, correlating with earlier prosthesis fitting post-transtibial amputation.[28,29] Whichever post-operative dressing is used, the physiatrist should ensure that all care team members, the patient, and their family members are familiar with proper management to reduce the risk of complications that might impede wound healing.

Depending on the institutional structure, the patient's post-operative pain may be managed by the surgical team, acute pain management team, or physiatrist. Often, physiatrists are consulted post-amputation—they should work collaboratively with the primary pain management team to ensure a multimodal approach for post-operative, phantom limb, and/or comorbid pain conditions. Physical and occupational therapists (PTs and OTs) play key roles in the team-management of pain as they can explore various therapeutic regimens and modalities. It is also essential to involve rehabilitation psychologists as pain can have an impact on mood (and visa-versa), and consequently, rehabilitation. A review of post-amputation pain management is beyond the scope of this article; however, this information can be found in "Pain After Amputation: A Clinical Review" in this issue.

In anticipation of post-operative discharge, the physiatrist will help determine the next most appropriate setting for ongoing rehabilitation, be it inpatient rehabilitation (IPR), subacute rehabilitation (SAR), or home with outpatient services. A diagnosis of limb-loss is a qualifying condition for the Medicare 60% rule for IPR and individuals with new major amputation benefit from the interdisciplinary care and frequent medical monitoring offered at IPR. In addition to overseeing the larger rehabilitation plan, physiatrists in IPR help manage medical comorbidities, coexisting injuries, wounds, pain, social integration, and mood disorders. Regarding post-operative rehabilitation venues, elderly individuals with major lower limb dysvascular amputations who go to IPR are more likely to survive 12 months postamputation and to be fit with a prosthesis and are less likely to be admitted to the hospital for non-amputation-related conditions, than those discharged to skilled nursing facility or home.[30] It is important to consider IPR for individuals with upper limb amputation as well as these patients are more likely to be successful prosthesis users if they have early post-amputation intervention with an experienced team, and if they are fit with a temporary prosthesis within 30 days of amputation.[31,32] When deciding on the discharge plan, the physiatrist should consider the patient's comorbid conditions, concomitant injuries, amputation level, home setup, and level of deconditioning. Cognitive impairment —whether from traumatic brain injury, microvascular disease, dementia, polypharmacy, or delirium—may be comorbid and may affect recommendations with regards to rehabilitation setting. Such patients may benefit from a longer course of less intensive rehabilitation offered at SAR, rather than IPR.

The individual's psychological recovery must also be considered as rates of depression are high among new PwLL.[33] Patients should be offered rehabilitation psychology services to help adjust to new challenges—anecdotally, many more patients are agreeable to this referral than will explicitly ask. Patient should also be offered services to connect with the greater limb-loss community—one such option is the Amputee Coalition, a national nonprofit organization for individuals with limb-loss or limb differences. It offers various services, including pairing individuals with certified peer mentors and maintaining a database of local support groups.[34] Many larger institutions and communities have local groups or meet-ups that should be explored.

No matter where the individual receives post-amputation rehabilitation, the physiatrist should work with the PTs, OTs, and nursing to ensure steps are taken to reduce the risk of contracture formation, optimize muscle strengthening, endurance, and proprioception. In the post-operative phase, individuals with lower limb-loss generally use a wheelchair for mobility and will work toward a walker or crutches. Assuring appropriate DME and addressing architectural and social barriers to home discharge are of upmost importance. Once the patient is ready to be discharged home, it is key to ensure rehabilitation referrals and physiatry follow-ups are in place.

PROSTHETIC RESTORATION: PRESCRIPTION AND CANDIDACY

Six-to-eight-weeks post-lower extremity amputation (or 4 weeks post-upper extremity amputation) is a sensible timeline to establish outpatient physiatric care. This interval takes into consideration expected healing rates and limb shaping/preparation, though should vary based on discharge setting, care needs, or complications at time of discharge. Early assessment should focus on wound healing, functional status and independence, safety, physical conditioning, and limb preparation for prosthesis use in applicable cases. **Box 1** proposes suggested elements to be included in an initial outpatient physiatric visit. Establishing rapport and the expectation for long-term follow-up is essential.

In patients for whom prosthesis use is expected, the goal should always be to initiate fitting and training as early as medically feasible. Literature suggests that early prosthetic fitting and training promotes lower rates of prosthesis abandonment, especially in upper limb amputees.[6,32,5,35] Prosthesis use is associated with improved mood and quality of life, and reduced rates of phantom limb pain.[33,36–39] Being able to walk with a prosthesis was noted to have had the "greatest positive impact on quality of life" in a recent systematic review.[40]

When prescribing a prosthetic device, it is valuable to communicate that all prosthetic solutions have trade-offs.[41] There is no "one-size-fits-all" product for every patient or situation. What might be advantageous in terms of function or appearance may entail compromises in other aspects (for instance, a hydraulic foot/ankle unit may improve gait on inclined surfaces, at the cost of reduced stability and durability). Achieving successful outcomes hinges on finding the right balance between the functionality of the prosthetic component and the patient's abilities and daily requirements. Given the multitude of commercially available componentry options, it is ideal to coordinate directly with a prosthetist when prescription or componentry changes are needed.

Prosthetic prescriptions require documentation to include a diagnosis and specific functional goals and justification. In the United States, functional justification following lower limb amputations necessitates use of Medical Functional Classification Levels, or K-levels, a numeric scale from 0 to 4 ranging from a projected non-ambulator to a high-level prosthesis user. This descriptor helps to communicate with payers and other providers the patient's projected functional level following prosthetic restoration and enables coverage for specific componentry. Following physiatric evaluation and prosthetic prescription, a detailed prescription is typically put together by the prosthetist and involves component specifications detailed via Healthcare Common Procedure Coding System (HCPCS) L codes.

Prosthesis Nonuse

Physicians take an oath to, "First, do no harm." Prosthetic devices are not without risks including, but not limited to, skin ulcerations (of both the residual and contralateral limbs) and injurious falls.[42–44] There is a lack of literature detailing situations in which prosthetic prescription is deemed inappropriate by the prescribing physician. However, this scenario is quite common, especially following TFA. In a 12-month

---

Box 1
Suggested elements of an outpatient limb-loss intake evaluation

History
- Post-operative
  - Interval wound healing and weight-bearing status
  - Mobility and functional status, care, and equipment needs
  - Limb protection/edema management, limb-shaping
- General health
  - Pain: residual and phantom limb, other musculoskeletal, and current management
  - Contralateral limb health and wound prevention
  - Comorbidities: cardiorespiratory and neurologic status, vision, hand function, cognition
- Psychosocial
  - Coping with disability, mental health history, support systems
  - Architectural setup and/or barriers, avocation/vocation

Physical examination
- Post-operative
  - Surgical site healing, edema, distal soft-tissue characteristics, sensitivity, sensation
  - Residuum shape and size measurements (length, distal and proximal circumference)
  - Lower extremity: strength, range of motion (ROM)/contracture (ankle, knee, and hip)
  - Upper extremity: strength, ROM/contracture (the shoulder girdle may power prosthesis)
- General Health
  - Contralateral limb health, strength, ROM, sensation
  - Unilateral stance time, hopping within parallel bars (*lower extremity limb loss*)
  - Neurologic: consider neurologic and visual screens if indicated
- Psychosocial
  - Depression, anxiety, and post-traumatic stress disorder screens (eg, Patient Health Questionnaire-9 [PHQ-9],Generalized anxiety disorder Questionnaire [GAD-7], Primary Care Post Traumatic Stress Disorder screen [PC-PTSD], respectively)

Counseling and planning
- Post-operative
  - Expected wound healing times, strategies, and/or referrals
  - Limb protection, shaping, and edema management (eg, compressive garments)
  - Safety strategies (eg, fall prevention, caregiver support)
- Rehabilitative
  - Initiate basic preparatory home exercises (eg, sit-to-stands, gentle ROM) or consider physical/occupational therapy referral
  - Contralateral limb protection (eg, diabetic shoes, custom accommodative inserts, podiatry referral, and education on contralateral amputation rates)
  - Education on prosthetic/gait rehabilitation timelines *if applicable*
  - Psychosocial offerings: Local support groups, peer support, psychology referral
  - Pain management
- Prosthetic restoration
  - Projected prosthetic users:
    - Identification of preferred Certified Prosthetist/Orthotist
    - If wound is healed, specific prosthetic prescription and wearing schedule (**Fig. 2**)
  - Projected non-users:
    - Discussion of current barriers, expectations, targets for candidacy, and alternatives to prosthesis use

---

longitudinal study, fewer than 25% of transfemoral amputees achieved community mobility, and only 50% achieved household mobility, suggesting that even with prosthetic restoration, many with TFAs are unable to walk sufficiently.[45] Like all medical prescriptions, risks and benefits must be considered and shared prior to prescription and this responsibility falls aptly on the prescribing physiatrist. The goal of ambulating with a prosthesis is nearly ubiquitous following lower limb amputation, which can lead to challenging conversations when prescription is not deemed safe or practical. It may be helpful to frame lower limb prostheses as "mobility tools" rather than replacement limbs. While this tool offers certain advantages (upright mobility, cosmesis, tasks involving the reaching of high surfaces, etc.), it is also the riskiest tool: raising the center of gravity predisposes to falls; it may promote wounds in both the residual limb and contralateral limb; it requires a high amount of energy expenditure and thus may not be feasible in those with compromised cardiopulmonary systems; and, it is time consuming and costly.[22,42,43] Some individuals may benefit from a TTA "transfer prosthesis" if walking is not feasible; however, transfemoral prostheses are not beneficial for transfers[46] and therefore should not be prescribed for this purpose. Many patients with reduced likelihood of bipedal ambulation may meet their functional goals through wheelchair mobility, assistive devices (ADs), home modifications, and social support. In the authors' experience, honest discussion regarding the risk-to-benefit ratio of prosthesis use is best had early and, in such cases, sensitivity is crucial to maintain rapport and patient engagement. Moreover, clearly defining specific requirements for prosthesis prescription and usage—such as the ability to hop the length of the parallel bars—can sometimes serve as motivating factors for individuals who are borderline candidates for prosthetic intervention, or self-evidence of poor-candidacy for those who cannot.

Once an initial prosthesis has been fabricated and delivered, the rehabilitation process continues via PT and/or OT referrals. This should be specific and targeted toward the patient's current level of function, short-term and long-term goals, and current setting (outpatient, rehabilitation facility, etc.). In the likely scenario that there is some time delay between prosthesis delivery and the initiation of PT, a "wearing schedule" should be provided to ease the patient into use; a sample is shown in **Fig. 2**. Early, unsupervised use of a prosthesis may result in pain, wounds, and injurious falls.

Once someone is fit with a prosthesis, they typically work toward using the least restrictive AD and some will be able to ambulate without an AD. Even if able to walk, most individuals will benefit from having a wheelchair as a backup means of mobility due to inevitable complications or comorbidities. Individuals with unilateral upper limb-loss may continue to use adaptive equipment, with or without a prosthesis, and most will adapt to perform tasks unilaterally. Early counseling regarding functional progression and physical changes should also be offered at this stage. A young, healthy individual with a more distal amputation is expected to ambulate sooner, more confidently, and without ADs, as compared to older, more medically complex individuals with higher level amputations. Physiatrists should continue to support, encourage, and to normalize struggles and setbacks through what may be many months of rehabilitation.

LONG-TERM CARE

PwLL should receive lifelong interdisciplinary care led by a physiatrist.[47,48] Outpatient follow-up visits should be patient-centered and goal-focused, including treatment of both prosthesis-related concerns and comorbid conditions. More specifically, discussion should include prosthetic fit and function and overall mobility, as well as broader concerns including pain, skin health, sweat management, DME needs, psychosocial adjustment, community re-integration, and in applicable scenarios, contralateral foot care. This approach not only provides patients a comprehensive hub for "all things amputation," but should aim to increase the long-term adherence to prosthesis usage.

Wearing Schedule & Recommendations
Days 1-3: Wear the prosthesis for a maximum of 1 hour at a time, with up to 15min of that standing and/or short distance walking as advised in clinic. These amounts are maximums and need not all be done at once. Examine the limb after every hour of wearing, and/or after every 15 minutes of standing or walking.
Days 3-7: If there were no problems after the maximums from Day 1-3 were reached, then the new maximums are 3 hours of wearing, and up to 30 minutes of that standing and/or walking. If the maximums were not reached on Day 1, then do not increase the wearing and standing/walking times until the maximum can be reached without significant problems.
Beyond 1 week: If there is no persistent pain or redness, the wearing time can be increased by 30 minutes per day and the standing/walking time increased by 10 minutes per day.
General considerations:
1. If in doubt about a problem, or if a new wound or blister develops, discontinue use of the prosthesis and call us. 2. Red or pink discoloration indicates pressure and may be normal if non-painful, and if it fades within 15 minutes. 3. All walking at this point should be supervised. Please only walk with the aid of a walker for now, in the home on level surfaces, or until you receive the recommended therapy. 4. Always wear your prescribed diabetic footwear, even in the home (if prescribed / recommended in clinic). 5. The above wearing times are guidelines only: you do not have to meet these maximums on any given day, but you should not exceed them without discussion with your provider. 6. Check your skin and the fit of the prosthesis every hour of use during the first two to four weeks. 7. For now, wear the shrinker any time that the prosthesis is not on to control any swelling problems that may arise.

Fig. 2. Suggested initial prosthesis wearing schedule.

Socket fit is noted as a top priority for patients in multiple large surveys[49,50] and as such, should be evaluated at every visit. A poorly fitting socket will inevitably lead to pain, skin or soft tissue breakdown, gait changes, and/or functional decline, with potential downstream effects including mental health decline and prosthesis abandonment.[51] Early visits may be as frequent as everyone to 3 months, gradually spacing out as limb volume stabilizes and prosthesis use (or nonuse) becomes more consistent. The initial prosthesis will be subject to frequent adjustments due to maturation of the soft tissue in the naive residual limb as well as changes in strength and gait patterns. Typically, this starts with simple sock-ply adjustment followed by interior socket wall padding; when these measures have been maximized and the patient continues to experience complications from poor fit, a new socket should be prescribed. The time to a sock re-fit may vary; in a study multiple new sockets were required in the initial 3 years in TTA amputees, and lower extremity prosthesis refit every 2 years on average.[52] In a Veterans Affairs (VA) study (which may not reflect civilian practices), new prescriptions for upper extremity prostheses were needed every 3.5 years.[53] All prosthetic componentry is prone to wear and breakdown. Issues with the interface (eg, gel liners) may contribute to pain or skin lesions. Malfunctioning hardware including sockets, prosthetic feet, or knees may culminate in catastrophic failure and falls. Componentry should be closely inspected at regular intervals, with careful note of manufacturer warranties and servicing recommendations; close involvement and discussion with the patient's prosthetist is important.

Functional prosthesis usage is a goal for patients and practitioners alike; however, usage is not universal and abandonment rates are higher than one might expect. Documented rates of prosthesis use may vary from 27% to 56% for upper limb prostheses and 49% to 95% for lower limb prostheses.[54] Those with upper limb-loss report high rates of abandonment, with larger studies suggesting rates approaching 50%.[6,7] Reasons for prosthetic abandonment vary among upper and lower limb amputees; however, patients predominantly report lack of comfort and poor function as common causes, with secondary issues being weight and lack of sensory feedback.[55] Patients were more likely to abandon devices when they had poorer device satisfaction scores at baseline or had low-intensity usage.[53] In another large survey, among patients who were current users, only 43% were satisfied with prosthesis.[52] Taken together, these numbers suggest a high number of unsatisfied prosthesis users often due to discomfort or poor functioning, which may lead to limited use and/or abandonment. This highlights the importance of regularly scheduled visits incorporating prosthetic adjustments, prescription alterations, and therapeutic interventions to keep patients safe and comfortable in their prostheses and able to work toward functional goals.

Access to prosthetic care and components varies among the civilian and veteran populations in the United States. Most VA systems of care provide access without yearly or lifetime caps. Civilian care may be limited, and as "DME," often incur annual and lifetime caps of $500 to 3000 versus $10,000, respectively.[56] Medicare covers 80% of costs that are considered "reasonably necessary to restore normal function in day-to-day activities"; however, the remaining 20% may be financially prohibitive for some patients. This may limit patients' access to high-technology devices and decrease the frequency of new prescriptions. To address this disparity, prosthetic parity motions have been started in several different states. Data show that access to care can improve function, quality of life, and return to work rates, while reducing overuse injuries, gait alterations, and subsequent amputation (with an overall decrease health care costs).[56]

Lifelong care should incorporate periodic discussion on functional goals and the effects of aging, as functional mobility and prosthesis use will decline with age.[54] Prosthetic prescription adjustments, therapy intervention, and/or new DME may be needed to address these changes. Pain, skin care (including sweat management), and the psychosocial effects of limb-loss need to be address periodically. In a large survey of patients with upper limb-loss, 85% of respondents had some pain (42% with pain interfering with ability to use a prosthesis); 50% of respondents cited hyperhidrosis as a primary complaint.[57] "Skin problems" have a high prevalence in prosthesis users, ranging 40% to 74%.[58,59] Further exploration of these topics can be found in other titles within this issue.

ADDITIONAL CONSIDERATIONS
The Interdisciplinary Team

Paramount to physiatric practice is "the team." Though beyond the scope of this article, it is worth mentioning the importance of an interdisciplinary model in limb-loss rehabilitation. In addition to the patient and physician, this team may include a certified prosthetist orthotist, PTs and/or OTs, rehabilitation psychologists, social workers, wound care specialists, surgeons, and family members. Each member brings unique expertise to address the various aspects of limb-loss, ensuring a holistic approach to recovery and prevention of secondary complications. It should be assembled early, preferably pre-amputation, to ensure timely and appropriate rehabilitation expectations.[60,61] Literature suggests improved outcomes for PwLL when incorporating an interdisciplinary rehabilitation team.[62,63] As such, it is an approach modeled by the Department of VA, Department of Defense, and several other countries including the Netherlands and Australia.[64,65]

Physiatric Training

While Physical Medicine and Rehabilitation (PM&R) residency programs do provide more exposure to amputee rehabilitation compared to other medical specialty programs, the availability of specialized amputation rehabilitation training varies significantly. In a survey conducted in 2013 by Elias et. Al, fewer than 60% of surveyed PM&R residencies have dedicated amputee/prosthetics rotations or faculty involved in amputee research.[66] There now exist at least 4 PM&R fellowship opportunities to gain 1 or 2 years of specialty training in the care of individuals with limb loss.[67–69]

SUMMARY

Having a designated team leader is crucial for any event or situation that involves a team of professionals. Physiatrists' expertise in functional assessment and forecasting, biomechanics, pain management, and therapeutic techniques, are unique amongst health care professionals and are ideally suited for leading this team. Management should span the entire spectrum of care, from pre-amputation onward. By deconstructing the phases of limb-loss rehabilitation and exploring evidence-based practices, one can better understand and integrate optimal care for these complex patients.

CLINICS CARE POINTS

- Preservation of functional limb length at the time of amputation is essential for optimizing functional outcomes, though there are caveats to this principle.
- Use of rigid removable dressings post-operatively correlates with earlier prosthesis fitting post-transtibial amputation.
- Elderly individuals with major lower limb dysvascular amputations who go to inpatient rehabilitation have improved prosthetic fitting and survival rates as compared to those who receive less intensive rehabilitation services.
- Early prosthetic fitting and training promotes lower rates of prosthesis abandonment.
- Prosthesis use is associated with improved mood and quality of life, and reduced rates of phantom limb pain.
- Pain, skin conditions, hyperhidrosis, and psychosocial dysfunction are common and should be addressed in long-term follow-up.

DISCLOSURES

None of the authors have any commercial or financial conflicts of interest and any funding sources.

REFERENCES

1. Herrera-Moreno D, Carvajal-Ovalle D, Cueva-Nuñez MA, et al. Body image, perceived stress, and resilience in military amputees of the internal armed conflict in Colombia. Int J Psychol Res 2018;11(2):56–62.

2. Zidarov D, Swaine B, Gauthier-Gagnon C. Quality of life of persons with lower-limb amputation during rehabilitation and at 3-month follow-up. Arch Phys Med Rehabil 2009;90(4):634–45.
3. Ziegler-Graham K, MacKenzie EJ, Ephraim PL, et al. Estimating the prevalence of limb loss in the United States: 2005 to 2050. Arch Phys Med Rehabil 2008;89(3): 422–9.
4. Czerniecki JM, Turner AP, Williams RM, et al. The development and validation of the AMPREDICT model for predicting mobility outcome after dysvascular lower extremity amputation. J Vasc Surg 2017;65(1):162–71.e3.
5. Salminger S, Stino H, Pichler LH, et al. Current rates of prosthetic usage in upper-limb amputees - have innovations had an impact on device acceptance? Disabil Rehabil 2022;44(14):3708–13.
6. Biddiss EA, Chau TT. Upper limb prosthesis use and abandonment: a survey of the last 25 years. Prosthet Orthot Int 2007;31(3):236–57.
7. Carey SL, Lura DJ, Highsmith MJ, et al. Differences in myoelectric and body-powered upper-limb prostheses: Systematic literature review. J Rehabil Res Dev 2015;52(3):247–62.
8. Dillingham TR, Pezzin LE, MacKenzie EJ. Limb amputation and limb deficiency: epidemiology and recent trends in the United States. South Med J 2002;95(8): 875–83.
9. Varma P, Stineman MG, Dillingham TR. Epidemiology of limb loss. Phys Med Rehabil Clin 2014;25(1):1–8.
10. Crowe CS, Impastato KA, Donaghy AC, et al. Prosthetic and orthotic options for lower extremity amputation and reconstruction. Plast Aesthetic Res. 2019;2019.
11. Low EE, Inkellis E, Morshed S. Complications and revision amputation following trauma-related lower limb loss. Injury 2017;48(2):364–70.
12. Wang C, Mai L, Yang C, et al. Reducing major lower extremity amputations after the introduction of a multidisciplinary team in patient with diabetes foot ulcer. BMC Endocr Disord 2016;16(1):38. Published 2016 Jul 7.
13. McDermott K, Fang M, Boulton AJM, et al. Etiology, Epidemiology, and Disparities in the Burden of Diabetic Foot Ulcers. Diabetes Care 2023;46(1):209–21.
14. Everett E, Mathioudakis N. Update on management of diabetic foot ulcers. Ann N Y Acad Sci 2018;1411(1):153–65.
15. Wilken JM, Roy CW, Shaffer SW, et al. Physical Performance Limitations After Severe Lower Extremity Trauma in Military Service Members. J Orthop Trauma 2018; 32(4):183–9.
16. Bedigrew KM, Patzkowski JC, Wilken JM, et al. Can an integrated orthotic and rehabilitation program decrease pain and improve function after lower extremity trauma? Clin Orthop Relat Res 2014;472(10):3017–25.
17. Aman M, Biglari B, Thielen M, et al. An Algorithm for Elective Amputation Combined with Targeted Muscle Reinnervation in Complex Regional Pain Syndrome-A Perspective. J Personalized Med 2022;12(7):1169. Published 2022 Jul 19.
18. Geertzen JHB, Scheper J, Schrier E, et al. Outcomes of amputation due to long-standing therapy-resistant complex regional pain syndrome type I. J Rehabil Med 2020;52(8):jrm00087. Published 2020 Aug 24.
19. Bell JC, Wolf EJ, Schnall BL, et al. Transfemoral amputations: is there an effect of residual limb length and orientation on energy expenditure? Clin Orthop Relat Res 2014;472(10):3055–61.
20. Resnik L, Borgia M, Cancio J, et al. Understanding Implications of Residual Limb Length, Strength, and Range-of-Motion Impairments of Veterans With Upper Limb Amputation. Am J Phys Med Rehabil 2022;101(6):545–54.

21. Penn-Barwell JG. Outcomes in lower limb amputation following trauma: a systematic review and meta-analysis. Injury 2011;42(12):1474–9.
22. Göktepe AS, Cakir B, Yilmaz B, et al. Energy expenditure of walking with prostheses: comparison of three amputation levels. Prosthet Orthot Int 2010;34(1):31–6.
23. Gaine WJ, McCreath SW. Syme's amputation revisited: a review of 46 cases. J Bone Joint Surg Br 1996;78(3):461–7.
24. Morse BC, Cull DL, Kalbaugh C, et al. Through-knee amputation in patients with peripheral arterial disease: a review of 50 cases. J Vasc Surg 2008;48(3):638–43.
25. Franchin M, Palermo V, Iannuzzi C, et al. A predictive score for 30-day survival for patients undergoing major lower limb amputation for peripheral arterial obstructive disease. Updates Surg 2021;73(5):1989–2000.
26. Aulivola B, Hile CN, Hamdan AD, et al. Major lower extremity amputation: outcome of a modern series. Arch Surg 2004;139(4):395–9.
27. Samuelsen BT, Andrews KL, Houdek MT, et al. The Impact of the Immediate Postoperative Prosthesis on Patient Mobility and Quality of Life after Transtibial Amputation. Am J Phys Med Rehabil 2017 Feb;96(2):116–9.
28. Smith DG, McFarland LV, Sangeorzan BJ, et al. Postoperative dressing and management strategies for transtibial amputations: a critical review. J Rehabil Res Dev 2003;40(3):213–24.
29. Churilov I, Churilov L, Murphy D. Do rigid dressings reduce the time from amputation to prosthetic fitting? A systematic review and meta-analysis. Ann Vasc Surg 2014;28(7):1801–8.
30. Dillingham TR, Pezzin LE. Rehabilitation setting and associated mortality and medical stability among persons with amputations. Arch Phys Med Rehabil 2008;89(6):1038–45.
31. Atkins D. Adult upper limb prosthetic training. atlas of limb prosthetics: surgical, prosthetic, and rehabilitation principles, 277–293. 2002. Available at: http://www.oandplibrary.org/alp/chap11-01.asp.
32. Malone JM, Fleming LL, Roberson J, et al. Immediate, early, and late postsurgical management of upper-limb amputation. J Rehabil Res Dev 1984;21(1):33–41.
33. Singh R, Ripley D, Pentland B, et al. Depression and anxiety symptoms after lower limb amputation: the rise and fall. Clin Rehabil 2009;23(3):281–6.
34. Amputee Coalition - Learn about amputation & prosthetic care & request support for people living with limb loss, their families, caregivers and clinicians who care for amputees. Amputee Coalition. Available at: https://www.amputee-coalition.org/.
35. Gaine WJ, Smart C, Bransby-Zachary M. Upper limb traumatic amputees. Review of prosthetic use. J Hand Surg Br. 1997;22(1):73–6.
36. Durmus D, Safaz I, Adıgüzel E, et al. The relationship between prosthesis use, phantom pain and psychiatric symptoms in male traumatic limb amputees. Compr Psychiatr 2015;59:45–53.
37. Horgan O, MacLachlan M. Psychosocial adjustment to lower-limb amputation: a review. Disabil Rehabil 2004;26(14–15):837–50.
38. Erlenwein J, Diers M, Ernst J, et al. Clinical updates on phantom limb pain. Pain Rep 2021;6(1):e888.
39. Wheaton LA. Neurorehabilitation in upper limb amputation: understanding how neurophysiological changes can affect functional rehabilitation. J NeuroEng Rehabil 2017;14(1):41.
40. Davie-Smith F, Coulter E, Kennon B, et al. Factors influencing quality of life following lower limb amputation for peripheral arterial occlusive disease: A systematic review of the literature. Prosthet Orthot Int 2017;41(6):537–47.

41. Passero T. Devising the prosthetic prescription and typical examples. Phys Med Rehabil Clin 2014;25:117–32.
42. Hafner BJ, Smith DG. Differences in function and safety between Medicare Functional Classification Level-2 and -3 transfemoral amputees and influence of prosthetic knee joint control. J Rehabil Res Dev 2009;46(3):417–33.
43. Izumi Y, Satterfield K, Lee S, et al. Risk of reamputation in diabetic patients stratified by limb and level of amputation: a 10-year observation. Diabetes Care 2006; 29(3):566–70.
44. Miller WC, Speechley M, Deathe B. The prevalence and risk factors of falling and fear of falling among lower extremity amputees. Arch Phys Med Rehabil 2001; 82(8):1031–7.
45. Davies B, Datta D. Mobility outcome following unilateral lower limb amputation. Prosthet Orthot Int 2003;27(3):186–90.
46. Highsmith MJ, Kahle JT, Carey SL, et al. Kinetic asymmetry in transfemoral amputees while performing sit to stand and stand to sit movements. Gait Posture 2011;34(1):86–91.
47. Meier RH 3rd, Heckman JT. Principles of contemporary amputation rehabilitation in the United States, 2013. Phys Med Rehabil Clin 2014;25(1):29–33.
48. Donaghy AC, Morgan SJ, Kaufman GE, et al. Team Approach to Prosthetic Prescription Decision-Making. Curr Phys Med Rehabil 2020;8:386–95.
49. Legro MW, Reiber G, del Aguila M, et al. Issues of importance reported by persons with lower limb amputations and prostheses. J Rehabil Res Dev 1999;36(3): 155–63.
50. Klute GK, Kantor C, Darrouzet C, et al. Lower-limb amputee needs assessment using multistakeholder focus-group approach. J Rehabil Res Dev 2009;46(3): 293–304.
51. MacKenzie EJ, Bosse MJ. Factors influencing outcome following limb-threatening lower limb trauma: lessons learned from the Lower Extremity Assessment Project (LEAP). J Am Acad Orthop Surg 2006;14(10 Spec No.):S205–10.
52. Dillingham TR, Pezzin LE, MacKenzie EJ, et al. Use and satisfaction with prosthetic devices among persons with trauma-related amputations: a long-term outcome study. Am J Phys Med Rehabil 2001 Aug;80(8):563–71.
53. Resnik L, Borgia M, Biester S, et al. Longitudinal study of prosthesis use in veterans with upper limb amputation. Prosthet Orthot Int 2021 Feb;45(1):26–35.
54. Raichle KA, Hanley MA, Molton I, et al. Prosthesis use in persons with lower- and upper-limb amputation. J Rehabil Res Dev 2008;45(7):961–72.
55. Smail LC, Neal C, Wilkins C, et al. Comfort and function remain key factors in upper limb prosthetic abandonment: findings of a scoping review. Disabil Rehabil Assist Technol 2021 Nov;16(8):821–30.
56. Etter K, Borgia M, Resnik L. Prescription and repair rates of prosthetic limbs in the VA healthcare system: implications for national prosthetic parity. Disabil Rehabil Assist Technol 2015;10(6):493–500.
57. Davidson J. A survey of the satisfaction of upper limb amputees with their prostheses, their lifestyles, and their abilities. J Hand Ther 2002;15(1):62–70.
58. Koc E, Tunca M, Akar A, et al. Skin problems in amputees: a descriptive study. Int J Dermatol 2008;47(5):463–6.
59. Dudek NL, Marks MB, Marshall SC, et al. Dermatologic conditions associated with use of a lower-extremity prosthesis. Arch Phys Med Rehabil 2005;86(4): 659–63.
60. Esquenazi A. Amputation rehabilitation and prosthetic restoration. From surgery to community reintegration. Disabil Rehabil 2004;26(14–15):831–6.

61. Keszler MS, Wright KS, Miranda A, et al. Multidisciplinary Amputation Team Management of Individuals with Limb Loss. Current Physical Medicine and Rehabilitation Reports 2020;8:118–26.
62. Johannesson A, Larsson GU, Ramstrand N, et al. Incidence of lower-limb amputation in the diabetic and nondiabetic general population: a 10-year population-based cohort study of initial unilateral and contralateral amputations and reamputations. Diabetes Care 2009;32(2):275–80.
63. Lim TS, Finlayson A, Thorpe JM, et al. Outcomes of a contemporary amputation series. ANZ J Surg 2006;76(5):300–5.
64. Geertzen J, Van Der Linde H, Rosenbrand K, et al. Dutch evidence-based guidelines for amputation and prosthetics of the lower extremity: rehabilitation process and prosthetics. Part 2. Prosthet Orthot Int 2015;39:361–71.
65. Model of amputee rehabilitation in south australia statewide rehabilitation clinical network contents. 2012. Available at: http://gifpa.apfisio.pt/gifpa/wp-content/ uploads/bsk-pdf-manager/4_GOVERNMENT_OF_SOUTH_AUSTRALIA-MODEL_ OF_AMPUTEE_REHABILITATION_IN_SOUTH_AUSTRALIA.
66. Elias JA, Morgenroth DC. Amputee care education in physical medicine and rehabilitation residency programs. Am J Phys Med Rehabil 2013;92:157–62.
67. Amputation Rehabilitation Fellowship. UW Medicine | Rehabilitation Medicine. Available at: https://rehab.washington.edu/education/fellowships/amputation-rehabilitation-fellowship. [Accessed 4 December 2023].
68. Prosthetics and Orthotics - Spaulding Rehab. Spauldingrehab.org. 2023. Available at: https://spauldingrehab.org/conditions-services/prosthetics-orthotics. [Accessed 4 December 2023].
69. Amputee and Musculoskeletal Medicine Fellowship - Department of Physical Medicine and Rehabilitation - VCU School of Medicine. pmr.vcu.edu. Available at: https:// pmr.vcu.edu/education/amputee-and-musculoskeletal-medicine-fellowship–/. [Accessed 4 December 2023].

Prostheses and Rehabilitation Principles in Pediatric Limb Deficiency

Yunna L. Sinskey, MD[a], Mary Catherine Spires, MD[b],*

KEYWORDS

- Pediatric phantom pain • Pediatric limb difference and deficiency
- Pediatric prosthetics • Congenital limb deficiency • Pediatric Limb Loss
- Pediatric prosthetic rehabilitation

KEY POINTS

- Physiatrists are experts in leading multidisciplinary teams caring for patients with pediatric limb differences.
- Pediatric patients with limb differences are otherwise no different from other children and need the care and support of a multidisciplinary team to maximize their potential.
- Parent and caregiver education is key in the care of children with limb differences.
- Frequent assessment of the psychosocial health of the child and the family is encouraged, including asking about bullying.

INTRODUCTION

Pediatric limb loss or limb deficiency is uncommon in the United Sates at incidence of 1 per 1943 live births per year, with a ratio of 2:1 upper to lower extremity.[1] Causes include congenital limb deficiency, and less frequently, limb loss secondary to trauma, cancer, or other illnesses. Vascular disruption, particularly as seen in amniotic band syndrome, is the leading suspect in the multifaceted and intricate causes of congenital limb loss, warranting further exploration of its precise mechanisms and potential interplay with other contributing factors.[2] Lawn mower–related injuries are the leading cause of major amputations in children under the age of 10.[2] Congenital limb loss and differences correlate with the embryologic development of the upper and lower limb, which occurs approximately 4 to 8 weeks after fertilization.[3] Although some associations have been identified, detailed underlying mechanisms of limb deficiency require further research.[4] The presence of limb deficiency is often not recognized

[a] Department of Rehabilitation Medicine, University of Washington & VA Puget Sound Health Care System (VAPSHCS), Seattle, WA 98108, USA; [b] Department of Physical Medicine and Rehabilitation, University of Michigan, 325 East Eisenhower Parkway, Suite 200, Ann Arbor, MI 48108, USA
* Corresponding author.
E-mail address: mcspires@med.umich.edu

Phys Med Rehabil Clin N Am 35 (2024) 707–724
https://doi.org/10.1016/j.pmr.2024.05.005 **pmr.theclinics.com**

before birth. Early recognition remains challenging, with prenatal ultrasound detection rates for upper extremity anomalies as low as 42%.[5]

Tailoring Care for Children with Limb Difference: The Role of Physical Medicine and Rehabilitation

Children with limb difference present unique challenges for health care professionals. Physicians trained in Physical Medicine and Rehabilitation (PM&R) are uniquely equipped to navigate these complexities. Physiatrist's comprehensive understanding of musculoskeletal health, growth and development, and rehabilitation empowers them to provide holistic care throughout the child's journey.

This journey is filled with dynamic needs. As the child develops, potential issues like overuse injuries, skin complications from prosthetic use, and psychological adjustments can arise. PM&R specialists expertly address these diverse challenges. They carefully assess each child's individual circumstances, recognizing that optimal prosthetic restoration is not a one-size-fits-all solution. Additionally, they assess whether children with limb deficiency, single limb or multiple deficiencies can benefit from adaptive equipment. For instance, children with multiple limb deficiencies or neurodevelopmental disorders may benefit from alternative interventions, such as a wheelchair, to achieve mobility and self-care goals.

Early collaboration is crucial. Typically, by the time a PM&R specialist encounters a child with congenital limb deficiency, initial investigations to determine whether the condition is part of a syndrome have already begun. Awareness of associated syndromes, particularly prevalent in upper extremity limb deficiencies, is critical for the PM&R clinician. Careful history and physical examination form the foundation, but further diagnostic workup may be necessary, especially in cases like radial longitudinal deficiency. Studies, such as echocardiograms, renal ultrasounds, hematologic studies, peripheral blood smears, spine radiographs, and even chromosomal challenge tests for suspected Fanconi anemia, may be needed.

By providing this nuanced and individualized approach, PM&R specialists play a vital role in optimizing outcomes for children with limb deficiency. This expertise ensures that each child receives the right support and care, at the right time, to navigate the challenges and embrace the possibilities of their unique journey.

PARENTS AND CAREGIVERS

In optimizing prosthesis use for children with limb difference, parental and caregiver involvement is crucial. They play a primary role in shaping the child's acceptance and utilization of the prosthesis, impacting both the timing and frequency of use. Comprehensive parental and caregiver education regarding available prosthetic options is essential. This should include a balanced discussion of both the functional and aesthetic advantages and limitations of each option.

Physician assessment should extend beyond the child and include the expectations and priorities of the parents/caregivers. For instance, parents/caregivers may prioritize cosmesis over function in the child with upper extremity deficiency. They may prefer a prosthesis that looks as "normal as possible." However, a body-powered "hook" terminal device often facilitates better function by allowing the user to see what they are manipulating, compared with a more lifelike body-powered prosthetic hand, which may impede the line of sight of the object they are manipulating. Some parents and caregivers may find the appearance of the hook terminal device unacceptable and prefer the anatomic-appearing hand.

PSYCHOSOCIAL CONSIDERATIONS

Attitudes of parents and caregivers, childhood interactions, social experiences, interactions with health care providers, and chronologic and developmental age impact a child's perception of their limb difference and self-esteem.[6]

It is important for physicians and other providers to foster the strengths of the parents/caregivers and to specifically acknowledge the challenges they face raising a child with a disability. Referral to support services may be needed. Providers must be attuned to signs of child neglect or abuse. As with any child, the provider is legally required to report suspected abuse to the appropriate legal channels.

Financial resources are a concern for many families. Parents/guardians need to know their financial obligations and be aware of their medical insurance plan coverage. The physician and the rehabilitation team can provide documentation of medical necessity and provide supporting information for appeal processes if services are denied. Social work may assist regarding financial assistance that is available. For example, in the State of Michigan, children with special health care needs can be enrolled in the Children's Special Health Care Services program within the Michigan Department of Health and Human Services, which is part of Title V of the Federal Social Security Act.

During follow-up care, the provider is advised to assess the psychosocial health of the child and the family, including socioeconomic stressors and access to care. Involvement of mental health providers is vital for children and families displaying concerning interactions and/or maladaptive behaviors. Families can also be advised of relevant resources that are available to them locally. **Table 1** provides examples of available resources.

The literature shows that children with a disability, such as limb differences or limb deficiency, experience bullying at a higher rate than their peers.[6] The physician is advised to encourage and support parents/caregivers to reach out to the school or setting where bullying is a concern. Participation in activities outside of school, consistent with the child's interests, have been shown to reduce incidence of bullying and improved self-esteem.[7] Sports, camps, art and social activities, and other extracurricular activities promote inclusion, physical fitness, and self-esteem.

EDUCATIONAL IMPLICATIONS

Parents should be advised of the educational opportunities for children with disabilities. Children with disabilities are guaranteed the right to a Free Appropriate Public Education through the Individuals with Disabilities Education Act (IDEA). This federal law defines the specific requirements and details that specify that the education of a child with a disability must be tailored to mitigate or eliminate the barriers to a child's education and learning and must occur in the least restrictive environment.

There are 2 separate age groups addressed in this law. Part C addresses services for ages 0 to 3 years, whereas Part B addresses students with disabilities ages 3 through 21 years. Some states provide this service beyond age 21. A child must have one of the 13 disabilities[8] as outlined in the IDEA to qualify for services within the public school system. Disabilities relevant to those with limb loss or differences may include orthopedic impairment, multiple disabilities, and other health impairment.

Public school systems have a responsibly to identify and evaluate children who may have a disability that impedes a child's education. If parents have concerns, they have the legal right to request an evaluation through their school district. An evaluation includes gathering information regarding their child's current functioning to determine whether they meet criteria for one of the disability categories outlined in IDEA. If the

Table 1
Resources available for pediatric amputee care for families and clinicians

Category	Resource	Description	Web Site
Family & Children Support	Amputee Coalition	Supports children and adults with limb loss through education, advocacy, and programs like the Work Force Development Program. Often, they can provide contact with local peer support groups for families and individuals	https://www.amputee-coalition.org/
	Children Having Infant Limb Deficiency (CHILD)	Facebook group for families of children with limb differences	https://m.facebook.com/swawrzynRN/
Children's Camps & Activities	Adventure Amputee Camp	Camp for children with limb differences focusing on outdoor adventures	https://adventureamputeecamp.org/
	Amputee Blade Runners	Provides prosthetic legs for running to children with limb differences	https://amputeebladerunners.com/
	Amputee Coalition Youth Camp	Camp for children with limb differences to connect with peers, explore new experiences, and build confidence	https://www.amputee-coalition.org/events-programs/youth-camp/
	Camp No Limits	Camp for children with limb loss and limb differences offering a variety of activities	https://www.nolimitsfoundation.org/about
	Challenged Athletes Foundation	Provides camps and clinics for children and adults with disabilities; offers grants for sports equipment	https://www.challengedathletes.org/athletes/
	Hands to Love	Annual camp for children with upper limb and hand differences	https://www.handstolove.org/
	Lucky Fin Project	Provides adaptive swim fins and other resources for children with limb differences	https://luckyfinproject.org/
	Move United	Offers sports camps and clinics for children and adults with disabilities	https://moveunitedsport.org/
Professional Resources	Association of Children's Prosthetic-Orthotic Clinics (ACPOC)	Supports professionals working with children with musculoskeletal differences	https://acpoc.org/
	American Academy of Physical Medicine and Rehabilitation (AAPM&R)	Provides resources and education for professionals in physical medicine and rehabilitation	https://www.aapmr.org/

child meets the criteria, special education services are provided as outlined in an individualized education plan (IEP). For children 3 years and older, the parent or guardian should contact their local public elementary school and express the potential impacts of their child's disability and request an evaluation. For children less than 3 years, parents or guardians must contact the early intervention program in their public school system.

For children who have a disability but do not qualify for an IEP, a 504-accommodation plan may be appropriate. These are based on protections outlined in Section 504 of the Rehabilitation Act of 1973. A 504 plan outlines accommodations needed to ensure academic success and access to his or her learning environment.

SURGERY

Children born with a malformed limb may benefit from surgery. Factors to be considered in the development of the surgical plan include consideration of optimal bone length, impact of growth plates, needed soft tissue coverage, and proximal stability.[9] For example, when determining the length of the residual limb, the clinician must be mindful of the potential growth and resulting final length difference compared with the contralateral limb. When the residual limb length is too short, the availability of different prosthesis components becomes limited.

Distal bony overgrowth is often problematic in children with amputation who have not undergone joint disarticulation. Bony overgrowth may contribute to poor prosthetic fit, wounds at the site of overgrowth, and pain, and consequently, limits prosthesis use and function. Bony overgrowth requires revision 50% of the time in metaphyseal-level amputations and 45% in diaphyseal amputations.[10]

Fibular hemimelia is one of the more common congenital long bone deficiencies and, because of premature partial physis closure or partially delayed growth, may result in various deformities, including genu valgus.[11] A relatively simple procedure, such as medial distal femoral physeal stapling, can allow correction of deformity over time while still allowing immediate prosthesis use.[11]

PROSTHESIS FITTING AND REHABILITATION PRINCIPLES

Prosthetic prescription and fabrication for children require balancing scientific principles with individual needs. A "one-size-fits-all" approach does not work. Many diverse factors impact prosthetic prescription and fabrication, including amputation level, residual limb characteristics, cognitive/developmental age, family goals, financial resources, and medical literacy. Some children may not benefit from a prosthesis. For example, some children with bilateral arm deficiency use their feet to play and may be able to function at similar or even higher levels without the prosthesis.[12]

Once a child is deemed a candidate for a prosthesis, early and comprehensive family involvement becomes crucial. Parents, siblings, extended family, and caregivers need to be actively engaged in understanding the role of the prosthesis in the child's development to maximize success. Empowering families with knowledge builds confidence in their decision making, especially during the child's formative years. Although the clinical team provides education, training, and support, parents and caregivers are key to assuring consistent and daily use.

Typically, children require more frequent prosthetic adjustments than adults because of their growth patterns and developmental needs.[13] Longitudinal bone growth exceeding circumferential growth necessitates more frequent lengthening or alignment adjustments compared with socket refits. Active play also contributes to increased wear and tear, leading to repairs and replacements. Depending on individual growth and activity levels, adjustments may be needed every few months.[14] Bony overgrowth can be accommodated in most socket designs, but may occasionally requires surgical intervention.[10]

Clinical experience shows that preschoolers need new prostheses nearly yearly, whereas school-aged children require them every 12 to 18 months, and teenagers require them every 18 to 24 months.[14] To minimize socket replacement, various growth-accommodating strategies exist. Prosthetists can use removable growth liners, initially fabricating the sockets to fit over multiple sock layers or use flexible inner sockets. For longitudinal changes, heel lifts on the contralateral shoe in unilateral lower limb cases can compensate for asymmetric lower extremity growth.

PROSTHESIS FITTING IN UPPER LIMB DEFICIENCY

Fitting upper limb prostheses in children follows a developmental approach. In unilateral forearm deficiency, initial fitting typically occurs around 6 months when infants achieve independent sitting balance.[15] Studies suggest starting before 2 years can improve wearing patterns and skills compared with infants who were fitted between 2 and 5 years of age.[16] In infants with bilateral upper limb deficiency for whom prosthesis use is recommended, the initial prosthesis should be fitted after independent walking is established, as the prosthesis makes it more difficult to crawl, move about on the floor, and pull to stand.[14]

The decision to go with a hook or a hand is unique to every patient. Many families with young children request a small passive anatomic hand or mitt for appearance purposes compared with a hook (**Fig. 1**).[13,15] If the terminal device on the initial prosthesis is passive, such as a mitt or hand, they do not provide active grasp or prehensile function, although it does allow for a second point of contact and some object manipulation. A hook will allow prehension. Although hands offer greater aesthetics, they tend to be less functional than hooks and are heavier in weight.[13] Also, the lateral fingers, primarily digits 4 and 5, tend to prevent the child from picking up smaller and flatter objects compared with the hook.[13] Some clinicians think that including an activated terminal device as part of the first prosthesis is beneficial. This approach allows the child to volitionally drop an object, an early developmental skill. A rattle, or other similar toy, can be placed in the terminal device and draw the child's attention to the prosthesis. Initially, because the prosthesis does not provide tactile feedback, the infant may ignore the prosthesis.

Recommendations for adding active terminal devices vary, but are generally added when a child is wearing the prosthesis full-time, follows simple two-step instructions, and is able to use the cable for simple grasp and release functions.[17] This typically

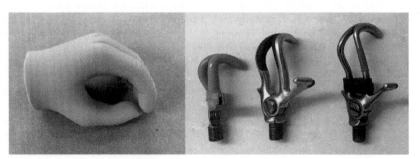

Fig. 1. Anatomic-appearing infant prosthetic hand (*left*) and various models of pediatric hook-style prosthetic hands (*right*).

occurs between 10 and 18 months but may be introduced later if cognitive development indicates.[17] Pediatric occupational or physical therapists are important for successful training, requiring close collaboration with parents and children.

Although varied by practice, the initial active terminal device is typically a body-powered device (**Fig. 2**) owing to its lighter weight and durability compared with a myoelectric prosthesis. Awareness of cause and effect is the most-used indicator for readiness for activation.[15] The addition of an active terminal device allows the child to use building blocks and simple toys similar to the developmental stages of a child without limb deficiency. Frequent visits with the prosthetist may be needed after the addition of an active terminal device, as proper harness fit is critical to operate the device in a growing child.

Timing of myoelectric transition varies depending on practice style. A myoelectric prosthesis may be added at age of 1 year per some clinicians.[18] A myoelectric prosthesis is heavier than a body-powered option and is a factor. Weight can be added to the current prosthesis to help the child accommodate to the added weight.

Between 4 and 5 years of age, depending on cognitive, physical, and social development, children with a transhumeral limb deficiency may be considered candidates for an elbow unit and/or a passive wrist rotation unit, which would allow positioning the hand in pronation or supination.[17] The limb length and length of the componentry impact the timing and fitting of these prosthetic additions.

At 5 to 6 years of age, children can typically grasp fragile objects without damage, begin to learn independent donning/doffing the prosthesis, keep the prosthesis clean, and notify parents/caregivers if they have skin breakdown or pain, or if the prosthesis is not working properly.

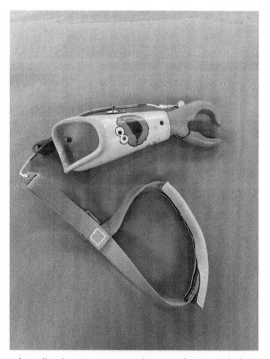

Fig. 2. Body-powered pediatric upper extremity prosthesis with harness and voluntary-closing terminal device.

As children develop diverse interests in activities like swimming, running, weightlifting, or playing an instrument, activity-specific terminal devices (**Fig. 3**) provide new possibilities. Activity-specific devices can improve independence, satisfaction with the prosthesis, and body image, which has been linked to enhanced cognitive performance in amputees.[19] Children who previously struggled with accepting or using their prosthesis may demonstrate a renewed interest in a prosthesis because of new activity interests. The principles discussed above are summarized pictorially in **Fig. 4**.

PROSTHESIS FITTING IN LOWER LIMB DEFICIENCY

In unilateral lower limb deficiency, the first prosthesis is fitted once the infant starts showing interest in pulling up to stand, which is typically around 7 to 12 months of age. Fitting too early can impede the infant's efforts to roll, particularly supine to prone. The prosthesis increases sitting balance and aids the infant's attempt to pull to stand, increasing weight-bearing symmetry and equalizing bilateral leg length. Infants who have upper and lower extremity deficiencies generally do better when fitted with lower limb prostheses first to develop sitting and sitting balance. In addition, this approach lessens the chance of overwhelming the child and family by fitting both the upper and lower extremity prosthesis at the same time. The initial lower extremity prosthesis is typically fabricated with a solid-ankle cushioned heel (SACH) foot, as it is lightweight and durable. Parents are advised to use rubber-soled shoes for increased traction.

A lower extremity prosthesis distributes weight on areas of the lower limb that are not naturally weight-bearing surfaces. Consequently, protecting the child's skin from the socket is important. Building skin and soft tissue tolerance to weight bearing occurs with gradual increases in wear time.

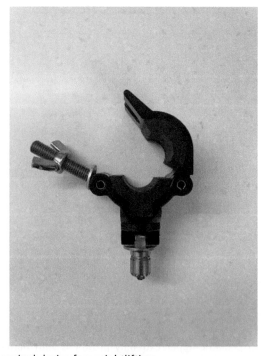

Fig. 3. Adaptive terminal device for weightlifting.

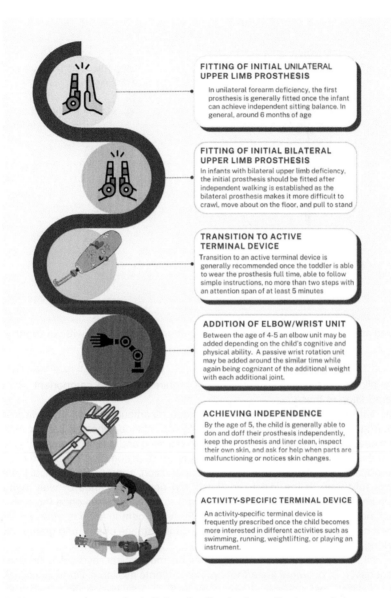

Fig. 4. Upper extremity prosthesis fitting timeline in the pediatric population.

Many children with below-knee amputations, both unilateral and bilateral, do not require assistive devices for independent ambulation.[20] When children are around 2 years old, they start running and jumping, and an asymmetric running gait emphasizing propulsion through the sound side is evident. Parents should be reassured that this is normal for a child that uses a prosthesis.

As the child grows, they may have various prosthetic components added that they did not qualify for earlier because of the dimensions, size, and characteristics of the specific prosthetic component. For example, the initial SACH foot may be changed to an energy-storing/return foot or a dynamic response foot as an appropriate child

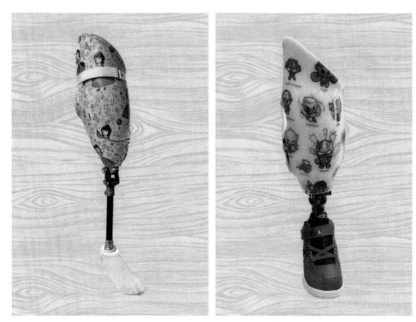

Fig. 5. Pediatric prosthesis for above-knee amputation with (*left*) and without (*right*) knee unit.

size is available. The manufacturer's weight requirements and component size can limit the addition of these.

Infants with above-knee amputations or knee disarticulation may benefit from a jointless (**Fig. 5**) or manual locking knee initially for balance, whereas some clinicians include a knee joint for early mobility, including crawling and pulling to stand.[21] Adding a knee to the prosthesis requires that there is room to accommodate a knee component. Introducing a prosthetic knee requires supervision, appropriate physical therapy, and close follow-up. If the initial prosthesis did not have a knee or was manually locked, a knee joint is typically added around 3 to 4 years of age once the child has achieved independent ambulation (see **Fig. 5**). A polycentric knee is often preferred because it has a smaller build height, stability during stance phase, and greater clearance during swing phase.[22]

Once children reach a specific weight/height, mechanical, hydraulic, pneumatic, microprocessor, or powered knee/foot options become available. Drawbacks include increased weight, cost, and adjustment complexity.[13] Activity-specific prostheses like running blades are an option based on a child's interest, but affordability can be a challenge. Lower limb prosthetic fitting principles are summarized pictorially in **Fig. 6**.

PROSTHESIS ACCEPTANCE AND REJECTION

The reasons behind prosthesis rejection are not always understood. Studies show that children who began wearing their prosthesis before the age of 2 or within 6 months after amputation were less likely to reject their prosthesis.[16,23] Acceptance and interest in a prosthesis may wax and wane depending on the developmental age and the child's interest in various activities. A child who was previously uninterested in a prosthesis often develops an interest in cosmesis and a wish to wear a prosthesis. In

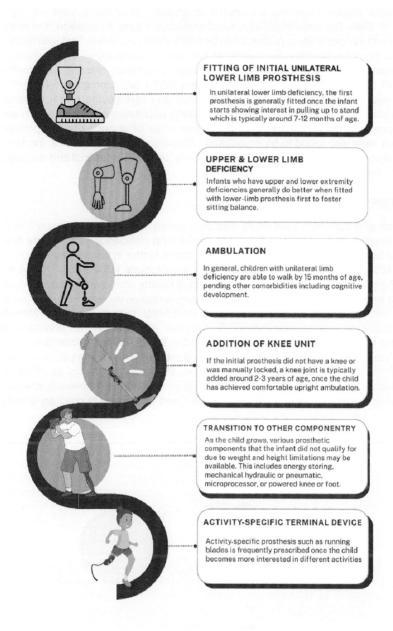

FITTING OF INITIAL UNILATERAL LOWER LIMB PROSTHESIS

In unilateral lower limb deficiency, the first prosthesis is generally fitted once the infant starts showing interest in pulling up to stand which is typically around 7-12 months of age.

UPPER & LOWER LIMB DEFICIENCY

Infants who have upper and lower extremity deficiencies generally do better when fitted with lower-limb prosthesis first to foster sitting balance.

AMBULATION

In general, children with unilateral limb deficiency are able to walk by 15 months of age, pending other comorbidities including cognitive development.

ADDITION OF KNEE UNIT

If the initial prosthesis did not have a knee or was manually locked, a knee joint is typically added around 2-3 years of age, once the child has achieved comfortable upright ambulation.

TRANSITION TO OTHER COMPONENTRY

As the child grows, various prosthetic components that the infant did not qualify for due to weight and height limitations may be available. This includes energy storing, mechanical hydraulic or pneumatic, microprocessor, or powered knee or foot.

ACTIVITY-SPECIFIC TERMINAL DEVICE

Activity-specific prosthesis such as running blades is frequently prescribed once the child becomes more interested in different activities

Fig. 6. Lower extremity prosthesis fitting timeline in pediatric population.

addition, their interest in participation in sports, or other activities involving upper extremity function, increases. An upper extremity prosthesis with an adaptive terminal device specific for the desired activity may further facilitate engagement in social activities.

Existing studies report varying compliance with prosthesis use in children, but compliance appears to be higher with lower extremity prostheses, mirroring adults, with some studies reporting successful prosthesis acceptance rates as high as 89%,[24,25] likely because of obvious functional advantages. In addition, the use and wear of a lower extremity prosthesis can be more easily disguised. For lower extremity prostheses, rejection rates are highest at the most proximal levels of amputation.[16]

In upper extremity amputees, studies suggest common reasons for prosthesis rejection are lack of improvement in function (53%) and discomfort (49%).[26] The mean rejection rates for body-powered (45%) and myoelectric (35%) prostheses were found to be significantly higher in pediatric populations compared with adults (body-powered, 26%; electric, 23%).[27] Higher rates of upper extremity prosthesis rejection were also found to be associated with parental disappointment, inadequate parental involvement in treatment, and dissatisfaction with emotional and social guidance by the clinical team.[28]

PHANTOM PAIN AND MANAGEMENT

Although phantom limb pain (PLP) was considered rare in children, recent studies have revealed its presence even in congenital limb deficiency with the prevalence ranging from 3.7% to 20%.[29,30] The occurrence is higher in trauma-related amputations (12%–83%)[29,30] and oncology-related amputations (48%–90%).[31,32] In these latter 2 groups, the onset of PLP typically occurs shortly after amputation, often within the first week.[16,17] Although the exact mechanisms remain unclear, PLP likely involves both central (cortical reorganization) and peripheral factors (neuroma formation, increased sympathetic sensitivity).[32,33] Surgical management of phantom pain, including the recent development of Regenerative Peripheral Nerve Interface and Targeted Muscle Reinnervation, are becoming potential options for the pediatric populations.[34–37] A more extensive discussion on PLP can be found in "Pain after Amputation: A Clinical Review," found in this issue. Although research specifically examining the link between PLP management and self-image in children is lacking,

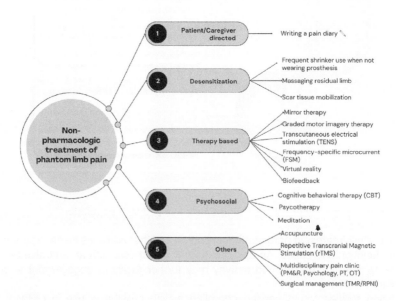

Fig. 7. Nonpharmacologic treatment options of PLP management in pediatric population.

Table 2
Common pharmacologic treatment options for phantom limb pain management in pediatric population

Pharmacologic Class	Examples	Adverse Effects	Comments
Nonsteroidal anti-inflammatory drugs (NSAIDs)/Acetaminophen	Ibuprofen Diclofenac Ketorolac Acetaminophen	Gastrointestinal distress, bleeding, acute kidney injury Hepatic injury from Acetaminophen	Renal dosing adjustment needed for NSAIDs Hepatic dosing adjustment needed for Acetaminophen NSAIDs contraindicated in patients with asthma, rhinitis, and nasal polyps Caution using Aspirin in the pediatric population. Ketorolac IM available if unable to tolerate oral medications
Anticonvulsant	Gabapentin Pregabalin	Drowsiness, dizziness, visual blurring	Renal dosing adjustment needed for both medications Both available in liquid form
Serotonin noradrenaline reuptake inhibitor (SNRI)	Duloxetine	Nausea, dizziness, drowsiness	For patients > age 7 Renal dosing adjustment needed Contraindicated in patients with glaucoma and in hepatic impairment. Has delayed-release sprinkle capsule
Tricyclic antidepressant	Amitriptyline Nortriptyline	Dry mouth, drowsiness, confusion, orthostatic hypotension, constipation, urinary retention, weight gain, arrhythmia	Contraindicated in patients with glaucoma and significant cardiovascular disease
Opioids	Tramadol Codeine Oxycodone	Constipation, sedation, seizures, ataxia	Only consider short term when other options fail May lower seizure threshold. Watch for hepatotoxicity when in use in conjunction with Acetaminophen

evidence from adult studies suggests that effective PLP management is crucial, as it can contribute to positive body image and increased prosthesis satisfaction.[38] This highlights the importance of further investigation in the pediatric population to further understand and effectively address these potential consequences (see **Fig. 6**).

Pediatric PLP management often incorporates modified versions of adult treatment options. Specific considerations regarding developmental stage, growth, and potential side effects necessitate adaptations in pediatric practice. Detailed treatment strategies tailored for children are presented in **Fig. 7** and **Table 2**.

FUTURE DIRECTION IN PEDIATRIC AMPUTEE CARE

Three-dimensional (3D) printing is a promising innovative technology in prosthetics care (**Fig. 8**), enabling the fabrication of complex, customizable sockets with significantly easier and faster production compared with traditional methods. This translates to fewer clinic visits for patients, enhancing accessibility and convenience. 3D printed prostheses hold particular promise for children with limb loss owing to several key advantages. First, their lighter weight offers improved comfort and ease of use, making them more child friendly. Second, the unmatched customizability empowers children to personalize their prostheses with chosen styles and colors, fostering a sense of ownership and acceptance. Third, the rapid production turnaround minimizes wait times, ensuring children can access essential mobility aids quickly. Notably, these prostheses can serve as transitional devices, easing the acclimatization process and ultimately increasing the likelihood of long-term prosthetic use, a crucial concern for young patients. Furthermore, diverse open-source 3D printed upper limb designs are readily available online, expanding access for patients, researchers, and prosthetists alike (eg, National Institutes of Health 3D Web site). In upper extremities, the ease of customization facilitates improved upper-limb symmetry and allows for specific thickness adjustments to optimize for comfort, function, and even bimanual coordination.[39]

Beyond enhancing individual care, 3D printing offers a cost-effective solution for health care systems by reducing production expenses and labor demands. This makes it a particularly attractive option for rural or developing areas lacking access to conventional prosthetic technology. However, challenges remain. One key concern is the limited durability of some printed materials, which may not withstand the active lifestyles of children. This has limited the widespread adoption of 3D printed prostheses for lower limbs. Recent studies, however, demonstrated that a 3D printed pylon with polylactic acid polymer had enough strength under stress and exceeded the requirements of the standard of metallic pylons in lower limb prostheses.[40] Although

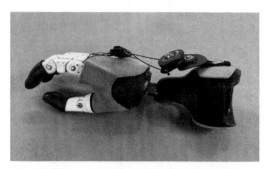

Fig. 8. Prosthetic hand with silicone inner liner, 3D printed outer frame, and College Park M fingers.

incorporation of new printable materials may address durability concerns, it could also inflate costs and limit accessibility.[41] Therefore, future research and development should prioritize the creation of robust yet affordable materials to fully unlock the potential of 3D printing in prosthetics for all populations.

SUMMARY

Pediatric patients with limb differences present unique challenges, necessitating meticulous care orchestrated by a physiatrist-led multidisciplinary team. Addressing the nuanced needs of this specialized cohort involves comprehensive measures, such as syndromic evaluation, informed decision making in prosthetic selection, careful identification and management of PLP, and the provision of holistic support. Essential components encompass parental/caregiver education and regular psychosocial assessments. Continued innovation and research are needed to enhance the functional and aesthetic potential of prostheses for pediatric patients with limb differences.

CLINICS CARE POINTS

- When assessing a child with congenital limb deficiency, initiate a workup to ascertain any potential syndromic associations. For example, radial longitudinal deficiencies may require additional diagnostic evaluations.
- Extracurricular activities aligned with a child's interests outside of school are effective in reducing bullying incidents and enhancing self-esteem.
- The Individuals with Disabilities Education Act guarantees children with disabilities the right to Free Appropriate Public Education, specifying tailored education in the least restrictive environment.
- Determining the appropriate prosthesis for each child requires informed decision making, which considers amputation level, length, shape, medical comorbidities, cognitive and physical development, family acceptance and socioeconomics and understanding of prosthetic restoration, and habilitation.
- Phantom pain, previously underestimated in prevalence, may manifest in children with congenital limb deficiency as well as in children with acquired limb loss.
- Various pharmacologic and nonpharmacologic approaches are available to mitigate pediatric phantom limb pain.

DISCLOSURE

None.

REFERENCES

1. CDC. Data & statistics on birth defects | CDC. Centers for Disease Control and Prevention; 2023. Available at: https://www.cdc.gov/ncbddd/birthdefects/data.html. [Accessed 21 November 2023].
2. Characteristics of Pediatric Traumatic Amputations Treated in Hospital Emergency Departments: United States, 1990–2002 | Pediatrics | American Academy of Pediatrics. Available at: https://publications.aap.org/pediatrics/article-abstract/116/5/e667/68051/Characteristics-of-Pediatric-Traumatic-Amputations?redirectedFrom=fulltext. [Accessed 28 November 2023].

3. Carlson BM. Human Embryology and Developmental Biology. 7th Edition. Amsterdam, Netherlands: Elsevier Inc; 2024.

4. Therapontos C, Erskine L, Gardner ER, et al. Thalidomide induces limb defects by preventing angiogenic outgrowth during early limb formation. Proc Natl Acad Sci 2009;106(21):8573–8. https://doi.org/10.1073/pnas.0901505106.

5. Alrabai HM, Farr A, Bettelheim D, et al. Prenatal diagnosis of congenital upper limb differences: a current concept review. J Matern Fetal Neonatal Med 2017; 30(21):2557–63. https://doi.org/10.1080/14767058.2016.1256989.

6. M P. Systematic Review: Bullying Involvement of Children With and Without Chronic Physical Illness and/or Physical/Sensory Disability-a Meta-Analytic Comparison With Healthy/Nondisabled Peers. J Pediatr Psychol 2017;42(3). https://doi.org/10.1093/jpepsy/jsw081.

7. Extracurricular Activities and Bullying Among Children and Adolescents with Disabilities | Maternal and Child Health Journal. Available at: https://link.springer.com/article/10.1007/s10995-019-02866-6. [Accessed 21 November 2023].

8. Sec. 300.8 Child with a disability. Individuals with Disabilities Education Act. Available at: https://sites.ed.gov/idea/regs/b/a/300.8. [Accessed 4 January 2024].

9. Griffet J. Amputation and prosthesis fitting in paediatric patients. Orthop Traumatol Surg Res OTSR 2016;102(1 Suppl):S161–75. https://doi.org/10.1016/j.otsr.2015.03.020.

10. O'Neal ML, Bahner R, Ganey TM, et al. Osseous Overgrowth After Amputation in Adolescents and Children. J Pediatr Orthop 1996;16(1):78.

11. Boakes JL, Stevens PM, Moseley RF. Treatment of genu valgus deformity in congenital absence of the fibula. J Pediatr Orthop 1991;11(6):721–4. https://doi.org/10.1097/01241398-199111000-00004.

12. Palisano R, Orlin M, Schreiber J. Campbell's Physical Therapy for Children. 6th edition. New York, USA: Elsevier; 2022.

13. Kanas JL, Prostheses. In: Abzug JM, Kozin SH, Zlotolow DA. The pediatric upper extremity, 2015, Springer; New York, USA, 1835–1856. , doi:10.1007/978-1-4614-8515-5_85.

14. Spires MC, Kelly BM, Davis AJ. Prosthetic restoration and rehabilitation of the upper and lower extremity. New York, USA: Demos Medical Publishing; 2013.

15. Shaperman J, Landsberger SE, Setoguchi Y. Early Upper Limb Prosthesis Fitting: When and What Do We Fit. JPO J Prosthetics Orthot 2003;15(1):11.

16. Meurs M, Maathuis CGB, Lucas C, et al. Prescription of the First Prosthesis and Later use in Children with Congenital Unilateral Upper Limb Deficiency: A Systematic Review. Prosthet Orthot Int 2006;30(2):165–73. https://doi.org/10.1080/03093640600731710.

17. Molnar GE, Alexander MA. In: Pediatric rehabilitation. 3rd edition. Hanley & Belfus; 1999. Available at: http://bvbr.bib-bvb.de:8991/F?func=service&doc_library=BVB01&doc_number=009280759&line_number=0001&func_code=DB_R ECORDS&service_type=MEDIA. [Accessed 8 January 2024].

18. Peterson JK, Prigge P. Early Upper-Limb Prosthetic Fitting and Brain Development: Considerations for Success. JPO J Prosthetics Orthot 2020;32(4):229. https://doi.org/10.1097/JPO.0000000000000320.

19. Gozaydinoglu S, Hosbay Z, Durmaz H. Body image perception, compliance with a prosthesis and cognitive performance in transfemoral amputees. Acta Orthop Traumatol Turcica 2019;53(3):221–5. https://doi.org/10.1016/j.aott.2019.03.014.

20. Burgess EM. Amputation Surgery and Rehabilitation: The Toronto Experience. JAMA 1982;247(20):2835–6. https://doi.org/10.1001/jama.1982.03320450067049.

21. Krajbich JI, Pinzur MS, Potter BK, et al. Atlas of amputations and limb deficiencies: surgical, prosthetic, and rehabilitation principles. Lippincott Williams & Wilkins; 2023.

22. Gard SA, Childress DS, Uellendahl JE. The influence of four-bar linkage knees on prosthetic swing-phase floor clearance. JPO J Prosthetics Orthot 1996;8(2):34.

23. Biddiss EA, Chau TT. Multivariate prediction of upper limb prosthesis acceptance or rejection. Disabil Rehabil Assist Technol 2008;3(4):181–92. https://doi.org/10.1080/17483100701869826.

24. Boonstra AM, Rijnders LJM, Groothoff JW, et al. Children with congenital deficiencies or acquired amputations of the lower limbs: Functional aspects. Prosthet Orthot Int 2000;24(1):19–27. https://doi.org/10.1080/03093640008726518.

25. Vannah WM, Davids JR, Drvaric DM, et al. A survey of function in children with lower limb deficiencies. Prosthet Orthot Int 1999;23(3):239–44. https://doi.org/10.3109/03093649909071640.

26. Wagner LV, Bagley AM, James MA. Reasons for Prosthetic Rejection by Children With Unilateral Congenital Transverse Forearm Total Deficiency. JPO J Prosthetics Orthot 2007;19(2):51–4. https://doi.org/10.1097/JPO.0b013e3180421539.

27. Biddiss EA, Chau TT. Upper limb prosthesis use and abandonment: A survey of the last 25 years. Prosthet Orthot Int 2007;31(3):236–57. https://doi.org/10.1080/03093640600994581.

28. Prosthesis rejection in children with a unilateral congenital arm defect - K Postema, V van der Donk, J van Limbeek, et al, 1999. https://journals.sagepub.com/doi/10.1177/026921559901300308?url_ver=Z39.88-2003&rfr_id=ori:rid:crossref.org&rfr_dat=cr_pub%20%200pubmed. Accessed January 10, 2024.

29. Wilkins KL, McGrath PJ, Finley GA, et al. Phantom limb sensations and phantom limb pain in child and adolescent amputees. Pain 1998;78(1):7–12. https://doi.org/10.1016/S0304-3959(98)00109-2.

30. Melzack R. Phantom limbs in people with congenital limb deficiency or amputation in early childhood. Brain 1997;120(9):1603–20. https://doi.org/10.1093/brain/120.9.1603.

31. Krane EJ, Heller LB. The prevalence of phantom sensation and pain in pediatric amputees. J Pain Symptom Manage 1995;10(1):21–9. https://doi.org/10.1016/0885-3924(94)00062-P.

32. Smith J, Thompson JM. Phantom Limb Pain and Chemotherapy in Pediatric Amputees. Mayo Clin Proc 1995;70(4):357–64. https://doi.org/10.4065/70.4.357.

33. Diers M, Fuchs X, Bekrater-Bodmann R, et al. Prevalence of Phantom Phenomena in Congenital and Early-Life Amputees. J Pain 2023;24(3):502–8. https://doi.org/10.1016/j.jpain.2022.10.010.

34. Zuo KJ, Willand MP, Ho ES, et al. Targeted Muscle Reinnervation: Considerations for Future Implementation in Adolescents and Younger Children. Plast Reconstr Surg 2018;141(6):1447. https://doi.org/10.1097/PRS.0000000000004370.

35. Kubiak CA, Kemp SWP, Cederna PS. Regenerative Peripheral Nerve Interface for Management of Postamputation Neuroma. JAMA Surg 2018;153(7):681–2. https://doi.org/10.1001/jamasurg.2018.0864.

36. Woo SL, Kung TA, Brown DL, et al. Regenerative Peripheral Nerve Interfaces for the Treatment of Postamputation Neuroma Pain: A Pilot Study. Plast Reconstr Surg – Glob Open 2016;4(12):e1038. https://doi.org/10.1097/GOX.0000000000001038.

37. Kubiak CA, Kemp SWP, Cederna PS, et al. Prophylactic Regenerative Peripheral Nerve Interfaces to Prevent Postamputation Pain. Plast Reconstr Surg 2019;144(3):421e. https://doi.org/10.1097/PRS.0000000000005922.

38. Beisheim-Ryan EH, Hicks GE, Pohlig RT, et al. Body image and perception among adults with and without phantom limb pain. PM&R 2023;15(3):278–90. https://doi.org/10.1002/pmrj.12750.

39. Copeland C, Reyes CC, Peck JL, et al. Functional performance and patient satisfaction comparison between a 3D printed and a standard transradial prosthesis: a case report. Biomed Eng Online 2022;21:7. https://doi.org/10.1186/s12938-022-00977-w.

40. Tavangarian F, Proano C, Zolko C. Performance of Low-Cost 3D Printed Pylon in Lower Limb Prosthetic Device, In: TMS 2019 148th annual meeting & exhibition supplemental proceedings. The minerals, metals & materials series, 2019, Springer International Publishing; New York, USA,1207–1215, doi:10.1007/978-3-030-05861-6_115.

41. Vujaklija I, Farina D. 3D printed upper limb prosthetics. Expet Rev Med Dev 2018; 15(7):505–12. https://doi.org/10.1080/17434440.2018.1494568.

Amputation Surgery
Review of New and Emerging Techniques

Rachel C. Hooper, MD[a],*, Brian Kelly, DO[b], Paul S. Cederna, MD[c,d], Geoffrey Siegel, MD[e]

KEYWORDS

- Major limb amputation • Targeted muscle reinnervation
- Regenerative peripheral nerve interface • Ossteointegrated implants

KEY POINTS

- Major limb amputation is a reconstructive procedure that requires careful consideration of the management of the residual muscle, bone, nerves, and soft tissue envelope.
- Targeted muscle reinnervation and regenerative peripheral nerve interface are adjunctive peripheral nerve procedures that are used to treat and prevent symptomatic neuromas, as well as provide high fidelity control of myoelectric prosthetics.
- Early communication with physical medicine and rehabilatiion physician as well as prosthetists is key to successful functional outcomes.

INTRODUCTION

Related to trauma, peripheral vascular disease, oncologic, infectious, and congenital conditions, major upper and lower limb amputation may become necessary as the primary treatment or salvage for other failed procedures. The history of major limb amputation surgery and subsequent prosthetic limbs for cosmesis and function is fascinating. There is archaeologic evidence dating back to ancient Egypt that people had limb amputation surgeries, wore prosthetics, and were even buried with their previously ablated limb.[1] Interestingly, historic surgical technique guides and descriptions of the fundamental surgical techniques are relatively unchanged over the centuries and American Civil War era texts remain recognizable with modern texts.[2] Although

[a] Section of Plastic Surgery, Department of Surgery, University of Michigan Medical School, 1500 East Medical Center Drive, Ann Arbor, MI, USA; [b] Division of Orthotics and Prosthetics, Department of Physical Medicine and Rehabilitation, University of Michigan Medical School, 3808 Medical Science Building, Ann Arbor, MI 48109, USA; [c] Department of Biomedical Engineering; [d] Department of Surgery, University of Michigan Medical School, 3808 Medical Science Building, Ann Arbor, MI 48109, USA; [e] Division of Musculoskeletal Oncology, Department of Orthopedic Surgery, University of Michigan Medical School, 3808 Medical Science Building, Ann Arbor, MI 48109, USA
* Corresponding author. Michigan Medicine, 2130 Taubman Center, SPC 5340, Ann Arbor, MI 48109-5340.
E-mail address: hooperra@med.umich.edu

Phys Med Rehabil Clin N Am 35 (2024) 725–737
https://doi.org/10.1016/j.pmr.2024.06.001
pmr.theclinics.com
1047-9651/24/© 2024 Elsevier Inc. All rights reserved, including for text and data mining, AI training, and similar technologies.

surgical techniques have not changed appreciably, modern medicine has evolved for the betterment of its patients, perhaps most drastically in the lower complication and mortality rates.[3] Other chapters in this text will highlight the functional benefits and limitations, but it is important to know that from a purely surgical standpoint, bony amputations can occur at any level of any bone depending on the underlying pathology, necessitating the surgery. This section will focus on the surgical advancements in bone-related techniques of the trans-tibial, trans-femoral, trans-radial, trans-humeral, and shoulder disarticulation levels.

Generalized Principles of Amputation Surgery

It has been dogmatic that a flat bony cut without sharp edges is necessary, and that the length of the residual limb should be long enough to maintain the best moment arm of muscle balance, but shortened sufficiently to allow for the prosthesis' distal joints to be equal in height to the contralateral native joint.[4] Approaches to the stabilization of the residual muscles have been debated; the muscles can be sutured directly to the bone in the myodesis technique, or opposing muscles can be sutured to each other via myoplasty. Distal muscle stabilization likely improves post-operative rehabilitation potential, but there are no studies comparing it to amputation without distal muscle stabilization.[5] It is also important for the surgeon to recognize and counsel the patient that their proximal muscles will atrophy, and bone mineral density will decrease after amputation. This may influence long-term functional outcomes, specifically in adjacent joint range-of-motion and limb muscle strength, especially in older patients.[6]

Importance of Peripheral Nerves Following Amputation

Transected peripheral nerves undergo disorganized proliferation, which can lead to symptomatic neuromas as the nerve undergoes axonal regeneration and attempts to reinnervate a target organ. Aberrant proliferation of nerve ends leads to symptomatic neuromas that contribute to painful light touch, pressure, or extremes of temperature of the residual limb; patients may also experience electricity, burning, dysesthesias, phantom limb pain, and sensation. Female sex, lower educational status, and traumatic etiology of amputation are associated with higher rates of phantom limb pain; specifically, 50% to 90% of amputees experience postamputation residual or phantom limb pain and 25% will develop chronic pain from symptomatic neuromas.[7–10]

After amputation, multimodal pain regimens are necessary to address the various aspects of pain (sharp, neuropathic, spasm-related, and phantom). Several prophylactic and therapeutic surgical approaches to the prevention of symptomatic neuromas following amputation have been described, including nerve caps, suture ligature, transposition of the nerve into nerve muscle and bone, or traction neurectomy; however, these approaches were rarely successful.[11] In addition to treatment and prevention of neuromas, the ability to successfully control a prosthetic is of critical importance to amputee patients. Because nerve management following major upper and lower extremity amputation has implications on quality of life, residual function, and prosthesis use, there has been increased attention to this aspect of the procedure.[8]

There is no consensus on the optimal surgical management of peripheral nerves following major limb amputation. Currently, 2 major surgical techniques are available to treat or prevent symptomatic neuromas: (1) Targeted muscle reinnervation (TMR) and (2) Creation of regeneration peripheral nerve interfaces (RPNI). Both techniques were developed for advanced myoelectric prosthesis control and were incidentally noted to produce significant improvement among patients with symptomatic neuromas. Both TMR and RPNI can be performed in a prophylactic manner at the time of index amputation, or for therapeutic purposes if a patient has had an amputation and later develops a symptomatic neuroma. We will describe the techniques and evidence for the use of TMR and RPNI in the treatment and prevention of symptomatic neuromas, as well as for advanced myoelectric prosthesis control.

Adjunctive Peripheral Nerve Procedures Following Major Limb Amputation

Targeted muscle reinnervation

TMR has been performed since 2004 and was first described in a shoulder disarticulation patient; the pectoralis major was separated into its 3 components and the musculocutaneous, median, and radial nerves were used for targeted reinnervation of the various components.[12] Although originally designed for advanced prosthesis control, it is now widely performed for major upper and lower extremity amputations, preferably at the time of index amputation; however, these can be performed in a delayed fashion.[12] The procedure is performed under general anesthesia. The major peripheral nerves are transected proximally to healthy fascicles ("amputated donor nerves") but kept as long as possible to achieve a tension-free anastomosis.[13] Next attention is turned to identification of the donor motor nerve of the targeted muscle. Because the recipient nerves must be stimulated during surgery, regional blocks and muscle relaxants should be avoided; nerve blocks for postoperative pain can be performed following coaptation.[13] Targeted motor nerves are stimulated with low amplitude nerve stimulation to ensure appropriate muscle function. After identification of the appropriate target, an end-to-end nerve coaptation is performed. Because there is often a mismatch between recipient and donor nerves, a cuff of adjacent muscle is often used to cover the neurorrhaphy.[9] It is critical that the targeted muscle have all other neural input eliminated to avoid muscle "confusion".[13] Additionally, when TMR is performed with the intention of prosthetic control, it is important that there is interposition of tissue between the targeted muscles to avoid "cross-talk" from signals during electromyographic amplification.[12]

Regenerative peripheral nerve interface

The RPNI was originally conceived as an approach to utilize residual nerve signals to power neuroprosthetics; however, this technology was also found to be effective in the treatment of symptomatic neuromas.[14] After establishing feasibility and effectiveness of the RPNI in animal models, RPNI surgery was introduced in amputee patients at the University of Michigan in 2013.[14–17] RPNIs allow the transected ends of regenerating nerves to reinnervate an autologous muscle graft as an end-organ. These procedures can be performed under general or regional anesthesia.

Because there is no need for nerve transfer or identification of donor motor nerves with this procedure, muscle relaxants can be used at the discretion of the anesthesiologists. The proximal end of a cut peripheral nerve is carefully identified and cut back to healthy fascicles. If performed at the time of amputation, the amputation specimen can be used for the harvest of autologous skeletal muscle grafts; however, if the amputation specimen is not suitable, a separate incision can be made in the limb to harvest muscle graft. Grafts are typically 30 mm long x 15 mm wide x 5 mm thick and harvested in the direction of the muscle fibers.[14] Graft length and width can be adjusted based on the nerve being wrapped, but the thickness should remain the same. If the graft is too thick, the muscle graft will not revascularize and regenerate and the patient is at risk for the formation of symptomatic neuroma.[15]

Intrafascicular dissection of large mixed motor and sensory peripheral nerves are required to separate nerves into their component fascicles to improve axon-to-denervated muscle fiber ratios.[14,15] Once the peripheral nerve and muscle graft are prepared, the nerve is implanted into the muscle graft. First, the epineurium of nerve is sutured to the epimysium in center of the muscle graft, aligned with the direction of the muscle fibers. Additional sutures are placed to ensure the nerve is securely attached to the muscle graft. Next, the muscle graft is used to wrap the nerve circumferentially and sutures are placed to the secure the muscle to itself around the nerve. Like TMR, RPNI can treat and prevent symptomatic neuromas following nerve injury or amputation. Additionally, RPNIs afford advanced prosthetic control and sensory feedback like TMR.[14,15] Because it avoids the need to dissect donor motor nerves and perform nerve-to-nerve transfer, RPNI is conceptually and technically simpler than TMR and performed by general, vascular, and orthopedic surgeons.[14,15]

Trans-tibial Amputations and Adjunctive Nerve Procedures

The Ertl technique is a controversial advancement first described in 1981 to allow for an end-bearing residual limb by creating a bony bridge between the tibia and fibula.[18] This works off the theory that an end-bearing residual limb would allow for better non-prosthetic mobility such as seen with through-knee amputations without their inherent difficulties in prosthesis fitting.[19] Small biomechanic studies have suggested that the Ertl technique facilitates an amputees' ability to better negotiate curbs, as well as contribute to a faster sit-to-stand task suggesting these patients have more muscle power.[20,21] However, a prospective randomized controlled study comparing Ertl to non-Ertl trans-tibial amputation is currently ongoing, but early results suggest that the Ertl has a higher complication rate and may not support major clinical gains.[22] Equal in importance to surgical modifications are the expansion of indications for trans-tibial amputations. There is growing supportive evidence that in certain distal lower extremity traumatic situations, trans-tibial amputation should no longer be considered a failure or last resort, but rather as a primary surgical option offering comparatively quicker return to function and better long-term outcomes.[23]

Following trans-tibial amputations, the tibial, common peroneal, saphenous, and sural nerves are identified in the surgical field and protected. The sural and saphenous nerves are also prepared for RPNI at the surgeons' discretion; they are in the subcutaneous tissues running with the lesser and greater saphenous nerves, respectively. When RPNI of saphenous and sural sensory nerves are performed, care should be taken to avoid having them at the weight-bearing portion of the residual limb. When TMR is being performed, the residual soleus and lateral gastrocnemius muscles are identified, and the motor nerves are stimulated to confirm activity in these targeted muscles. The motor nerves are transected, and the tibial and common peroneal nerves are sutured to the motor branches of the soleus and lateral gastrocnemius muscles respectively in an end-to end manner using microsurgical techniques.[8] Alternatively, when a dual incision approach is used, the common peroneal is separated into its component superficial and deep branches; the tibial, superficial, and deep peroneal nerves are directly sutured to the motor branches emanating from soleus, peroneus longus, and tibialis anterior, respectively.[8]

When RPNI is being considered, the transected tibial, superficial peroneal, and deep peroneal nerves are identified in the posterior, lateral, and anterior compartment, respectively (**Fig. 1**). In certain instances, the surgeon may elect to identify the common peroneal nerve more proximally at the level of the fibular head and perform an interfascicular dissection to separate the component deep and superficial peroneal nerves.[10,14,15] The nerves are transected sharply to healthy fascicles. Muscle grafts are harvested from healthy skeletal muscle, and the nerves are individually wrapped using autologous muscle grafts (see **Fig. 1**). Following creation of the RPNI, it is buried within the respective muscle compartment.

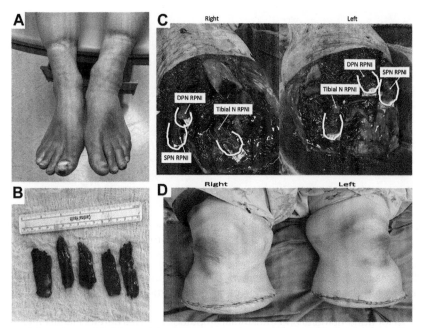

Fig. 1. (*A*) Patient with bilateral lower extremity PVD and rest pain requesting bilateral transtibial amputations. (*B*) Free muscle grafts harvested from the amputation specimen. (*C*) Intraoperatively, the SPN (superficial peroneal nerve), DPN (deep peroneal nerve) and Tibial nerve are implanted into free muscle grafts on the right and left. (*D*) Closure of bilateral lower extremity transtibial amputation.

Trans-femoral Amputations and Adjunctive Nerve Procedures

When trans-femoral amputation is indicated, the tibial, common peroneal, saphenous, and posterior cutaneous nerve of the thigh are identified for TMR or RPNI. If an interval operation is planned, a posterior approach is used, with the patient in a prone position. The sciatic nerve is identified between the residual biceps femoris and semitendinosus muscles and separated into its respective branches. For the purposes of TMR, the tibial nerve is coapted to a motor branch of the semitendinosus and the common peroneal is sutured to a branch of the biceps femoris.[8] When RPNI is performed, the individual branches of the sciatic nerve are implanted into autologous muscle grafts (**Fig. 2**). An additional incision is required to access the saphenous nerve; it is identified between the gracilis and sartorius muscles. Once identified the saphenous nerve is sutured to a motor branch of the vastus medialis during TMR or implanted into a muscle graft during RPNI.[8]

Trans-humeral and Trans-radial Amputations and Adjunctive Nerve Procedures

Following trans-humeral amputations, the median and ulnar nerves are identified and preserved anteriorly, and the radial nerve is identified posteriorly. For TMR, the recipient motor nerves include the branches of the short head of the biceps, the branch to brachialis and the branch to the lateral head of the triceps. Coaptation of the median and ulnar nerves is performed to the short head biceps and brachialis branches, respectively and the radial nerve is coapted to the branch of the lateral head of the triceps.[8] For transradial amputees, the median and ulnar nerves are identified in the

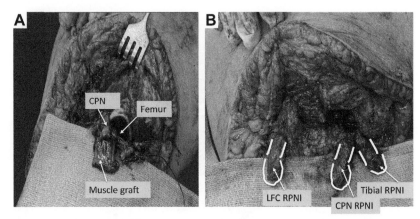

Fig. 2. (A) Trans-femoral amputation with identified common peroneal nerve (B) RPNI of the LFC (lateral femoral cutaneous nerve), CPN (common peroneal nerve) and Tibial nerve.

distal forearm and cubital tunnel, respectively. The median nerve is sutured to the anterior interosseus nerve or branch of flexor digitorum superficialis; the ulnar nerve is sutured to the branch of the flexor carpi ulnaris.

RPNI for trans-humeral and transradial amputees involves careful identification and protection of the median, ulnar, and superficial radial nerves in the distal residual limb. Trans-humeral amputation involves the identification of the median, ulnar, and radial nerves in the upper arm (Fig. 3). Intrafascicular dissection of each mixed peripheral

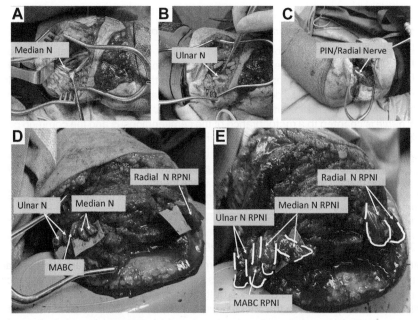

Fig. 3. Trans-humeral Amputation with identification of the (A) median (B) ulnar and (C) radial nerves. Intrafasicular dissection is performed to identify (D) grouped fascicles which are (E) implanted into free muscle grafts.

nerve is performed to provide appropriate fascicular match to autologous free muscle graft (see **Fig. 3**). For transradial amputations, the median nerve is identified in the volar compartment between the flexor digitorum superficialis and profundas muscles; the ulnar nerve is identified traveling along the ulnar artery just radial to the flexor carpi ulnaris tendon. The superficial radial nerve is identified as it exits the brachioradialis fascia. The median and ulnar nerve can be dissected into its grouped fascicles and sequentially implanted into a free muscle graft.

Shoulder Disarticulation and Adjunctive Nerve Procedures

Branches from the brachial plexus, including the median, ulnar, radial, and musculo-cutaneous nerves are identified for adjunctive nerve procedures at the time of shoulder disarticulation or following amputation if a symptomatic neuroma develops. For TMR, the pectoralis major and latissimus dorsi can be used as the donor targets.[8] When the pectoralis major is used, careful dissection down to the sternal and clavicular heads of the pectoralis is performed to identify the medial and lateral pectoral nerves. The thoracodorsal nerve is identified deep to the latissimus muscle. Typical nerve transfers for TMR in this region involves musculocutaneous nerve to the clavicular head pectoralis branch, median nerve to sternal head, ulnar nerve to lower sternal branch of pectoralis, and radial nerve to thoracodorsal nerve.

Similarly, for RPNI following shoulder disarticulation, the branches of the brachial plexus are identified and protected. Intrafascicular dissection is typically performed for the median, ulnar, and radial nerves with each set of grouped fascicles implanted into an autologous muscle graft.[24]

Rehabilitation Following Targeted Muscle Reinnervation and Regenerative Peripheral Nerve Interface

Comprehensive care of amputee patients involves a multidisciplinary team of surgeons (orthopedic/general/plastic/vascular), prosthetists or orthotists, physiatrists, and physical or occupational therapists.[25,26] Wounds are allowed to heal in the usual fashion with suture and drain removal at the surgeon's discretion. Compression garments and residual limb contouring are used in preparation for prosthetic fitting. Early fitting and integration of prosthesis is critical for upper extremity amputees because decline in prosthetic wear compliance decreases after the 3rd postoperative month if not already introduced.[26] Lower extremity amputees may require additional time before initiating contouring and training related to wound healing challenges, particularly with peripheral vascular disease patients.

Outcomes Following Targeted Muscle Reinnervation and Regenerative Peripheral Nerve Interface

TMR and RPNI have both demonstrated the ability to prevent and treat symptomatic neuromas. In a case series of 22 trans-tibial amputations treated with TMR performed at the index operation, the participants reported a decline in phantom limb pain from 72% at 1 month to 13% at 6 months, which was significant compared to the historic controls.[9] In a blinded prospective randomized control trial examining the outcomes of TMR versus neurectomy and standard treatment among 28 upper and lower major limb amputees, the investigators found decreased phantom and residual limb pain among the TMR patients.[7]

Upper extremity amputees that wish to with myoelectric prosthetics, rely on electromyography (EMG) signals from a pair of antagonistic muscles to perform a specific movement; however, among amputees with transradial or trans-humeral where both elbow and hand motion are desired, the patient would require a "switch mode" that facilitates the use of the device for both elbow and hand function.[12] This can be cumbersome and difficult to learn, contributing to prosthetic abandonment. For patients who have undergone TMR that wish to use a myoelectric upper extremity prosthetic, the divided peripheral nerves reinnervate residual muscles to provide control signals. Reinnervation occurs 3 to 9 months following the procedure.[13] An intense neurorehabilitation program using EMG-feedback is necessary to learn how to activate specific signals. The TMR signals must be spatially separated for appropriate recording using standard EMG surface electrodes; this process may require multiple visits to the prosthetists for optimization.[13] Following TMR, the targeted muscle is reinnervated by donor motor neurons of the amputated nerve; this leads to muscle control by a separate cortical area of the brain.[13] Traditional amputee patients are typically able to achieve 2 prosthetic functions; however, trans-humeral and glenohumeral amputees who undergo TMR can achieve 6 and 5 individual and intuitive myoelectrical signals, respectively.[13]

Several studies have demonstrated the utility of RPNI for the treatment and prevention of symptomatic neuromas. In a retrospective study, comparing lower extremity patients that underwent prophylactic RPNI compared to historic controls, patients who underwent RPNI experienced a significant decrease in symptomatic neuroma and phantom limb pain at the 1-year time point.[15] For upper extremity amputees, RPNI has demonstrated the ability to provide high fidelity motor efferent signals for prosthetic control following implantation of indwelling electrodes for amplification of EMG signals.[15] Ultrasonography of upper extremity RPNI demonstrated subregion specific contraction when patients were asked to perform specific volitional phantom limb movements.[15] Amputations were performed at the transradial, transhumeral, and forequarter level and patients underwent RPNI creation followed by implantation of indwelling bipolar electrodes for amplification of EMG signal. Signal recording detected individual finger flexion, extension, abduction, and adduction in a phantom hand and each individual patient was able to make a fist, point, and extend fingers.[15]

Transcutaneous Osseointegrative Implants

Perhaps the most exciting surgical advancement in major limb amputations is the advent of osseointegration (OI). OI is the implantation of a load-bearing transcutaneous metal implant into which the adjacent bone fuses (**Fig. 4**). This concept has been around since the 1950's and has been most studied in the realm of dental implants.[27] This technique has successfully transitioned its utility to upper and lower limb amputation patients who have difficulty wearing traditional socket prosthetics. The OI-affixed prosthetic limb quickly locks into the trans-cutaneous metal implant to give the wearer a plug-and-play type limb that has the benefits of end-bearing with associated proprioception. This transition has been a slowly evolving process with the first transfemoral OI cases performed in the 1970s, but unfortunately all failed due to development of osteomyelitis.[28] Since those early discouraging results, advancements in soft tissue handling techniques have improved outcomes; however, it should be noted that every study mentions infection as a significant risk or complication of the OI procedure, but infections are usually superficial and treated conservatively and rarely life-threatening.[29–32]

OI implants for major extremity amputees come in 2 general forms: screw-type and press-fit. To date, only the screw-type implant has Food and Drug Administration (FDA) approval in the United States, but the press-fit implants are being used in compassionate-use and experimental cases as part of a forthcoming and expectant FDA approval process. The screw-type implant requires a 2-stage surgical approach with at least a 3-month timeframe between surgeries. This allows for appropriate time

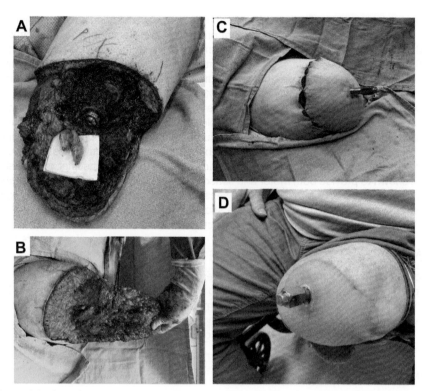

Fig. 4. (*A*) Above knee amputation with preparation of sciatic nerve for RPNI and placement of osteointegrated prosthesis (*B*) Completion of RPNIs (*C*) Flap closure over osteointegrated implant and immediate intraoperative appearance (*D*) Fully healed AKA with osteointegrated device.

for bony fixative ingrowth to the implant, as well as recognizing the necessity for delicate soft-tissue handling techniques to promote both wound healing and minimize shear stresses at the cutaneous-implant junction. The goal is for the skin to adhere to the distal cut end of the bone and minimize soft tissue motion with activity, which has contributed to the diminished rate of deep infections in these OI cases. The press-fit implants have the benefit of being performed in a single stage surgery, but with less regimented consideration for soft tissue handling techniques. There has not yet been a head-to-head study comparing outcomes in both classes of implants and a direct comparison of the 2 implant types is beyond the scope of this chapter.

Focusing first on studies of lower extremity amputation levels, early 1-year follow-up for trans-femoral and trans-tibial OI showed performance improvement compared with traditional socket-suspended prosthetics.[33] A separate 2-year follow-up study for transfemoral OI showed high overall survival (92%) combined with enhanced prosthesis use and mobility, fewer patient complaints, and improved patient quality of life indices compared with traditional socket-suspended prosthesis.[34] A small cohort of transfemoral OI with mean follow-up of 11.4 years shows OI allows for prolonged usage and improves quality of life compared with conventional prostheses.[35]

There have been concerns that upper extremity prostheses place transhumeral OI implants under supraphysiologic stresses, especially in torsional loads, at the bone-implant interface.[36] The upper extremity is not weight-bearing and not subjected the same sort of compressive forces that promote increases in bone mineral density and subsequent strength as the lower extremity.[6] More studies need to be performed to determine the clinical relevance of these stresses in a non-weight bearing extremity, but clinical studies have shown that trans-humeral OI improves quality of life and function with 2- and 5-year survival rates of 83% and 80%, respectively.[37,38]

OI for major limb amputations, like all state-of-the art technology, is costly, but in the situation of the transfemoral amputee unable to mobilize with traditional prostheses, OI improves quality of life and ability to productively function and contribute to society and so these patients reap the maximum benefit and cost-effectiveness of the device.[39,40] Future advancements in trans-humeral OI and neuromuscular prostheses have shown to provide both motor and sensory feedback to the user with little training other than daily use, and this increased sensory acuity and effectiveness in work and other activities of daily living.[41] So it is a short jump to assume that trans-humeral OI will 1 day provide similar societal cost-effectiveness.

SUMMARY

Appropriate management of peripheral nerves during upper and lower extremity amputation surgery is critically important to pain outcomes and overall quality of life in these individuals. At each major level of amputation, the regional motor and sensory nerves can be readily identified and managed with TMR or RPNI for durable pain control or advanced prosthetic control. These adjunctive procedures should be offered to all major limb amputee patients.

CLINICS CARE POINTS

- Today, surgeons have an expanded armamentarium in the management of amputee patients including surgical techniques for the treatment and prevention of symptomatic neuromas and the use of OI implants.
- TMR and RPNI have demonstrated the ability for advanced prosthetic control and should be considered as part of the treatment algorithm for amputee patients cared for by a multidisciplinary team.

DISCLOSURE

The authors have no financial disclosures.

REFERENCES

1. Thurston AJ. Paré and prosthetics: the early history of artificial limbs. ANZ J Surg 2007;77(12):1114–9. PMID: 17973673.
2. Barnes J.K., editor. The medical and surgical history of the war of the rebellion (1861-1865). 1873. Washington, DC: United States Printing Office; 1870-1888.
3. van Netten JJ, Fortington LV, Hinchliffe RJ, et al. Early Post-operative Mortality After Major Lower Limb Amputation: A Systematic Review of Population and Regional Based Studies. Eur J Vasc Endovasc Surg 2016;51(2):248–57. Epub 2015 Nov 14. PMID: 26588994.
4. Geertzen JHB, de Beus MC, Jutte PC, et al. What is the optimal femur length in a trans-femoral amputation? A mixed method study: Scoping review, expert

opinions and biomechanical analysis. Med Hypotheses 2019;129:109238. https://doi.org/10.1016/j.mehy.2019.109238. Epub 2019 May 23. PMID: 31371086.

5. Fabre I, Thompson D, Gwilym B, et al. Surgical Techniques of, and outcomes after, Distal Muscle Stabilisation in Transfemoral Amputation; A systematic review and narrative synthesis. Ann Vasc Surg 2023;S0890-S5096(23):00656-8. Epub ahead of print. PMID: 37802139.

6. Finco MG, Kim S, Ngo W, et al. A review of musculoskeletal adaptations in individuals following major lower-limb amputation. J Musculoskelet Neuronal Interact 2022;22(2):269-83. PMID: 35642706; PMCID: PMC9186459.

7. Dumanian GA, Potter BK, Mioton LM, et al. Targerted Muscle Reinnervation Treats Neuroma and Phantom Pain in Major Limb Amputees. A Randomized Trial. Ann Surg 2019;270:238-46.

8. Janes LE, Fracol ME, Dumananian GA, et al. Targeted Muscle Reinnervation for the Treatment of Neuroma. Hand Clin 2021;37:345-59.

9. Bowen JB, Ruter D, Wee C, et al. Targeted Muscle Reinnervation Technique in Below-Knee Amputation. Plast Recontr Surg 2019;143:309-12.

10. Kubiak CA, Adidharma W, Kung TA, et al. Decreasing Postamputation Pain with the Regenerative Peripheral Nerve Interface. Ann Vasc Surg 2022;79:421-6.

11. Dellon AL, Mackinnon SE. Treatment of Painful Neuroma by Neuroma Resection and Muscle Implantation. Plas Recon Surg 1986;77:427-38.

12. Ryan DJ, Ayalon O, Hacquebord J. Targeted muscle reinnervation (TMR) and other consideration in upper extremity amputation. Bull Hosp Jt Dis 2022;80:25-30.

13. Bergmeister KD, Salminger S, Aszmann OC. Targeted Muscle Reinnervation for Prosthetic Control. Hand Clin 2021;37:415-24.

14. Kubiak CA, Kemp SWP, Cederna PS. Regenerative peripheral nerve interface for management of postamputation neuroma. JAMA Surgery 2018;153:681-2.

15. Kubiak CA, Kemp SWP, Cederna PS, et al. Prophylactic regenerative peripheral nerve interfaces to prevent postamputation pain. Plas Reconstr Surgery 2019; 144:421e-30e.

16. Kung TA, Langhals NR, Martin DC, et al. Regenerative peripheral nerve interface viability and signal transduction with an implanted electrode. Plast Reconstr Surg 2014;133(6):1380-94.

17. Woo SL, Kung TA, Brown DL, et al. Regenerative peripheral nerve interfaces for the treatment of postamputation neuroma pain. Plast Reconstr Surg Glob Open 2016;4(12):e1038.

18. von Ertl JW. Die Versorgung von Amputationsstümpfen durch Osteo-Myoplastik nach v. Ertl [The care of amputation stumps by osteo-myeloplastic according to v. Ertl]. Z Plast Chir 1981;5(3):184-9. German. PMID: 7029943.

19. Panhelleux B, Shalhoub J, Silverman AK, et al. A review of through-knee amputation. Vascular 2022 Dec;30(6):1149-59. Epub 2021 Nov 29. PMID: 34844469; PMCID: PMC9660278.

20. Ferris AE, Christiansen CL, Heise GD, et al. Biomechanical analysis of curb ascent in persons with Ertl and non-Ertl transtibial amputations. Prosthet Orthot Int 2020 Feb;44(1):36-43. Epub 2019 Nov 12. PMID: 31713462.

21. Ferris AE, Christiansen CL, Heise GD, et al. Ertl and Non-Ertl amputees exhibit functional biomechanical differences during the sit-to-stand task. Clin Biomech 2017 May;44:1-6. Epub 2017 Feb 22. PMID: 28273496.

22. Bosse MJ, Morshed S, Reider L, et al. METRC. Transtibial Amputation Outcomes Study (TAOS): Comparing Transtibial Amputation With and Without a Tibiofibular

Synostosis (Ertl) Procedure. J Orthop Trauma 2017;31(Suppl 1):S63–9. PMID: 28323804.

23. Major Extremity Trauma Research Consortium (METRC). Outcomes Following Severe Distal Tibial, Ankle, and/or Mid/Hindfoot Trauma: Comparison of Limb Salvage and Transtibial Amputation (OUTLET). J Bone Joint Surg Am 2021; 103(17):1588–97. https://doi.org/10.2106/JBJS.20.01320. PMID: 33979309.

24. Vu PP, Vaskow AK, Irwin ZT, et al. A Regenerative Peripheral Nerve Interface Allows Real-Time Control of an Artificial Hand in Upper Extremity Amputees. Sci Transl Med 2020;12:eaay2857.

25. Smurr LM, Gulick K, Yancoek MK, et al. Managing the Upper Extremity Amputee: A Protocol for Success. J Hand Therapy 2008;21:160–76.

26. Meier RH, Melton D. Ideal Functional Outcomes for Amputation Levels. Phys Med Rehabil Clin N Am 2014;25:199–212.

27. Brånemark PI. Osseointegration and its experimental background. J Prosthet Dent 1983 Sep;50(3):399–410. PMID: 6352924.

28. Mooney V, Schwartz SA, Roth AM, et al. Percutaneous implant devices. Ann Biomed Eng 1977 Mar;5(1):34–46. PMID: 851262.

29. Hoellwarth JS, Tetsworth K, Oomatia A, et al. Association Between Osseointegration of Lower Extremity Amputation and Mortality Among Adults. JAMA Netw Open 2022;5(10):e2235074. https://doi.org/10.1001/jamanetworkopen.2022. 35074. PMID: 36227599; PMCID: PMC9561949.

30. Overmann AL, Forsberg JA. The state of the art of osseointegration for limb prosthesis. Biomed Eng Lett 2019;10(1):5–16. PMID: 32175127; PMCID: PMC7046912.

31. Li Y, Brånemark R. Osseointegrated prostheses for rehabilitation following amputation : The pioneering Swedish model. Unfallchirurg 2017;120(4):285–92. PMID: 28229193; PMCID: PMC5371647.

32. Li Y, Felländer-Tsai L. The bone anchored prostheses for amputees - Historical development, current status, and future aspects. Biomaterials 2021;273:120836. https:// doi.org/10.1016/j.biomaterials.2021.120836. Epub 2021 Apr 19. PMID: 33894405.

33. Atallah R, van de Meent H, Verhamme L, et al. Safety, prosthesis wearing time and health-related quality of life of lower extremity bone-anchored prostheses using a press-fit titanium osseointegration implant: A prospective one-year follow-up cohort study. PLoS One 2020;15(3):e0230027. PMID: 32150598; PMCID: PMC7062258.

34. Brånemark R, Berlin O, Hagberg K, et al. A novel osseointegrated percutaneous prosthetic system for the treatment of patients with transfemoral amputation: A prospective study of 51 patients. Bone Joint Lett J 2014;96-B(1):106–13 [Erratum appears in Bone Joint J 2014;96-B(4):562. PMID: 24395320].

35. Matthews DJ, Arastu M, Uden M, et al. UK trial of the Osseointegrated Prosthesis for the Rehabilitation for Amputees: 1995-2018. Prosthet Orthot Int 2019;43(1): 112–22. Epub 2018 Aug 16. PMID: 30112981.

36. Taylor CE, Drew AJ, Zhang Y, et al. Upper extremity prosthetic selection influences loading of transhumeral osseointegrated systems. PLoS One 2020;15(8): e0237179. PMID: 32760149; PMCID: PMC7410272.

37. Jönsson S, Caine-Winterberger K, Brånemark R. Osseointegration amputation prostheses on the upper limbs: methods, prosthetics and rehabilitation. Prosthet Orthot Int 2011;35(2):190–200. PMID: 21697201.

38. Tsikandylakis G, Berlin Ö, Brånemark R. Implant survival, adverse events, and bone remodeling of osseointegrated percutaneous implants for transhumeral amputees. Clin Orthop Relat Res 2014;472(10):2947–56. PMID: 24879569; PMCID: PMC4160502.

39. Handford C, McMenemy L, Kendrew J, et al. Improving outcomes for amputees: The health-related quality of life and cost utility analysis of osseointegration prosthetics in transfemoral amputees. Injury 2022;53(12):4114–22. Epub 2022 Oct 17. PMID: 36333155.

40. Overmann AL, Aparicio C, Richards JT, et al. Orthopaedic osseointegration: Implantology and future directions. J Orthop Res 2020;38(7):1445–54. Epub 2020 Jan 13. PMID: 31876306.

41. Ortiz-Catalan M, Mastinu E, Sassu P, et al. Self-Contained Neuromusculoskeletal Arm Prostheses. N Engl J Med 2020;382(18):1732–8 [Erratum appears in N Engl J Med 2022;387(21):2008. PMID: 32348644].

Dermatologic Conditions Following Limb Loss

Shaliz Aflatooni, BS[a], Kate Beekman, BS[a], Kerry Hennessy, MD[b],
Michael Jason Highsmith, PhD, DPT, CP[c,d],
Jeffrey T. Heckman, DO[e,f], Peter R. Shumaker, MD[g],
Chad M. Hivnor, MD[h], Thomas M. Beachkofsky, MD[i],*

KEYWORDS

- Lower extremity amputation • Prosthesis user • Prosthetics • Rehabilitation
- Skin pathology

KEY POINTS

- Compared to upper extremity prosthesis users, lower extremity prosthesis users face heightened skin injury risks.
- Close contact between the residual limb and the prosthesis can compromise skin integrity through increased perspiration, friction, and shearing forces.
- Crucial preventive measures include properly fitting prostheses with annual prosthesis consultations and daily hygiene of the residual limb and socket site.
- Treatment options, both non-procedural and procedural, are available for preventing and managing skin-related complications.

[a] Morsani College of Medicine, University of South Florida, 560 Channelside Drive, Tampa, FL 33602, USA; [b] Department of Dermatology and Cutaneous Surgery, Morsani College of Medicine, University of South Florida, 13330 USF Laurel Drive, Tampa, FL 33612, USA; [c] Orthotic, Prosthetic & Pedorthic Clinical Services (OPPCS) Program Office (12RPS4), Rehabilitation & Prosthetic Services, US Department of Veterans Affairs, 810 Vermont Avenue Northwest, Washington, DC 20420, USA; [d] School of Physical Therapy & Rehabilitation Sciences, Morsani College of Medicine, University of South Florida, 3515 East Fletcher Avenue, Tampa, FL 33613, USA; [e] Morsani College of Medicine, University of South Florida, 12901 Bruce B. Downs Boulevard, MDC 55, Tampa, FL 33612, USA; [f] James A. Haley Veterans' Hospital & Clinics, 13000 Bruce B. Downs Boulevard, Mailstop-117 Tampa, FL 33612, USA; [g] Dermatology Department, US Department of Veterans Affairs, Veterans Administration San Diego Healthcare System, 3350 La Jolla Village Drive, Suite 111B, San Diego, CA 92161, USA; [h] Dermatology Department, US Department of Veterans Affairs, South Texas Veterans Health Care System, 7400 Merton Mentor Drive, San Antonio, TX 78229, USA; [i] Dermatology Department, US Department of Veterans Affairs, James A. Haley Veterans' Hospital, 12210 Bruce B Downs Boulevard, Building 111H, Tampa, FL 33612, USA
* Corresponding author. Dermatology Department, James A. Haley Veterans' Hospital, 12210 Bruce B. Downs Boulevard, Tampa, FL 33612.
E-mail address: thomas.beachkofsky@va.gov

Phys Med Rehabil Clin N Am 35 (2024) 739–755
https://doi.org/10.1016/j.pmr.2024.06.002
1047-9651/24/Published by Elsevier Inc.

INTRODUCTION

Following partial limb loss, individuals are at an elevated risk of dermatoses involving their residual limbs and amputation sites, primarily attributed to damage inflicted upon cutaneous, musculoskeletal, and vascular structures, as well as impaired lymphatic drainage.[1] The unspecialized nature of the skin and variable postsurgical changes render it less resilient to the heightened compressive and shear forces, increased temperature and moisture experienced within the socket of a prosthesis. Consequently, this susceptibility can lead to skin irritation, which, when coupled with inadequate hygiene practices and an ill-fitting prosthesis, can exacerbate the development of various skin pathologies. Notably, individuals with a history of immunosuppression, diabetes mellitus, or peripheral vascular disease face an even greater risk of skin breakdown at the residual limb, heightening their susceptibility to opportunistic infections.[1]

Dermatoses in patients with limb loss and prosthetic limb use often occur among patients without a prior history of dermatologic disease.[2] Prosthetic limb use is associated with skin injury from 3 primary etiologies (often in combination) including maceration, friction, and pressure. Many studies have reported a high prevalence rate of dermatoses at the residual limb site ranging from 34% to 75%.[3–5] A 6 year retrospective chart review of prosthetic limb users demonstrated ulcers, irritations, inclusion cysts, calluses, and verrucous hyperplasia to be the 5 most commonly encountered dermatologic diagnoses, accounting for 80% of skin lesions.[6] Herein we seek to provide a comprehensive review of the dermatologic disorders that affect patients with limb loss and provide state-of-the-art management options.

CONSIDERATIONS REGARDING AMPUTATION SITE AND TYPE OF PROSTHESIS
Amputation Etiology

Amputation can result from traumatic injury or the sequelae of various medical conditions such as vascular disease, cancer, and infection. Patients who undergo nontraumatic amputations, especially those with conditions like peripheral vascular disease, diabetes mellitus, or malignancy, are more likely to experience both macrovascular and microvascular complications. In a study involving 220 patients with peripheral vascular disease, 22% (53 of 244 limbs) progressed to major amputation by 365 days.[7] In addition to medical comorbidities, a patient's age and nutritional status may also influence the development of secondary dermatoses. Aging skin is linked to a prolonged and impaired wound healing process, increasing susceptibility to infection and scarring.[8] Additionally, elderly patients may exhibit decreased flexibility and range of motion necessary for proper skin care as well as other activities of daily living.

Amputation Location

The location of the amputation may also impact the risk of dermatoses. Transtibial amputations are the most common type of major amputation and can be difficult to fit into a prosthesis due to bony prominences from the residual tibia and fibula (**Fig. 1**).[6] In a study of 828 lower extremity amputations, transtibial residual limbs were 4 times more likely than transfemoral residual limbs to demonstrate dermatologic pathology ($P<.01$).[4] For individuals with a transfemoral amputation, skin near the distal femur is most commonly associated with dermatoses, followed by the groin.[6] In contrast to lower extremity prosthesis users, upper extremity prosthesis users may be less dependent on the prosthesis itself for daily mobility tasks, such as walking. Thus, the dermatoses seen in upper extremity prosthesis users may be less commonly associated with maceration, friction, and pressure-induced injuries.

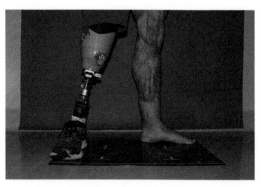

Fig. 1. Patient donning custom prosthesis after transtibial amputation.

TYPES OF PROSTHETIC AND SUSPENSION SYSTEMS

A prosthetic limb is composed of multiple components, each with a specific purpose to enhance function and mobility. The complexity of these components varies based on the type of prosthetic limb, the amputation level, and the individual's unique requirements. The key elements of a prosthetic limb include the socket, the suspension system, and the components (ie, knee, foot, etc.). The socket serves as the interface between the prosthesis and the residual limb, while the suspension system ensures that the prosthetic limb remains securely in place on the residual limb when unweighted, particularly during swing phase in walking. Suction suspension systems may use vacuum technology to establish a reliable seal between the socket and the residual limb. By removing air from the socket through a 1 way valve, negative pressure is created, enhancing stability. Alternatively, locking suspension systems employ mechanical mechanisms, such as a pin and lock system, to provide a secure attachment.

Some users opt for a gel liner suspension system, which provides comfort, suspension, and protection to the user. The conforming property of certain gel liner materials helps reduce pressure points and friction. Combining different suspension methods, such as a gel liner with a locking mechanism, can be advantageous for achieving a more secure and comfortable fit.[9] Prosthetic sleeves, made of neoprene or silicone, secure the connection between the residual limb and prosthetic socket. The sleeve is worn over the residual limb to create friction and a secure seal. Prosthetic sleeves may serve as primary suspension, enhance socket fit, and potentially reduce the need for additional suspension components. However, sleeves may also be used as auxiliary suspension.

DERMATOLOGIC CONDITIONS ASSOCIATED WITH LIMB LOSS

Prosthetic consultation and collaborative management in these cases are vital. The patient should have, at minimum, an annual visit with the multidisciplinary team to assure optimal prosthetic limb fit, alignment, function, and overall health (**Fig. 2**). Patients should also be advised to meet with their prosthetist as needed at the first sign of skin issues or progressive skin changes (**Table 1**).

FRICTIONAL DISEASES

Prolonged friction and pressure can induce adventitious bursae within the subcutaneous connective tissue. Clinically, these bursae present as well-defined, transilluminant,

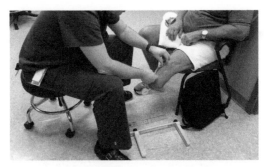

Fig. 2. Prosthetist assessing transtibial limb volumetrics for socket fit in a routine annual visit.

and fluctuant masses. Bursae can manifest as either aseptic or septic in nature. Preventative measures include ensuring properly fitted prosthetic sockets and customized designs and interfaces, such as liners or gel cups, to reduce friction and lower the risk of complications.[10]

SKIN AND SOFT TISSUE INFECTIONS

Maceration, friction, and pressure in combination with existing comorbidities may increase a patient's risk of skin and soft tissue infections (SSTIs). The introduction of a prosthetic device at the vulnerable residual limb site may alter the local microbiome, impacting wound healing and increasing the risk of SSTIs (**Fig. 3**). Prolonged prosthesis contact with the residual limb can lead to excessive skin moisture through increased perspiration and lack of evaporation. Fungal infections, such as *Tinea corporis,* may present as annular, erythematous scaling plaques, while yeast infections may appear as well-defined erythema with maceration and satellite pustules. These fungal infections may commonly occur in the groin in transfemoral level prosthesis users, and in the mid-thigh and the popliteal fossa in transtibial level prosthesis users.

Postoperative bacterial infections are a concerning complication following major lower limb amputations, potentially leading to reamputation and additional limb shortening. A retrospective study of 231 patients revealed that 7.3% experienced residual limb infections, emphasizing the significance of prophylactic measures including antibiotics.[11] A boil, or furuncle, is a bacterial skin abscess, typically *Staphylococcus aureus*, that commonly forms in a hair follicle. Furuncles present as tender erythematous nodules that may become fluctuant overtime with surrounding erythema and edema. For furunculosis management and prevention, chlorhexidine 4% antimicrobial skin cleanser is recommended 2 to 3 times per week to reduce pathologic microbes.[12] Proper wound care and vigilant surgical-site monitoring are essential in preventing complications like abscess formation and ensuring a successful wound healing process after surgery.[10]

FOLLICULITIS, SECONDARY HYPERHIDROSIS

Folliculitis, or inflammation of hair follicles, presents as erythematous pruritic papules and pustules and is exacerbated by factors like friction, bacterial infection, and high humidity within the socket. Gel liners and prosthetic limbs contribute to a local increase in skin temperature resulting in secondary hyperhidrosis. Hyperhidrosis poses challenges in prosthetic limb fit and function and can lead to tissue maceration and

Table 1
Common dermatologic disorders diagnosed at the residual limb due to prosthetic limb use

Diagnosis	Cause	Presentation, Signs, and Symptoms	Treatment
Allergic Contact Dermatitis	• Allergy or sensitivity to materials used in prosthetic components	• Pruritic, well-demarcated erythematous papules and plaques	• Recognize and avoid allergen contact • Substitute allergen for a different prosthetic material • Utilizing a silicone sleeve and gel liners infused with oil or aloe vera
Acroangiodermatitis	• Proliferation of fibroblasts and small vessels attributed to a poorly fitting suction prosthesis	• Erythematous papules, plaques, or nodules	• Elevation of the limb • Stump shrinker
Bursitis	• Prolonged friction, pressure, and irritation	• Distinct, well-defined, transilluminant, fluctuant masses	• Aseptic bursitis can be treated with complete prosthetic reset, elevation, ice, NSAIDs • Septic bursitis is treated with antibiotic therapy
Irritant Contact Dermatitis	• Overuse of abrasive skin cleansers • Chafing of the skin against the prosthetic socket • Prolonged exposure to moisture	• Pruritic, well-demarcated erythematous papules and plaques	• Avoiding abrasive cleansing agents • Utilizing a silicone sleeve and gel liners infused with oil or aloe vera
Secondary Hyperhidrosis	• Occlusive nature of the prosthetic liner and increased temperature within the socket	• Excess perspiration	• Topical aluminum ion-based antiperspirants • Preventive prosthetic removal and limb drying • Selected prosthetic componentry • Chemodenervation (ie, botulinum toxin) • Laser hair reduction • Microwave therapy

(continued on next page)

Table 1
(continued)

Diagnosis	Cause	Presentation, Signs, and Symptoms	Treatment
Ulcer	• Pressure and shear forces exerted on the residual limb at the prosthetic interface • Alteration to residual limb shape and volume can create a mismatch between the prosthetic socket and residual limb	• Erythematous open lesion that can extend from the epidermis to the fascia depending on severity	• Early-stage ulceration without comorbidities, the patient may continue prosthetic use • Unload pressure intolerant areas; reestablish optimal load distribution • Prosthetic discontinuance is recommended for patients with multiple comorbidities that delay healing • Specialty wound care including surgical debridement • Vacuum-assisted suction suspension
Fungal Infection	• Warm and humid conditions	• Tinea infection may present as annular, erythematous scaling plaques • Yeast infection may present as well-defined macerated erythema with satellite pustules	• Antifungal medications • Prevention through hygiene education and practices
Verrucous Hyperplasia	• Stump lacks adequate support within the prosthetic socket, which causes distal fluid congestion	• Warty papules and plaques	• Adjusting the prosthetic socket to distribute pressure more evenly across the stump
Epidermoid Cysts	• Invagination of keratin into the dermis that typically occur moist, hair-bearing skin that is irritated by shear and stress forces	• Painful subcutaneous nodules with a central punctum	• Localized pressure relief • Surgical removal of cyst
Sinus Tracts	• Inflammation of the hair follicles from shear and stress forces can precipitate bacterial colonization creating abscesses • Abscesses may rupture leading to ulceration and secondary infection	• Painful opening or pore with discharge • Tender with erythema	• Localized pressure relief • Surgical removal of tract

Corns and Calluses	Skin thickening from pressure-induced hyperkeratosis	• Corns can consist of either firm papules with translucent central cores or often macerated papules • Calluses are broad keratotic plaques	• Cessation of prosthetic use as needed • Optimize prosthetic interface load distribution • Prevention using cotton and silk socks • Gentle debridement in office with curettage and at home with a pumice stone
Skin Malignancy	• Disruption of blood and lymphatic flow, altering immune response at stump site	• Discolored, large, asymmetric, and/or irregular lesion	• Biopsy and surgical removal • Other systemic oncologic therapies as indicated
Furunculosis	• Bacterial infection of hair follicle, typically Staphylococcus aureus	• Large, tender, erythematous pustules	• Incision and drainage of pustule • Antimicrobial skin cleanser • Prescribed antibiotics • Prosthetic pressure relief or cessation of prosthetic wear until resolved • Prevention through hygiene education and practices
Folliculitis	• Inflammation of hair follicles from friction, bacterial infection, or excessive humidity	• Erythematous, pruritic, and painful pustules	• Prosthetic pressure relief or brief cessation of the prosthesis • Topical antibiotic (if bacterial cause suspected) • Laser hair removal
Negative Pressure Hyperemia	• Decreased contact with the socket (ie, weight gain/loss, edema), creating lymphatic and circulatory congestion	• Edema, erythema, tenderness	• Acutely, brief cessation of prosthesis use • Socket replacement • Lifestyle modifications to manage weight • Medication to reduce fluid volume

Abbreviation: NSAID, nonsteroidal anti-inflammatory drug.

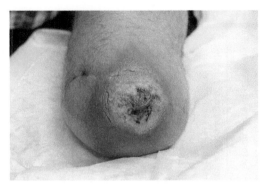

Fig. 3. Secondary infection due to infrequent washing and poor skin care.

frictional dermatitis, often necessitating liner and prosthetic limb removal. If not managed properly, severe, secondary hyperhidrosis can result in loss of suction and prosthetic limb instability potentially resulting in patient falls.

NEGATIVE PRESSURE CHANGES

Suction or vacuum suspension secures a prosthetic socket to a residual limb using a valve and/or pump system to create negative pressure. Compromised circulation at the residual limb site attributed to a poorly fitting suction prosthesis may cause proliferation of fibroblasts and small vessels, leading to acroangiodermatitis. Acroangiodermatitis is clinically characterized by painful erythematous papules, plaques, or nodules.[2,13]

Suboptimal prosthetic limb fit may also impede venous drainage, causing venous congestion, varicosities, edema, and painful ulcers. For example, rapid weight gain may prevent full donning and total contact in a negative-pressure environment. This may manifest as a tender erythematous patch on the residual limb, termed negative pressure hyperemia.[14] Immediate management includes brief cessation of prosthesis use for acute pain relief. However, comprehensive long-term strategies should be employed including reestablishing total contact with pads, socket replacement, lifestyle modifications, and volume control with a stump shrinker and limb elevation to reduce swelling.

ALLERGIC AND IRRITANT CONTACT DERMATITIS

Allergic contact dermatitis, characterized by pruritic, well-demarcated erythematous papules, and plaques, may be secondary to substances present at the prosthesis interface. Symptoms may be exacerbated by occlusion and moist conditions. Proper diagnosis involves determining whether the reaction is localized to the prosthesis contact area or extends elsewhere on the limb or body. Patch testing is crucial for diagnosis and management.[10] Irritant contact dermatitis of the residual limb can result from abrasive skin cleansers that damage the skin's barrier function or from occlusion of skin products that might be tolerated under typical circumstances, such as antiperspirants. Using a silicone sleeve can prevent sensitization, while gel liners with mineral oil or aloe vera condition the skin and enhance tolerance at the residual limb–prosthetic limb interface.

EPIDERMOID INCLUSION CYSTS AND SINUS TRACTS

Epidermoid cysts may also arise secondary to prosthesis use and are more commonly associated with traumatic amputation.[6] These painful subcutaneous nodules, formed by keratin invagination into the dermis, often develop in moist, hair-bearing skin irritated by shear and pressure. Without treatment, cysts and abscesses may rupture, causing ulceration, secondary infection, and sinus tract formation.[2] Prosthetic limb management involves localized pressure relief, and patients should be educated on managing perspiration during higher temperatures or increased activity.

PRESSURE INJURIES

The skin and underlying soft tissues of the residual limb are not adapted for load bearing and shearing forces. Reactive hyperkeratosis at pressure points can lead to the formation of corns and calluses. Corns can consist of either firm papules with translucent central cores (ie, hard corns, or "heloma durum") or painful, often macerated papules (ie, soft corns, or "heloma mole"). Calluses are broad keratotic plaques. Mild changes can be mitigated with gentle paring/debridement at home with files and pumice stones. Off-loading focal pressure with padding, socks, or other self-management strategies can be helpful but has limitations regarding restoration of overall optimal prosthetic limb fit. Prosthetists may need to evaluate the socket to optimize and restore total surface bearing, relieve high-stress areas, and enhance load distribution, addressing the underlying factors contributing to corns and calluses.

Ulcers, a common consequence of pressure and shear forces from prosthetic limb use, often result from changes in residual limb volume that lead to a poor fit between the socket and residual limb (**Fig. 4**). Use of a residual limb "shrinker" is a common intervention to mitigate volume increase. In one study involving 528 patients with lower extremity amputation, the primary complaint was ulcers.[6] Pressure sores, or decubitus ulcers, are particularly seen on bony prominences of the residual limb. Pressure sores are staged based on their severity. *Stage 1* is characterized by intact skin that may appear reddened, with damage limited to the epidermis. In *stage 2*, there is partial-thickness skin loss, with the damage extending into the dermis. In *stage 3*, the ulcer is classified as full-thickness skin loss, possibly exposing subcutaneous fat. In *stage 4*, there is skin loss extending through the fascia.[15] Higher rates of chronic ulcers are seen in patients with underlying conditions such as vascular insufficiency or diabetes mellitus, and it may be necessary to pause prosthetic limb use to promote

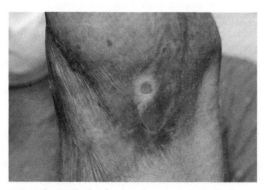

Fig. 4. Chronic ulceration due to lack of wound care and reluctance to stop wearing prosthetic limb and follow-up with therapy and prosthetics team.

healing.[2,6,14] Patients with early-stage ulceration who lack comorbidities may often continue prosthetic limb use. Furthermore, vacuum-assisted suction suspension prostheses may generally be used while managing wounds without negatively impacting wound healing.[16,17] Surgical intervention may be necessary in cases of chronic wounds.

A poorly fitting prosthesis can potentially trigger the development of verrucous hyperplasia. Verrucous hyperplasia arises from persistent residual limb edema and distal fluid congestion due to incomplete contact between the residual limb and the prosthesis socket.[1,2] Clinically, verrucous hyperplasia manifests as multiple irregular warty papules and plaques most often at the distal end of the residual limb. The edema is often attributed to venous or lymphatic stasis induced by prosthesis usage, particularly in cases involving prostheses with suction suspension. Fortunately, adjustments to the prosthetic socket aimed at distributing pressure more evenly across the residual limb may offer potential improvements in cases of verrucous hyperplasia.[1]

PAIN SYNDROMES

Individuals who have undergone amputation may continue to experience sensation of the missing limb continuously or intermittently. The perception of pain in the absent limb (ie, phantom limb pain) is a very common complication following amputation surgery. It may occur due to maladaptive brain plasticity and can range from mild to severe. Although not directly related to the skin, patients will often attribute their pain to their skin and seek therapy from dermatologists; therefore, it is of vital importance for providers to appropriately address these neuropathic complaints. Though trials to date on the treatment of phantom limb sensations and pain are of low-to-moderate quality, management may include pharmacotherapy such as gabapentin, ketamine, and morphine as well as nerve blocks, repetitive transcutaneous magnetic stimulation, and mirror therapy.[18]

TREATMENT

Dermatologic conditions in individuals with limb loss are typically managed rather than cured, and the available treatments often focus on symptom relief and control.

Non-procedural Interventions

Maintaining proper hygiene for the residual limb and prosthetic components is crucial to reduce the risk of dermatoses and promote comfort. Regular cleaning of the residual limb, prosthetic liner, and interior with a fragrance-free antibacterial cleanser prevents the accumulation of bacteria, sweat, and dead skin cells. A solution that creates a protective chemical barrier against bacteria can be used to deep clean prosthetic liners and reduce odors and irritation. In-clinic wound imaging techniques, such as devices that detect red or cyan fluorescence in clinically relevant levels of bacteria, may help guide wound cleaning, cautious debridement, dressing selection, and judicious use of antibiotics.[19] Wound imaging techniques can help guide wound care. In case of an active wound infection, refraining from prosthetic limb use until full healing is advisable. Commonly, patients are prescribed 2 liners for rotation, and patients are encouraged to communicate when their liners appear worn for prescription of liner replacement.

Fluctuations in residual limb volume can significantly impact the comfort and fit of a patient's prosthesis and influence mechanical pressure and shear stress. A decrease in volume concentrates stress on bony prominences, heightens discomfort, and increases the risk of skin irritation and breakdown. Conversely, increased volume hinders blood flow and nutrient delivery. Changes in limb volume in either direction can compromise fit. Typically, patients encounter a larger limb size in the morning with decreasing volume as the day progresses. However, individuals with vascular complications may experience the opposite trend. To adapt to these daily fluctuations, patients who use certain prostheses often resort to the addition or removal of socks. The addition of socks serves to increase interstitial fluid pressure, thereby reducing limb volume. Sock removal can lead to an increase in residual limb volume. A study on patients with transtibial amputation noted median absolute fluid volume changes of approximately 0.8% during a 30 min test session for sock addition or removal.[20] Thus, the prosthetic limb prescription must consider a patient's propensity for volume fluctuation and their potential compliance with self-maintenance practices. Innovative approaches to assist patients with compliance with self-maintenance limb volume practices have been developed and are commercially available.[21]

Chafing and hyperhidrosis may also be reduced by using a topical aluminum ion-based antiperspirant (ie, aluminum chloride, aluminum zirconium, and aluminum hydroxy bromide) on the residual limb.[21] These compounds block sweat ducts and decrease excess perspiration. However, they may also increase the risk of skin irritation/irritant contact dermatitis while concentrated under the prosthetic liner. Their occlusive effect on hair follicles may increase the propensity for folliculitis or furunculosis.[12] To maximize effectiveness, it is advised to apply the antiperspirant at night and wash the limb in the morning in order to remove residue while still allowing the aluminum ions to remain beneath the skin surface.[22]

In appropriate candidates, slow-healing ulcers and wounds may be treated with a vacuum-assisted suction socket (VASS) system, which helps to prevent the daily loss of residual limb volume and minimize skin irritation induced by shear stress.[23] This application of VASS systems remains controversial and is a developing strategy. Relative volume fluctuation, cognition, strength, and compliance are among characteristics evaluated in determining candidacy for VASS systems.

Procedural Interventions

In addition to effective daily maintenance and non-procedural interventions as needed, multiple minimally invasive procedures may be considered to improve prosthetic limb fit and comfort and to reduce the risk of skin complications.

Hair and Sweat Reduction

If the site is hair-bearing, a course of 3 to 6 laser hair reduction (LHR) treatments at 2 to 3 month intervals may be considered to reduce irritation, improve overall comfort, and decrease the risk of folliculitis and abscesses (**Fig. 5**). Maintenance treatments may be required periodically over months and years for any regrowth. Lasers of the appropriate wavelength are selected based on skin phototype to target pigmented hair follicles below the surface of the skin. In the experience of the authors, potential advantages of LHR in this setting include decreased skin friction and irritation especially at the top of the liner that is prone to rolling and movement, a more secure feel, and decreased folliculitis and skin infections. Patients also commonly report decreased subjective sweating, though this aspect of care requires further investigation. In one study, 20 patients with lower limb amputations using prosthetic limbs were administered a health-related quality of life (HRQOL) survey before and after an average of 3 treatments of LHR to their residual lower limbs. A statistically significant improvement in HRQOL was observed after LHR.[24]

Individuals with limb loss with persistent hyperhidrosis and increased moisture in the prosthesis socket despite antiperspirant use may be candidates for botulinum

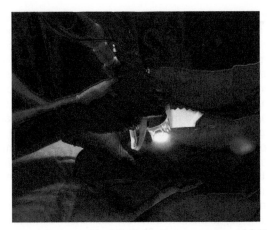

Fig. 5. Laser hair removal at the residual limb for the prevention of folliculitis.

toxin injections and microwave thermolysis. Botulinum toxin is approved for the treatment of axillary hyperhidrosis, and both botulinum toxins A and B have been investigated for the temporary management of hyperhidrosis in residual limbs (**Fig. 6**).[25–27] Microwave thermolysis (miraDry) is a nonsurgical energy-based device approved for axillary hyperhidrosis. Microwave energy heats tissue water targeting the water-rich eccrine glands in the dermis. Microwave thermolysis has also been studied for the long-term management of hyperhidrosis in residual limbs with efficacy reported for

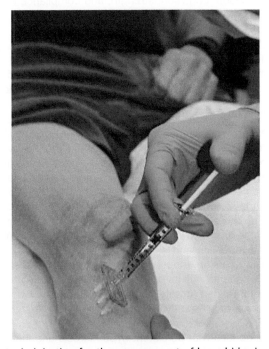

Fig. 6. Botulinum toxin injection for the management of hyperhidrosis.

up to 6 years after treatment.[28–30] Due to the variable anatomy associated with residual limbs, heat must be applied with caution in potentially compromised areas.

Scar Management

Scar management is a universal aspect of postamputation care regardless of the etiology, though amputations following trauma are more likely to be associated with other sequelae such as injuries at other sites, scar contractures, split-thick and full-thick skin grafts, and graft donor sites on residual limbs. Scar tissue lacks cutaneous adnexae (eg, follicles and eccrine glands) and is generally thinner and more fragile than normal skin. Therefore, scar tissue is even more susceptible to maceration, pressure, shear, and frictional forces associated with prosthetic limb use (**Fig. 7**). Scar treatment should adhere to a multi-modality approach including physical therapy, dermatologic surgery, and surgical consultation as appropriate. Conservative treatment includes therapeutic mobility exercises and various nonsurgical interventions such as massage, daily application of silicone-based scar treatment gel for raised scars, and the use of compression garments or bandages. Prosthetic liners likely have some built-in efficacy in terms of compression. Intralesional steroid injections with or without 5 fluorouracil can reduce scar hypertrophy.[31–33]

Lasers, especially ablative fractional lasers, should be considered a first-line treatment of debilitating and symptomatic scars.[34,35] Fractional lasers create a novel pattern of injury through the heating of tissue water characterized by relatively deep and narrow ablation/coagulation columns and wide spacing with abundant tissue sparing that facilitates rapid healing. Column depth and density are both selectable by the dermatologic surgeon. This results in a safe and well-tolerated recapitulation of the wound-healing cascade and long-term collagen remodeling to a more normal state over a course of treatment. More than simply improving visual characteristics such as erythema, dyspigmentation, and textural irregularity, a course of fractional laser treatment can improve scar pliability and durability and help restore function associated with scar contractures. Even if scar tissue does not cross a joint, increased time in the prosthesis and exercise tolerance with increased scar durability result in functional gains.

Ablative fractional laser therapy has also been associated with accelerated wound healing in chronic scar-associated wounds, including in patients with amputation.[36] Ablative fractional lasers (eg, 10,600 and 2940 nm) are associated with high water absorption and tissue ablation, while non-ablative fractional lasers (eg, 1550 and 1565 nm)

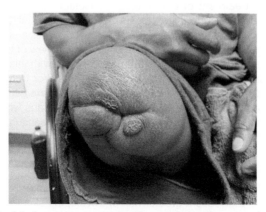

Fig. 7. Distal residual limb scar in a patient with transfemoral amputation.

are associated with moderate water absorption and tissue coagulation. Ablative fractional lasers generally have greater available penetration depth and are the primary choice for thicker scars, contractures, and wound healing, while non-ablative fractional lasers are effective for mild–moderate textural irregularity and dyspigmentation. Lasers that target hemoglobin, such as intense pulsed light and the 595 nm pulsed dye laser, are effective for the reduction of scar erythema, flattening of hypertrophic scars, and in managing symptoms such as itch.[34]

APPROACH TO EVALUATION OF CUTANEOUS MALIGNANCIES

Cutaneous malignancy postamputation may occur due to the site being an immunocompromised district or from a recurrence of previous malignancy. Immunocompromised districts are regional immune defects of the skin that occur after infections, malignancies, immune disorders, burns, radiation, vaccinations, or trauma. Amputation trauma creates a disruption of blood and lymphatic flow, resulting in a dysregulation of neuroimmune regulators and permanent alteration of the immune response at the site.[37,38] Squamous cell carcinomas, basal cell carcinomas, and lymphangiosarcoma have been documented following amputation.[1,39,40] The site may also be prone to the formation of Marjolin ulcers, a cutaneous malignancy that follows chronic healing wounds or scars.[40] Annual dermatologic and prosthetic assessments are recommended for early detection.

EVOLVING AREAS OF INTEREST

Osseointegration is an advanced reconstructive surgery for limb loss, offering an alternative to traditional socket-based prostheses. Osseointegration involves directly attaching bone to a metal implant, connected transcutaneously to a prosthetic limb and appendicular skeleton. This approach helps prevent skin injuries associated with traditional prosthetic limbs. Nevertheless, the percutaneous nature of the metal implant increases susceptibility to infection, and constant contact may cause irritation and potential breakdown. Improper loading can result in a lack of integration or loss of bony ingrowth in the implants overtime.[41,42] In addition to osseointegration, the use of improved imaging and 3 dimensional printing may accelerate the creation of prosthetic devices for patients in the future.

LIMITATIONS

The evaluation and treatment of dermatologic conditions following limb loss is an evolving area of study. The current literature is lacking in high-quality scientific studies, and there is a paucity of subject matter experts who work in this area of medicine. This study was limited by the inability to perform a systematic review of the literature. Additionally, most of the study authors gain primary experience with this topic through military medical experiences while serving on active duty and/or through service in the Veterans Health Administration. These experiences may create bias toward dermatologic conditions that may be more common to military veterans with limb loss. However, the multidisciplinary expertise provides a level of consensus experience in the management of skin issues in persons with limb loss and those who use prostheses.

SUMMARY

Persons with limb loss, and especially those who use artificial limbs, are subjected to abnormal exposures that pose a greater risk of developing skin issues than persons without amputation. It is important for any clinician providing care for persons with limb loss to have a foundational knowledge of potential issues and management approaches. A routine annual visit is recommended to assess skin health and prosthetic limb fit and function, and as needed to address unusual symptoms before chronic problems emerge. It is also recommended that the patient be educated to practice sound self-care, volume management, and hygiene. Multidisciplinary care is essential, and multiple minimally invasive dermatologic surgery procedures are available to help maximize cutaneous function and prosthetic limb fit and comfort.

CLINICS CARE POINTS

- Patients with lower extremity amputation are at increased risk of skin compromise due to greater dependence on prostheses for mobility tasks and increased shear and compression forces.

- Annual prosthetic consultations and multidisciplinary care, including dermatology and dermatologic surgery, can help ensure proper prosthetic limb fit and identify and mitigate developing skin issues.

- The residual limb skin is vulnerable to maceration, friction, and pressure-induced injuries due to close contact with the prosthesis interface.

- Proper hygiene of the residual limb site and socket, and preventative removal of the prosthesis when not required can help prevent infections and decrease secondary hyperhidrosis.

- Residual limb volume can impact the fit of the prosthesis and can often be managed with the addition or removal of additional socks, if recommended.

- LHR can be a helpful adjunctive therapy to improve the fit and comfort of prostheses (especially lower extremity) and reduce the incidence of complications such as folliculitis.

- Hyperhidrosis can be managed through an ascending ladder of care including proper hygiene, preventive prosthetic limb removal and drying, selection of prosthetic componentry, topical antiperspirants, LHR, injected botulinum toxin, and consideration for eccrine gland thermolysis.

- Scars and scar complications at the amputation site may be effectively managed through massage, mobility exercises, topical treatments, steroid injections, and various laser treatments such as fractional laser therapy.

DISCLOSURE

Contents of this study represent the opinions of the authors and not necessarily those of the US Department of Veterans Affairs, the University of South Florida, or any other academic or health care agency or institution. This project was unfunded. The authors declare no conflict of interest.

REFERENCES

1. Buikema KES, Meyerle JH. Amputation stump: Privileged harbor for infections, tumors, and immune disorders. Clin Dermatol 2014;32(5):670–7.
2. Meulenbelt H, Geertzen J, Dijkstra P, et al. Skin problems in lower limb amputees: an overview by case reports. J Eur Acad Dermatol Venereol 2007;21(2).
3. Yang NB, Garza LA, Foote CE, et al. High prevalence of stump dermatoses 38 years or more after amputation. Arch Dermatol 2012;148(11):1283.
4. Dudek NL, Marks MB, Marshall SC, et al. Dermatologic conditions associated with use of a lower-extremity prosthesis. Arch Phys Med Rehabil 2005;86(4):659–63.

5. Meulenbelt H, Geertzen J, Jonkman M, et al. Skin problems of the stump in lower limb amputees: 1. A clinical study. Acta Derm Venereol 2011;91(2):173–7.

6. Dudek NL, Marks MB, Marshall SC. Skin problems in an amputee clinic. Am J Phys Med Rehabil 2006;85(5):424–9.

7. Chan AS, Montbriand J, Eisenberg N, et al. Outcomes of minor amputations in patients with peripheral vascular disease over a 10-year period at a tertiary care institution. Vascular 2019;27(1):8–18.

8. Khalid KA, Nawi AFM, Zulkifli N, et al. Aging and wound healing of the skin: a review of clinical and pathophysiological hallmarks. Life Basel Switz 2022;12(12): 2142.

9. Kapp S. Suspension systems for prostheses. Clin Orthop 1999;361:55–62.

10. Pascale BA, Potter BK. Residual limb complications and management strategies. Curr Phys Med Rehabil Rep 2014;2(4):241–9.

11. de Godoy JMP, Ribeiro JV, Caracanhas LA, et al. Hospital infection after major amputations. Ann Clin Microbiol Antimicrob 2010;9:15.

12.. Highsmith MJ, Cummings S, Highsmith JT. Furunculosis in a transtibial amputee. Phys Med Rehabil Int 2014;1(3).

13. Virgili A, Trincone S, Zampino MR, et al. Acroangiodermatitis of amputation stump. Eur J Dermatol EJD 2003;13(4):402–3.

14. Highsmith JT, Highsmith MJ. Common skin pathology in LE prosthesis users. JAAPA Off J Am Acad Physician Assist 2007;20(11):33–6, 47.

15. Boyko TV, Longaker MT, Yang GP. Review of the current management of pressure ulcers. Adv Wound Care 2018;7(2):57–67.

16. Kahle JT, Orriola JJ, Johnston W, et al. The effects of vacuum-assisted suspension on residual limb physiology, wound healing, and function: a systematic review. Technol Innovat 2014;15(4):333–41.

17. Highsmith MJ, Kahle JT, Klenow TD, et al. Interventions to manage residual limb ulceration due to prosthetic use in individuals with lower extremity amputation: a systematic review of the literature. Technol Innovat 2016;18(2–3):115–23.

18. Richardson C, Kulkarni J. A review of the management of phantom limb pain: challenges and solutions. J Pain Res 2017;10:1861–70.

19. Price N. Routine fluorescence imaging to detect wound bacteria reduces antibiotic use and antimicrobial dressing expenditure while improving healing rates: retrospective analysis of 229 foot ulcers. Diagn Basel Switz 2020;10(11):927.

20. Sanders JE, Harrison DS, Allyn KJ, et al. How do sock ply changes affect residual-limb fluid volume in people with transtibial amputation? J Rehabil Res Dev 2012;49(2):241–56.

21. Innovation revolutionary: A solution to prosthetic socks management - VA News. 2022. Available at: https://news.va.gov/105705/innovation-revolutionary-a-solution-to-prosthetic-socks-management/. [Accessed 1 December 2023].

22. Hölzle E. Topical pharmacological treatment. Curr Probl Dermatol 2002;30:30–43.

23. Lannan FM, Powell J, Kim GM, et al. Hyperhidrosis of the residual limb: a narrative review of the measurement and treatment of excess perspiration affecting individuals with amputation. Prosthet Orthot Int 2021;45(6):477–86.

24. Traballesi M, Delussu AS, Fusco A, et al. Residual limb wounds or ulcers heal in transtibial amputees using an active suction socket system. A randomized controlled study. Eur J Phys Rehabil Med 2012;48(4):613–23.

25. Miletta NR, Kim S, Lezanski-Gujda A, et al. Improving health-related quality of life in wounded warriors: the promising benefits of laser hair removal to the residual limb–prosthetic interface. Dermatol Surg 2016;42(10):1182–7.

26. Charrow A, DiFazio M, Foster L, et al. Intradermal botulinum toxin type A injection effectively reduces residual limb hyperhidrosis in amputees: a case series. Arch Phys Med Rehabil 2008;89(7):1407–9.

27. Kern U, Kohl M, Seifert U, et al. Botulinum toxin type B in the treatment of residual limb hyperhidrosis for lower limb amputees: a pilot study. Am J Phys Med Rehabil 2011;90(4):321–9.

28. Lowe NJ, Glaser DA, Eadie N, et al. Botulinum toxin type A in the treatment of primary axillary hyperhidrosis: a 52-week multicenter double-blind, randomized, placebo-controlled study of efficacy and safety. J Am Acad Dermatol 2007; 56(4):604–11.

29. Glaser DA, Coleman WP, Fan LK, et al. A randomized, blinded clinical evaluation of a novel microwave device for treating axillary hyperhidrosis: the dermatologic reduction in underarm perspiration study. Dermatol Surg Off Publ Am Soc Dermatol Surg AI 2012;38(2):185–91.

30. Mula KN, Winston J, Pace S, et al. Use of a microwave device for treatment of amputation residual limb hyperhidrosis. Dermatol Surg Off Publ Am Soc Dermatol Surg AI 2017;43(1):149–52.

31. Kravitz SA, Lannan FM, Simpson MM. Long-term effectiveness of microwave thermoablation in persons with residual limb hyperhidrosis: a case series. Mil Med 2023;188(1–2):e417–20.

32. Puri N, Talwar A. The efficacy of silicone gel for the treatment of hypertrophic scars and keloids. J Cutan Aesthetic Surg 2009;2(2):104–6.

33. Sheng M, Chen Y, Li H, et al. The application of corticosteroids for pathological scar prevention and treatment: current review and update. Burns Trauma 2023; 11:tkad009.

34. Shah VV, Aldahan AS, Mlacker S, et al. 5-Fluorouracil in the treatment of keloids and hypertrophic scars: a comprehensive review of the literature. Dermatol Ther 2016;6(2):169–83.

35. Seago M, Shumaker PR, Spring LK, et al. Laser treatment of traumatic scars and contractures: 2020 International Consensus Recommendations. Lasers Surg Med 2020;52(2):96–116.

36. Buhalog B, Moustafa F, Arkin L, et al. Ablative fractional laser treatment of hypertrophic burn and traumatic scars: a systematic review of the literature. Arch Dermatol Res 2021;313(5):301–17.

37. Shumaker PR, Kwan JM, Badiavas EV, et al. Rapid healing of scar-associated chronic wounds after ablative fractional resurfacing. Arch Dermatol 2012; 148(11):1289–93.

38. Ruocco V, Brunetti G, Puca R, et al. The immunocompromised district: a unifying concept for lymphoedematous, herpes-infected and otherwise damaged sites. J Eur Acad Dermatol Venereol 2009;23(12):1364–73.

39. Karakozis S, Stamou SC, He P, et al. Carcinoma arising in an amputation stump. Am Surg 2001;67(5):495–7.

40. Scheman AJ, Kosarek CA. Purple nodules on the lower extremity following above-knee amputation. Angiosarcoma. Arch Dermatol 1988;124(2):263–4, 266-267.

41. Pekarek B, Buck S, Osher L. A comprehensive review on marjolin's ulcers: diagnosis and treatment. J Am Coll Certif Wound Spec 2011;3(3):60–4.

42. Overmann AL, Forsberg JA. The state of the art of osseointegration for limb prosthesis. Biomed Eng Lett 2020;10(1):5–16.

Postamputation Pain Management

Merideth Byl, DO, MBA[a,b], Jennifer Tram, MD[a,b],
Brandon Kalasho, DO[a,b], Sanjog Pangarkar, MD[a,b],
Quynh Giao Pham, MD[a,b,c],*

KEYWORDS

- Phantom limb pain • Postamputation pain • Residual limb pain • Perioperative pain
- Rehabilitation

KEY POINTS

- Postamputation pain may include residual limb pain (RLP) and phantom limb pain (PLP) and may develop into chronic pain in 30% to 80% of patients after amputation.
- RLP is pain localized to the remaining limb after amputation and may be caused by poor healing, infection, poor prosthetic fit, or neuropathic pain.
- PLP is pain distal to the amputation site and may arise from somatosensory cortical reorganization such that nociceptive stimulation of adjacent tissue in the proximal limb stimulates the perception of pain in the removed limb.
- Treatment of PLP may require pharmacologic agents including nonsteroidal anti-inflammatory drugs (NSAIDs), corticosteroids, anticonvulsants, antidepressants, opioids; rehabilitation including mirror therapy, somatosensory activity feedback, virtual reality; and interventional or surgical options including neuromodulation, targeted muscle reinnervation, and repetitive transcranial magnetic stimulation.
- Treatment of RLP may involve pharmacologic agents such as acetaminophen, NSAIDs, antidepressants/anticonvulsants, calcitonin, antihypertensives, opioids, N-methyl-D-aspartate antagonists, rehabilitation, psychological support, and integrative treatments.

INTRODUCTION

The earliest known documentation of phantom limb pain (PLP) occurs in military surgeon Ambroise Paré's *Ten Books of Surgery*, which was published in 1564.[1] Dr. Paré urged physicians to avoid dismissing complaints of phantom limb pain in postamputation

---

[a] Department of Physical Medicine & Rehabilitation, Greater Los Angeles Veteran Affairs HealthCare System, 11301 Wilshire Boulevard, Los Angeles, CA 90073, USA; [b] Division of PM&R, Department of Medicine, 200 UCLA Medical Plaza, Suite 420, Los Angeles, CA 90095, USA; [c] David Geffen School of Medicine at UCLA, 10833 Le Conte Avenue, Los Angeles, CA 90095, USA
* Corresponding author.
E-mail address: AngelaQuynh.Pham@va.gov

Phys Med Rehabil Clin N Am 35 (2024) 757–768
https://doi.org/10.1016/j.pmr.2024.06.003
1047-9651/24/© 2024 Elsevier Inc. All rights reserved, including those for text and data mining, AI training, and similar technologies.
pmr.theclinics.com

patients and hypothesized that phantom limb pain may occur because of proximal degeneration of damaged nerves.[1] Despite its early identification, the term phantom limb pain was not used until the 1860s, when neurologist Silas Weir Mitchell described amputation injuries from the Civil War.[2] At the time, phantom limb pain was primarily regarded as a psychological diagnosis, which further stigmatized patients already suffering from this painful condition.[2]

Despite advances in medical care and surgical techniques since the Civil War, post-amputation pain (PAP) is still one of the most common and challenging conditions for rehabilitation physicians. PAP is often used to describe several disorders, including PLP, phantom limb sensation (PLS), and residual limb pain (RLP). Chronic pain following amputation occurs between 30% and 80% of patients undergoing amputation surgery and may develop up to 2 decades after limb resection. The variation of prevalence rates for PLP and RLP in the literature is likely influenced by PAP, the heterogeneity of the patient population, and the reason for amputation (dysvascular, traumatic, or malignancy).[3]

PAP may resolve after surgery, but if pain persists beyond the time required for tissue healing, it is generally considered chronic in nature. RLP, which was historically referred to as stump pain, is pain limited to the remaining limb after amputation. This pain may be caused by tissue injury, such as inadequate healing, local infection, redundant tissue, poor prosthetic fit, or neuropathic pain (such as nerve entrapment in scar tissue or neuroma). Approximately 25% of persons with amputation will experience these symptoms within the first week of surgery.[4] In contrast, PLS involves non-painful perceptions in the absent limb.[5] In this article, the authors review the various factors related to PAP and current treatment options.

PAIN PHYSIOLOGY

Limb pain experienced by someone with an amputation can be explained by several processes. These include peripheral mechanisms, spinal cord mechanisms, and supraspinal mechanisms, which can occur alone or in combination. Pain related to peripheral mechanisms occurs via ectopic discharges from afferent nerves at the amputation site or dorsal root ganglia, increased sensitivity from a neuroma, or sympathetically maintained pain related to the surgical site. These ectopic discharges, which occur from spontaneous firing of injured nerves and/or neuromas at the amputation site, travel via afferent nerves to the central nervous system and alter pain perception. There is associated upregulation of voltage-gated sodium channels in the affected nerves, making them more sensitive and reactive to mechanical and chemical stimuli. Additionally, ectopic discharges are linked to upregulation of voltage-gated sodium channels in the dorsal root ganglia cells, which further contribute to postamputation sensory abnormality.[6]

There are 2 primary mechanisms contributing to pain at the spinal cord, anatomic reorganization, and central sensitization. Following peripheral nerve injury, anatomic reorganization occurs when degeneration of the unmyelinated C-fibers leads to sprouting of larger myelinated Aβ-fibers into lamina 1 and 2 of the Rexed laminae, contributing to the genesis of PLP. During central sensitization, dorsal horn cells receive excessive input from painful stimuli at the amputation site leading to hyperalgesia. In addition, excitatory amino acids, such as glutamic acid and aspartic acid, act on N-methyl-D-aspartate (NMDA) receptors and are theorized to contribute to hyperalgesia.[6]

Supraspinal mechanisms also contribute to the overall pain experience of someone with an amputation. Studies utilizing magnetoencephalograms reveal cortical reorganization in both humans and monkeys postamputation. Study participants demonstrated that after upper extremity amputation, the corresponding somatosensory cortex begins receiving information from other areas of the body. It is theorized that PLP can result from errors in the remapping.[6]

PERIOPERATIVE PAIN MANAGEMENT

Thoughtful perioperative pain management is important to reduce pain after amputation surgery. Regardless of the indication for surgery, the perioperative period can pose certain challenges both in the timing of treatments and obtaining timely insurance coverage for that care.[7] To this end, Enhanced Recovery After Surgery (ERAS) programs are designed to optimize patient understanding, employ opioid-sparing analgesics, standardize intraoperative anesthesia, promote early mobilization, and prevent nosocomial infections. The typical starting point in ERAS is education and expectation setting for pain control, including a discussion on acute pain control measures, presurgical anxiety, opioid utilization, and postsurgical mobilization.

In addition, regional anesthesia during surgery has sufficient evidence to promote its use in amputation care. The duration for maintaining the catheter after surgery as well as medications used during surgery may also have an impact on recovery and sensitization. As an example, the use of perioperative ketamine is controversial but still commonly employed.[8] In the surgical domain, meticulous soft tissue manipulation and judicious engagement of muscular structures through myodesis (deepest layer of muscle attached to the bone) or myoplasty (more superficial layers of muscle attached to each other) techniques may improve outcome. Intraoperatively, the conscientious placement of severed nerves within cushioned soft tissue may reduce potential complications arising from pressure or scar formation.

Further, during staged amputations, strategic planning can reduce anticipated complications, most notably, neuroma formation, which is an inevitable consequence of nerve transection. Placement of the transected nerve in cushioned, soft tissue away from areas of potential pressure or scarring can improve outcomes. Moreover, dysvascular amputations introduce a layer of complexity because of the need to identify the most distal location for viable tissue while maintaining limb length for eventual prosthetic fitting. Interventional methodologies may also be limited due to the need for anticoagulation due to comorbidities.[7]

RISK FACTORS AND PREDICTION OF POSTAMPUTATION PAIN

Certain considerations may be helpful in identifying risk factors associated with chronic PAP.

Genetics

The propensity for chronic pain may be inherited through the complex interplay between various genes and environmental factors.[9] Both human twin studies and animal models have demonstrated that approximately 30% to 70% of generalized chronic pain perception can be attributed to genetic factors.[10]

Psychological Factors and Disease States

Anxiety, depression, catastrophizing, perceptions of illness, inadequate coping strategies, a diminished sense of control, deficient social support, and heightened expectations have all been implicated in the development of chronic postsurgical pain.[11] Additionally, fibromyalgia, migraine, irritable bowel syndrome, irritable bladder, and Raynaud's syndrome have also been linked with chronic postsurgical pain.[12]

Preoperative Pain

Preoperative chronic pain, irrespective of its proximity to the surgical site, increases the likelihood of developing chronic postsurgical pain. This phenomenon likely stems from induction of central sensitization to pain.[13]

Preoperative Opioid Utilization

It has been well documented that extended opioid exposure can lead to either diminished antinociception or hyperalgesia. High doses of intraoperative mu-receptor agonists have been associated with heightened postoperative pain and increased morphine consumption.[14]

NEURAXIAL ANALGESIA, PHARMACOLOGIC MANAGEMENT, AND SURGICAL MANAGEMENT

Neuraxial analgesia has emerged as an integral element in perioperative pain management for amputation procedures. A recent investigation revealed that the administration of epidural analgesia 48 hours prior to amputation yielded a noteworthy reduction in PLP, an effect sustained up to 6 months postoperatively. Concordant findings in other studies underscore the advantages of epidural or systemic analgesia when administered more than 24 hours prior to surgery, particularly in mitigating PLP.[15]

The concept of preventive analgesia assumes the ability to modulate both the central and peripheral nervous systems during the perioperative timeframe. A notable approach involved the application of continuous peripheral nerve block employing a regional catheter initially positioned at the distal terminus of the sciatic nerve or posterior tibial nerve, subsequently advanced to a location just proximal to the level of amputation. This technique entails an initial bolus dose of local anesthetic succeeded by a sustained low-dose infusion, typically 0.25% bupivacaine at a rate of 5 to 8 mL/h. Advantages of this modality include early mobilization followed by expedited rehabilitation and consequent reduction of edema.[15]

Additionally, findings by Bach and colleagues[16] demonstrated the efficacy of a preoperative epidural approach not only in mitigating postoperative pain but also in diminishing the likelihood of subsequent PLP. Concurrent investigations have probed the effectiveness of combined pharmacologic agents, including bupivacaine, diamorphine, and clonidine, administered through epidural infusions to improve PLP.

These insights collectively contribute to the evolving landscape of neuraxial analgesia, substantiating its role in amputation care, with a particular emphasis on its temporal administration to help improve outcomes.[16]

RESIDUAL LIMB PAIN VERSUS PHANTOM LIMB PAIN

A national survey conducted in the United States in 2005 reported that 95% of persons with amputation experienced PLP or RLP.[17] While both pain responses may occur concurrently, it is important to recognize the distinction between residual limb and PLP. While RLP occurs at the surgical site or in the limb proximal to the surgical site, PLP occurs distal to the surgical site, in the absent limb.

PATHOPHYSIOLOGY OF RESIDUAL LIMB PAIN

RLP is more common in the immediate postsurgical phase and may be caused by the formation of scar or neuroma,[18] which leads to local inflammation, regenerative nerve sprouting, and increased afferent nociceptive transmission.[19] Poor prosthetic fitting may also contribute to RLP and can be identified during careful skin examination of the residual limb and identification of appropriate weight tolerant and weight intolerant areas.[19] Other causes of RLP include osteophyte formation, infection, and bursitis.[20] There is also evidence of centralization of the pain response through somatosensory cortex reorganization and dorsal horn reorganization in response to deafferentation of the limb.[19]

PREVALENCE, ETIOLOGY, AND RISK FACTORS OF RESIDUAL LIMB PAIN

List and colleagues reviewed the published literature between 2000 and 2020 and estimated the prevalence of RLP at 59% after lower extremity amputation.[21] Risk factors for the development of RLP include advanced age and amputation of the upper extremity. Additionally, cancer-associated and traumatic amputations have been associated with more severe forms of RLP.[22] Another study has suggested an association between osteoporosis, as measured by bone mineral density, and RLP.[20]

PHANTOM LIMB PAIN VERSUS PHANTOM LIMB SENSATION

PLP is characterized by pain distal to the amputation site and may develop after the immediate postsurgical phase. One study with nearly 100 participants identified 2 distinct periods, at 1 month postamputation and at 12 months postamputation, for the onset of PLP.[18] Common descriptors of PLP include a stabbing, burning, throbbing, or twisting pain, which is consistent with nerve injury-mediated pain.[18,23] PLS is different from PLP as patients experience non-painful perceptions in the absent limb accompanied by the illusion of "telescoping," wherein the distal portion of the limb feels closer to the site of amputation.

PATHOPHYSIOLOGY OF PHANTOM LIMB PAIN

PLP is classically thought to arise from supraspinal processes including somatosensory cortical reorganization such that the nociceptive stimulation of adjacent tissue in the proximal limb could stimulate pain in the removed limb.[19] For example, brain MRIs of patients post hand amputation have demonstrated that movement of the proximal limb will activate the same cortical areas that previously served the hand.[18,19] Risk factors for the development of PLP include female gender, concurrent RLP, and PAP levels.[18]

Given its complex pathophysiology, treatment of PLP may require pharmacologic agents including nonsteroidal anti-inflammatory drugs (NSAIDs), steroids, anticonvulsants, antidepressants, opioids; rehabilitation including mirror therapy, somatosensory activity feedback, virtual reality (VR); and interventional or surgical options including neuromodulation, targeted muscle reinnervation (TMR), repetitive transcranial magnetic stimulation. Treatment of PLP is challenging given varying individual responses to therapies and procedures.

PHARMACOLOGIC INTERVENTION: ACETAMINOPHEN/NONSTEROIDAL ANTI-INFLAMMATORY DRUGS

Paracetamol and NSAIDs are useful in reducing postoperative pain in general.[24] Although these drugs are among the most prescribed for the treatment of PLP,[25] they have not demonstrated efficacy in alleviating PLP.

PHARMACOLOGIC INTERVENTION: ANTIDEPRESSANTS/ANTICONVULSANTS

Tricyclic antidepressants (TCAs) are among the most commonly used medications for the treatment of PLP.[25] Amitriptyline is widely studied for its use in the treatment of neuropathic pain but its anticholinergic and potential cardiac side effects limit its use. In addition, there are mixed results in the literature regarding efficacy of TCAs in the treatment of PLP.[18,26] Some selective serotonin–norepinephrine reuptake inhibitors (SNRIs) have shown some efficacy in the management of PLP. Milnacipran has been successfully used in PLP.[27,28]

Gabapentin has commonly been used to manage neuropathic pain. Gabapentin's primary mechanism involves the potential inhibition of excitatory neurotransmitter release and a reduction in glutamate availability at both NMDA and non-NMDA receptors. However, its efficacy in addressing neuropathic pain is largely attributed to binding the α-2-delta subunit of voltage-dependent calcium channels.[28] Gabapentin has been shown in a placebo-controlled study to be effective in alleviating PLP.[29]

Topiramate, an anticonvulsant with multiple mechanisms of action (gamma-aminobutyric acid agonist, sodium channel blocker, and kainate antagonist), has been shown in a double-blinded randomized controlled trial to be effective in PLP.[30]

There is weak evidence in the literature to support the role of other pharmacologic agents including duloxetine, fluoxetine, clonazepam, pregabalin, and capsaicin in the treatment of PLP.[31]

PHARMACOLOGIC INTERVENTION: CALCITONIN

Multiple studies have demonstrated the analgesic properties of calcitonin. Mechanisms contributing to this effect involve modulation of Na + channels and serotonin receptor expression and are independent of its osteoclastic inhibitory function.[32] Salmon calcitonin has proven to be a valuable analgesic with respect to PLP. Current evidence supports the utilization of calcitonin for the treatment of acute onset PLP; however, there is conflicting evidence regarding its benefit in chronic PLP.[33]

PHARMACOLOGIC INTERVENTION: ANTIHYPERTENSIVES

There is no definitive evidence to support the use of clonidine, an alpha 2-adrenergic agonist, for treating PLP. Nonetheless, the drug is often used in this condition because peripheral alpha 2 adrenoceptors have been hypothesized to be involved in pain inhibition.[34]

PHARMACOLOGIC INTERVENTION: OPIOIDS

Opioids are effective in addressing PLP and may reduce cortical reorganization on neuromagnetic source imaging.[35] Although the administration of a pure mu opioid receptor agonist can reduce the intensity of PAP, overall functional activity and self-reported pain-related interference in ADLs do not seem to be impacted.[36] To reduce the likelihood of "opioid-induced hyperalgesia" and limit the overall morphine milligram equivalents, some authors have suggested using opioids with multimodal mechanisms of action.[37] One such drug is buprenorphine, which is a partial mu opioid receptor agonist/antagonist, kappa receptor antagonist, delta receptor antagonist, and opioid receptor-like 1 agonist.

A systematic review demonstrated that the best evidence for pharmacologic treatment of PLP includes intravenous (IV) ketamine or IV morphine during the perioperative phase (**Table 1**).[31] There is also some evidence to support the use of morphine or bupivacaine for short-term and long-term pain relief as well as the use of gabapentin for intermediate-term pain relief.[31] The use of long-term opioids for chronic noncancer pain is controversial and should include a discussion of the risks, benefits, and alternatives prior to initiation and on a regular basis to ensure safety.

		Phantom
Pharmacologic Agents	**Residual Limb Pain**	**Limb Pain**
Paracetamol	√	√a
NSAIDS	√	√a
Tricyclic Antidepressants		√a
Serotonin-norepinephrine Reuptake Inhibitors (milnacipran, duloxetine)		√
Anticonvulsants (gabapentin, topiramate, pregabalin, valproic acid)		√
Calcitonin		√
Alpha 2-adrenergic Agonist (clonidine)		√a
Opioids (morphine)	√	√ (acute PLP)
NMDA Antagonist (ketamine)	√	√
Corticosteroids		√
Anesthetic (bupivacaine)		√
Pregabalin		√
Benzodiazepine (clonazepam)		√a
Topicals (capsaicin)		√a

Table 1
Pharmacologic treatment for postamputation pain[b]

a Evidence of efficacy is lacking.
b These medications are not FDA approved specifically for PLP, PLS, RLP.

PHARMACOLOGIC INTERVENTION: N-METHYL-D-ASPARTATE ANTAGONIST

Ketamine acts as an NMDA antagonist, analgesic, and anti-inflammatory in sub-anesthetic doses.[38] Low-dose intravenous ketamine has been shown to be useful for the management of perioperative pain and is efficacious in reducing opioid consumption by 40%.[39] Oral formulations have also been shown to be effective and safe for postamputation surgical pain. It is yet to be seen if oral ketamine is effective in reducing the incidence of chronic PAP.[40] Memantine, an NMDA receptor antagonist, has also demonstrated efficacy in the reduction of acute PLP but not chronic PLP.

REHABILITATION

In addition to optimizing function in transfers and mobility, other goals of rehabilitation include contracture prevention and edema control, both of which can aid in mitigating RLP. An example of rehabilitation modalities used for edema control is an elasticated shrinker sock that promotes healing and aids in shaping of the residual limb.[41] Appropriate prosthetic prescription in conjunction with functional goals is crucial for early recovery. Appropriate strength training and conditioning of the remaining limbs are key to preventing compensatory mechanics that can lead to future pain conditions.[42] The use of transcutaneous electrical nerve stimulation (TENS) has been reported to be beneficial in pain management postamputation.[41]

One of the most effective rehabilitation therapies for the treatment of PLP is mirror therapy, which may help retrain neural perception pathways. In mirror therapy, patients use a mirror to sense the amputated limb moving as if the limb were still present and part of the body. Viewing the reflected image of an intact body part may help the brain reconcile the differences between the sense of where the body is and what the eyes perceive, thus reversing maladaptive cortical changes.[43] The literature suggests that there may be more benefit to mirror therapy in treating deeper somatic pain than superficial nociceptive pain.[43,44]

One randomized, sham-controlled trial demonstrated superiority of mirror therapy over covered mirror therapy and mental imagery therapy, suggesting that pain relief may be caused by activation of mirror neurons in the brain hemisphere opposite the side of the amputated limb.[45] In this study, the patient groups receiving only covered mirror therapy or imagery therapy initially did not experience significant pain relief but did experience pain relief when they were switched over to mirror therapy.[45]

Another rehabilitation therapy that may be efficacious in relieving pain is the use of a Sauerbruch prosthesis, which provides direct somatosensory feedback from the prosthetic hand. A purely cosmetic prosthesis does not provide any somatosensory or activity feedback. One study demonstrated that a Sauerbruch prosthesis is associated with a lower incidence of PLP compared to a standard cosmetic prosthesis.[46,47] This supports the theory that PLP is driven by maladaptive cortical reorganization and that reversal of these maladaptive cortical pathways via somatosensory feedback from a prosthetic may relieve PLP symptoms. Similarly, the use of a myoelectric prosthesis with the incorporation of somatosensory feedback has been demonstrated to reduce PLP and increase functionality of the prosthesis.[47]

PSYCHOSOCIAL INTERVENTION

Psychosocial factors that affect someone with an amputation include employment status change, alteration in body image, prosthesis use, and psychosocial adjustment.[48] Included in these factors is the potential for developing chronic pain, which can significantly impact multiple aspects of a person's life. Integrating psychological support into the rehabilitation process is important. An emphasis on acceptance of chronic pain, rather than the expectation of complete pain elimination, may help enhance coping mechanisms and improve quality of life. Understanding and addressing the psychosocial factors in someone with an amputation experiencing chronic pain require a comprehensive and individualized approach.

INTEGRATIVE APPROACH

Integrative treatments for chronic pain in patients with amputation include acupuncture, ultrasound, TENS, and massage therapy.[6] While acupuncture shows low efficacy, the literature supports use of mind–body therapies such as hypnosis, biofeedback, eye movement desensitization and reprocessing, and adjunctive relaxation techniques. Clinical data further support the utilization of mind–body therapies to ameliorate stress, fatigue, and depression.[48] These approaches contribute to a comprehensive care paradigm for amputation-related pain and disability.

Another novel approach in the management of PLP is VR. Studies have shown 50% to 90% reduction of PLP in those with amputation after treatment with immersive VR training during which the brain is led to believe that the missing limb is still intact, and its movement is controllable. However, these studies have limited participants and are in the early stages of technology. Additional clinical studies are needed to further explore the potential for VR in the management of PLP.[49]

PSYCHOLOGICAL INTERVENTIONS

There is mounting evidence for the effectiveness of mind–body interventions in the treatment of chronic pain. However, with the exception of mirror therapy, there are few studies dedicated to the efficacy of mind–body interventions such as hypnosis, guided imagery, relaxation techniques, and biofeedback for the relief of PAP. In addition, these studies have a small sample size and vary widely in the applications of mind–body techniques. Often, they also lack study replication and standardization. Reviews of these limited studies show promising results, and more research is needed to further explore these treatment options.[48]

INTERVENTIONAL/SURGICAL INTERVENTION

Generally, surgical and interventional options may be indicated for PLP refractory to conservative management. Neuromodulation via deep brain stimulation, spinal cord stimulators, dorsal root ganglion stimulators, or peripheral nerve stimulators attempts to modify maladaptive neuroplastic changes. Currently, there is a paucity of literature demonstrating the utility of these neurostimulation devices in chronic PLP[18] though there is some evidence for short-term benefit of repetitive transcranial magnetic stimulation. Other surgical options include the surgical removal of neuromas or areas of heterotopic ossification, which may contribute to RLP.[18] Upper extremity TMR is a surgical technique that may also help improve functionality of the myoelectric prosthesis described in the "rehabilitation" section.

SUMMARY

The management of amputation-related pain is a complex and challenging responsibility for rehabilitation clinicians and requires a collaborative and multidisciplinary approach. Despite advances in medical and surgical techniques, PAP is unfortunately still common but may improve with improvement in ERAS protocols and presurgical planning. At the present time, there is no Food and Drug Administration-approved treatment for PLP or RLP; however, traditional treatments including medication management, rehabilitation therapy, integrative approaches, and interventional therapies may improve outcomes when phenotypically driven. As such, employing a multimodal strategy that is patient-centered and addresses the physical, psychological, and social needs in postamputation care is essential for improving patient care.

CLINICS CARE POINTS

- Treatment of post-amputation pain requires a multimodal and multidisciplinary team approach.
- Residual limb pain occurs at the surgical site whereas phantom limb pain occurs distal to the surgical site, in the absent limb.
- Rational polypharmacy using medications with different mechanisms of action may improve post-amputation pain.
- NMDA antagonists, such as ketamine, are useful in acute but not chronic phantom limb pain.
- Mirror therapy is an effective treatment for phantom limb pain.
- Rapidly evolving changes in technology and peri-operative protocols may improve clinical outcomes in the future.

DISCLOSURE

None.

REFERENCES

1. Skuse A. Surgery and selfhood in early modern England: altered bodies and contexts of identity [Internet]. Cambridge (UK): Cambridge University Press; 2021. CHAPTER 6, Phantom Limbs and the Hard Problem. Available at: https://www.ncbi.nlm.nih.gov/books/NBK571301/.
2. Collins KL, Russell HG, Schumacher PJ, et al. A review of current theories and treatments for phantom limb pain. J Clin Invest 2018;128(6):2168–76. Epub 2018 Jun 1. PMID: 29856366; PMCID: PMC5983333.
3. Hanley MA, Jensen MP, Smith DG, et al. Preamputation pain and acute pain predict chronic pain after lower extremity amputation. J Pain 2007;8(2):102–9.
4. Buchheit T, Van de Ven T, Hsia HL, et al. Pain Phenotypes and Associated Clinical Risk Factors Following Traumatic Amputation: Results from Veterans Integrated Pain Evaluation Research (VIPER). Pain Med 2016 Jan;17(1):149–61. PMID: 26177330; PMCID: PMC6280998.
5. Srivastava D. Chronic post-amputation pain: peri-operative management - Review. Br J Pain 2017;11(4):192–202.
6. Jackson MA, Simpson KH. Pain after amputation. Contin Educ Anaesth Crit Care Pain 2004;4(1):20–3.
7. Kent ML, Hsia HLJ, Van de Ven TJ, et al. Perioperative Pain Management Strategies for Amputation: A Topical Review. Pain Med 2017;18(3):504–19.
8. Hayes C, Armstrong-Brown A, Burstal R. Perioperative intravenous ketamine infusion for the prevention of persistent post-amputation pain: a randomized, controlled trial. Anaesth Intensive Care 2004;32(3):330–8.
9. Clarke H, Katz J, Flor H, et al. Genetics of chronic post-surgical pain: a crucial step toward personal pain medicine. Can J Anaesth 2015;62(3):294–303. Epub 2014 Dec 4. PMID: 25471684.
10. Macgregor AJ, Andrew T, Sambrook PN, et al. Structural, psychological, and genetic influences on low back and neck pain: a study of adult female twins. Arthritis Rheum 2004;51:160–7.
11. Niraj G, Rowbotham DJ. Persistent postoperative pain: where are we now? Br J Anaesth 2011;107(1):25–9. Epub 2011 May 24. PMID: 21610014.
12. Pozek JP, Beausang D, Baratta JL, et al. The acute to chronic pain transition: can chronic pain be prevented? Med Clin North Am 2016;100(1):17–30.
13. Borsook D, Kussman BD, George E, et al. Surgically induced neuropathic pain: understanding the perioperative process. Ann Surg 2013;257(3):403–12. PMID: 23059501; PMCID: PMC3546123.
14. Koppert W, Schmelz M. The impact of opioid-induced hyperalgesia for postoperative pain. Best Pract Res Clin Anaesthesiol 2007;21(1):65–83.
15. De Jong R, Shysh AJ. Development of a Multimodal Analgesia Protocol for Perioperative Acute Pain Management for Lower Limb Amputation. Pain Res Manag 2018;2018:5237040.
16. Ypsilantis E, Tang TY. Pre-emptive analgesia for chronic limb pain after amputation for peripheral vascular disease: a systematic review. Ann Vasc Surg 2010; 24(8):1139–46. PMID: 20800987.
17. Ephraim PL, Wegener ST, MacKenzie EJ, et al. Phantom pain, residual limb pain, and back pain in amputees: results of a national survey. Arch Phys Med Rehabil 2005;86(10):1910–9. PMID: 16213230.
18. Modest JM, Raducha JE, Testa EJ, et al. Management of Post-Amputation Pain. R I Med J 2013;103(4):19–22. PMID: 32357588.

19. Hsu E, Cohen SP. Postamputation pain: epidemiology, mechanisms, and treatment. J Pain Res 2013;6:121–36. Epub 2013 Feb 13. PMID: 23426608; PMCID: PMC3576040.
20. Yazicioglu K, Tugcu I, Yilmaz B, et al. Osteoporosis: A factor on residual limb pain in traumatic trans-tibial amputations. Prosthet Orthot Int 2008;32(2):172–8. https://doi.org/10.1080/03093640802016316.
21. List EB, Krijgh DD, Martin E, et al. Prevalence of residual limb pain and symptomatic neuromas after lower extremity amputation: a systematic review and meta-analysis. Pain 2021;162(7):1906–13. PMID: 33470746.
22. Evans AG, Chaker SC, Curran GE, et al. Postamputation Residual Limb Pain Severity and Prevalence: A Systematic Review and Meta-Analysis. Plast Surg (Oakv) 2022; 30(3):254–68. Epub 2021 Jun 8. PMID: 35990396; PMCID: PMC9389065.
23. Bloomquist T. Amputation and phantom limb pain: a pain-prevention model. AANA J (Am Assoc Nurse Anesth) 2001;69(3):211–7. PMID: 11759564.
24. Macario A, Royal MA. A literature review of randomized clinical trials of intravenous acetaminophen (paracetamol) for acute postoperative pain. Pain Pract 2011;11:290–6.
25. Subedi B, Grossberg GT. Phantom limb pain: mechanisms and treatment approaches. Pain Res Treat 2011;2011:864605. Epub 2011 Aug 14. PMID: 22110933; PMCID: PMC3198614.
26. Robinson LR, Czerniecki JM, Ehde DM, et al. Trial of amitriptyline for relief of pain in amputees: results of a randomized controlled study. Arch Phys Med Rehabil 2004;85(1):1–6.
27. Nagoshi Y, Watanabe A, Inoue S, et al. Usefulness of milnacipran in treating phantom limb pain. Neuropsychiatr Dis Treat 2012;8:549–53. https://doi.org/10.2147/NDT.S37431.
28. Shimoyama M, Shimoyama N, Hori Y. Gabapentin affects glutamatergic excitatory neurotransmission in the rat dorsal horn. Pain 2000;85:405–14.
29. Bone M, Critchley P, Buggy DJ. Gabapentin in postamputation phantom limb pain: a randomized, double-blind, placebo-controlled, cross-over study. Reg Anesth Pain Med 2002;27(5):481–6.
30. Harden RN, Houle TT, Remble TA, et al. Topiramate for phantom limb pain: a time-series analysis. Pain Med 2005;6(5):375–8.
31. McCormick Z, Chang-Chien G, Marshall B, et al. Phantom limb pain: a systematic neuroanatomical-based review of pharmacologic treatment. Pain Med 2014; 15(2):292–305. Epub 2013 Nov 13. PMID: 24224475.
32. Yazdani J, Khiavi RK, Ghavimi MA, et al. Calcitonina como agente analgésico: revisão dos mecanismos de ação e das aplicações clínicas [Calcitonin as an analgesic agent: review of mechanisms of action and clinical applications]. Braz J Anesthesiol 2019;69(6):594–604.
33. Neumüller J, Lang-Illievich K, Brenna CTA, et al. Calcitonin in the Treatment of Phantom Limb Pain: A Systematic Review. CNS Drugs 2023;37(6):513–21. Epub 2023 Jun 1. PMID: 37261670; PMCID: PMC10276773.
34. Pertovaara A. Noradrenergic pain modulation. Prog Neurobiol 2006 Oct;80(2): 53–83. Epub 2006 Oct 9. PMID: 17030082.
35. Huse E, Larbig W, Flor H, et al. The effect of opioids on phantom limb pain and cortical reorganization. Pain 2001;90(1–2):47–55. PMID: 11166969.
36. Wu CL, Agarwal S, Tella PK, et al. Morphine versus mexiletine for treatment of postamputation pain: a randomized, placebo-controlled, crossover trial. Anesthesiology 2008;109(2):289–96. PMID: 18648238; PMCID: PMC2654208.

37. Srejic U, Banimahd F. Haunting of the phantom limb pain abolished by buprenorphine/naloxone. BMJ Case Rep 2021;14(2):e237009. PMID: 33608331; PMCID: PMC7896584.

38. Loix S, De Kock M, Henin P. The anti-inflammatory effects of ketamine: state of the art. Acta Anaesthesiol Belg 2011;62(1):47–58. PMID: 21612145.

39. Jouguelet-Lacoste J, La Colla L, Schilling D, et al. The use of intravenous infusion or single dose of low-dose ketamine for postoperative analgesia: a review of the current literature. Pain Med 2015;16(2):383–403. Epub 2014 Dec 19. PMID: 25530168.

40. Buvanendran A, Kroin JS, Rajagopal A, et al. Oral Ketamine for Acute Pain Management After Amputation Surgery. Pain Med 2018;19(6):1265–70.

41. Guest F, Marshall C, Stansby G. Amputation and Rehabilitation. Surgery (Oxford) 2019;37(2):102–5.

42. Klarich J, Brueckner I. Amputee Rehabilitation and Preprosthetic Care. Phys Med Rehabil Clin N Am 2014;25(1):75–91. Elsevier Inc.

43. Kim SY, Kim YY. Mirror therapy for phantom limb pain. Korean J Pain 2012;25(4):272–4. Epub 2012 Oct 4. PMID: 23091690; PMCID: PMC3468806.

44. Sumitani M, Miyauchi S, McCabe CS, et al. Mirror visual feedback alleviates deafferentation pain, depending on qualitative aspects of the pain: a preliminary report. Rheumatology (Oxford) 2008;47:1038–43.

45. Chan BL, Witt R, Charrow AP, et al. The Effect of Medical Marijuana Laws on Marijuana Use in the United States: Evidence from Recreational Marijuana Laws. N Engl J Med 2007;357:2206–7.

46. Weiss T, Miltner WH, Adler T, et al. Decrease in phantom limb pain associated with prosthesis-induced increased use of an amputation stump in humans. Neurosci Lett 1999 Sep 10;272(2):131–4. PMID: 10507559.

47. Dietrich C, Nehrdich S, Seifert S, et al. Leg Prosthesis With Somatosensory Feedback Reduces Phantom Limb Pain and Increases Functionality. Front Neurol 2018;9:270.

48. Moura VL, Faurot KR, Gaylord SA, et al. Mind-body interventions for treatment of phantom limb pain in persons with amputation. Am J Phys Med Rehabil 2012 Aug;91(8):701–14.

49. Rutledge T, Velez D, Depp C, et al. A virtual reality intervention for the treatment of phantom limb pain: development and feasibility results. Pain Med 2019. https://doi.org/10.1093/pm/pnz121.

Adaptive Sports and Recreation in Persons with Limb Loss/Limb Deficiency

Melissa J. Tinney, MD[a,b,*], Mary E. Caldwell, DO, CAQSM[c,1],
Eric M. Lamberg, EdD, PT, CPed[d,e,2]

KEYWORDS

- Adaptive sports • Para sports • Physical activity • Limb loss • Limb deficiency

KEY POINTS

- There are a multitude of adaptive sports programs for persons with limb loss/limb deficiency as a continuum of rehabilitation.
- There are specific biomechanical factors to consider when prescribing an activity-specific prosthesis and other adaptive sports equipment.
- There are clinical and safety considerations for the participation of a person with limb loss/limb deficiency in adaptive sports.
- Examining clinical outcomes in adaptive sports helps inform the quality and safety of participants and programs.
- To facilitate adaptive sports participation, one must consider the characteristics of the participant, the demands of the sport, and the design of the activity-specific prosthesis or equipment.

INTRODUCTION

Limb-deficient athletes can have a traumatic, illness-induced, or congenital amputation. Amputation is estimated to affect every 1 in 85 persons by 2050.[1] Society often assumes that limb loss/limb deficiency (LL/LD) equals disability; however, impairment and disability are not the same. Recall, disability is measured by the person themselves

[a] Department of Physical Medicine & Rehabilitation, University of Michigan, Ann Arbor, MI, USA; [b] Lieutenant Colonel Charles S. Kettles VA Medical Center, Ann Arbor, MI, USA; [c] Department of Physical Medicine & Rehabilitation, VCU Physical Medicine & Rehabilitation, Virginia Commonwealth School of Medicine, 1223 East Marshall Street, Box 980677, Richmond, VA 23298-0677, USA; [d] Department of Physical Therapy, Stony Brook University, 100 Nicolls Road, Stony Brook, NY 11794, USA; [e] American Amputee Soccer Association, Stony Brook, NY 11790, USA
[1] 3912 Kensington Avenue, Richmond, VA 23221, USA.
[2] 43 Roxbury Dr., Commack, NY 11725, USA.
* Corresponding author. 325 East Eisenhower Parkway, Ann Arbor, MI 48108.
E-mail addresses: majugo@med.umich.edu; melissa.tinney@va.gov

Phys Med Rehabil Clin N Am 35 (2024) 769–793
https://doi.org/10.1016/j.pmr.2024.06.004
1047-9651/24/Published by Elsevier Inc.

and what they perceive they "cannot" do.[2] The World Health Organization reports adults with disabilities, including a small portion of surveyed patients with amputation (<2% of the total population surveyed), have lower physical activity levels compared to adults without disability.[3] In the United States, over 40% of persons with disability are sedentary compared to 24% without disabilities.[4] As physical activity is linked to significant health benefits, adaptive sports give persons with LL/LD opportunities to participate and compete.[5,6] There are, however, multiple barriers to participation including financial, physical, emotional distress, motivation, community resources/access to training, lack of media coverage, and difficulty with travel and dependence on other people.[7–9] Building knowledge in adaptive sports programs helps facilitate a person with LL/LD go beyond activities of daily living and basic locomotion goals. Considering the participant, the demands of the activity, and the equipment/activity-specific prosthesis (ASP) required leads to successful participation in adaptive sports (**Fig. 1**).

CLASSIFICATION AND GOVERNANCE OF ADAPTIVE SPORTS

Each adaptive sport has a governing body, which determines the rules and regulations for the sport and the impairment types for eligibility to play the sport. There are 10 categories of eligible impairments: impaired muscle power, LD, leg length difference, short stature, hypertonia, ataxia, athetosis, impaired passive range of motion, vision impairment, and intellectual impairment.[10] Athletes must meet the minimum criteria for their impairment in order to participate. Some sports allow all levels of LL/LD (double/single/upper/lower) to participate, while others restrict, and this may vary at an international versus domestic level. Athletes are classified into competition groups based on their degree of activity limitation to compete against similar athletes. Eligible impairment and the sports' classification rules and regulations should be reviewed prior to an event as they are subject to change.[11]

There are currently 22 sanctioned Paralympic summer sports and 6 winter sports[12] (**Table 1**). Persons with LL/LD can participate in many of these sports as referenced.

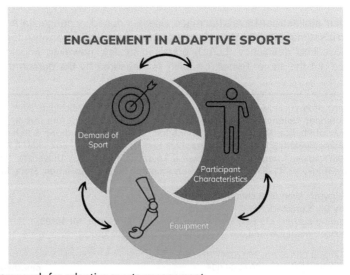

ENGAGEMENT IN ADAPTIVE SPORTS

Demand of Sport

Participant Characteristics

Equipment

Fig. 1. Framework for adaptive sports engagement.

Table 1
Current paralympic sports

Summer Sports	Governing Body
Para Archery[a]	World Archery
Para Athletics[a] (must use prosthetic on track, but on field use is optional)	International Paralympic Committee (IPC)
Para Badminton[a]	Badminton World Federation
Blind Football (must be almost fully or completely blind for international level)[b]	International Blind Sports Federation
Boccia[a]	Boccia International Sports Federation
Para Canoe[a]	International Canoe Federation
Para Cycling[a]	Union Cycliste Internationale
Para Equestrian[a]	International Federation for Equestrian Sports
Goalball(Must be legally blind for international level)[b]	International Blind Sports Federation
Para Judo (Blind Athletes)[b]	International Blind Sports Federation
Para Powerlifting[a]	IPC
Para Rowing[a]	World Rowing
Shooting Para Sport[a]	IPC and World Shooting Para Sport technical Committee and Management team
Sitting Volleyball[a]	World Para Volley
Para Swimming[a]	World Para Swimming/IPC
Para Table Tennis[a]	International Table Tennis Federation
Para Taekwondo[a]	World Taekwondo
Para Triathlon[a]	International Triathlon Union
Wheelchair Basketball[a]	International Wheelchair Basketball Federation
Wheelchair Fencing[a]	International Wheelchair and Amputee Sports Federation
Wheelchair Rugby[a]	International Wheelchair Rugby Federation
Wheelchair Tennis[a]	International Tennis Federation
Winter Sports	Governing Body
Para Alpine Skiing[a]	World Alpine Skiing
Para Nordic Skiing (Para biathlon and Para cross-country skiing)[a]	International Biathlon Union/International Ski and snowboard Federation
Para Ice Hockey[a] (lower limb loss only)	IPC/World Para Ice Hockey Technical Committee
Para Snowboard[a]	International Ski and Snowboard Federation
Wheelchair Curling [a](lower limb loss only)	Wheelchair Curling Federation

[a] Limb-deficient athletes can participate in this sport.
[b] It is not clear from the IPC Web site or Governing Body Web site whether blind athletes who also have an amputation are permitted to participate. Please note this information can change. Data from International Paralympic Committee.[12]

There are also many other activities and avenues for participation and competition not affiliated with the Paralympics, including the World Abilitysport Games, the Invictus Games, the US Veterans Administration Office of National Veterans Sports Programs and Special Events, and the Move United Sanctioned Competitions.[13–16]

TYPES OF ADAPTIVE SPORTS

Adaptive sport programs can be affiliated with hospital systems, nonprofit or for-profit organizations, disability advocacy groups, or through schools and universities. They can have affiliations with the governing bodies noted in **Table 1** and/or be a member of Move United, the largest nonprofit organization dedicated to growing adaptive sports programs in the United States.[17] Studying the risks and demands of different adaptive sports can help inform strategies for training such as pacing, event modification and protocols for when to suspend competition and when it may be unsafe for the athletes.[18] The sports discussed in this article are limited to common adaptive sports reviewed in the current literature.

Adaptive Golf

In the United States, adaptive golf is governed by the National Amputee Golf Association (NAGA). NAGA is supported by the Professional Golf Association and the United States Golf Association (USGA). To be eligible, a player must have an amputation at a major joint (wrist, elbow, shoulder, ankle, knee, or hip) or have total loss of the use of a limb or congenital LD.[19] Equipment required can vary from a rotator or torsion adapter in a lower extremity prosthesis, to a terminal device for an upper extremity prosthesis. If the participant is nonambulatory, he/she can utilize a single-rider golf cart and play seated.[20] Orthotic and prosthetic devices are now permitted in USGA competitions.[21] Adaptive golf research highlights rehabilitation with focus on weight-bearing on the prosthesis for golf, which can help assist with weight shifting needed when playing.[22] Development of adaptive golf putters is an example of team collaboration for creating new adaptive sports equipment[23] (**Fig. 2**).

Amputee Soccer

Amputee Soccer allows for individuals with upper LL/LD to participate as goalkeepers and use only one arm to save the ball. In addition, goalkeepers are restricted to a defined "goalie box." Individuals with lower LL/LD participate as field players. Lower limb prosthetic devices are not allowed; thus, field players must use forearm crutches and may only control and manipulate the ball with their non-amputated side. Contact of the ball with any portion of the LL/LD side or the forearm crutches is considered a handball. Amputee soccer requires a relatively small amount of adaptive equipment that improves access. In the United States, the sport is governed by the American Amputee Soccer Association[24] that is a member of US Soccer and the sole member from the United States to the international governing board, the World Amputee Football Federation. Research shows the sport requires upper body, core, and lower limb strength, cardiovascular[25,26] and muscular endurance, and requisite balance and co-ordination skills[27–29] (**Fig. 3**).

Para Athletics

Para athletics has the largest representation of athletes at the Paralympic summer games. Events include track, throwing, jumping, and the marathon. The rules of Paralympic track and field are similar to those of Olympic track and field events. Certain adaptations to the rules are made to accommodate certain disabilities.[30] There is a large variety of equipment needed for participation including racing wheelchairs, ASPs for running, jumping or throwing, and throwing frames. Research regarding heat illness incidence at the Para World Championships recorded low incidence of severe heat illness, although athletes with certain conditions including LL/LD have previously been thought to have less heat tolerance.

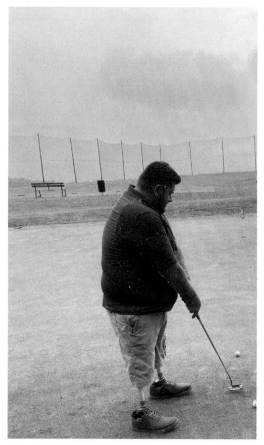

Fig. 2. Adaptive Golfer. (Credit: University of Michigan Adaptive and Inclusive Sports Experience.)

This highlighted need for acclimatization and countermeasure strategies for heat[31] (**Figs. 4–7**).

Para Cycling

Adaptive cycling includes road and track events. Depending on the event and athlete's impairment, different cycles including tandem bikes (blind cyclists with a pilot), bicycles, handcycles, and tricycles may be used. Velodrome (track) events often include time trials, tandem sprints, team sprint, and pursuit races. Road events include road races and time trials at varying distances depending on the cycle type. Athletes can compete with an ASP or not. There are different sports classes for handcycles (H), tricycles (T), bicycle (standard-C), and tandem.[32] Athletes with upper LL/LD often use a prosthetic terminal device that has an open/close function so they can reposition or they may use an elbow unit and attach it to their prosthetic socket, allowing them to lock/unlock it at various angles and reposition as needed.[33] The 2 primary handcycle designs used in Paralympic competition are one in kneeling position with the athlete's torso upright or leaning forward over the cranks or recumbent cycles where the athlete lies supine with cranks positioned above the chest.[34] Research has shown injuries in

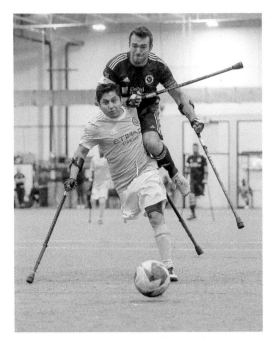

Fig. 3. Amputee soccer. (Credit-American Amputee Soccer Association (AASA). Photos By Brian Bayless.)

para cycling that include upper extremity as well as pelvic and lower limb, similar to able-bodied cyclists. Upper extremity mononeuropathies are also common in para cyclists[35] (**Figs. 8** and **9**).

Para Ice Hockey/Sled Hockey

In para ice hockey, all athletes must have a lower limb impairment. Athletes use a metal frame sled/sledge where the puck can go under it, protective gear and 2 sticks with a hooked blade, and pick on opposite ends. The puck is made of rubber. Protective gear includes a helmet with a face cage and protective body pads (shoulder, shin, elbow, padded gloves).[36] The customization of a sled can help with mobility as well as reduce pressure/friction, similar to a prosthetic socket. A certified prosthetist will fabricate the custom sled that is attached to a frame. During the 2002 Salt Lake Paralympic Winter Games, data showed that fracture injuries were high and accounted for 33% of injuries.[37] This necessitated rule changes to require leg protection and all sleds to be equidistant from the ice to prevent one sled from going up and over another in a collision.[34,38] Sled hockey continues to have a high rate of acute injury in the Winter Paralympic Games, including fractures, lacerations, and sprains.[39] Shoulder injuries have been reported as most common in community programs[40] (**Fig. 10**).

Para Skiing and Snowboarding

Para alpine and para nordic skiing include the typical Olympic events: team events, downhill, slalom, giant slalom, super-G, super combined, bi-athlon, and similar racing distances. There are sports classes for standing skiers (lower, upper, combined lower and upper), sit-skiers (must have leg impairment), and vision. If an athlete has one arm impairment, she/he can compete with one pole; versus both arms having impairments, then no poles.[41] There are 2 track, 3 track, 4 track skiing, mono-ski, and bi-ski. Mono-ski

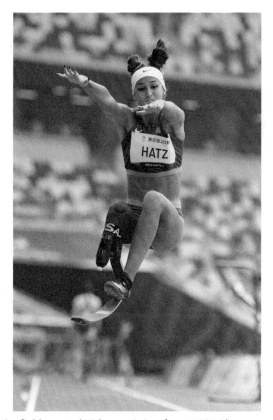

Fig. 4. Para athletics field event. (With permission from USOPC.)

was created for athletes with good upper body and core strength that can ski from a sit position. Bi-skiers also sit to ski but sit in a molded shell to give more core support. Two track skiing is tethered to a guide typically (visual or hearing-impaired athlete, or athlete with mild traumatic brain injury [TBI]) or can be traditional skiing. Three track is 1 ski and 2 handheld outriggers (standing). Four track is 2 skis and 2 handheld outriggers (standing). Athletes with upper LL/LD can opt to have the poles attached to their prosthesis directly to avoid clipping/unclipping. Athletes with lower LL/LD often detach their regular prosthetic foot and use an ankle adapter to allow direct contact of the ski to the prosthesis eliminating need for a boot.[33] There are specialized knee components that are designed for cold weather sports with adjustable resistance for knee flexion and hydraulic dampening (**Fig. 11**).

Para snowboarding includes snow-board cross, banked slalom, and giant slalom. Athletes are classified by impairments in their legs versus their arms. Many athletes with LL/LD compete with their prosthesis. Snowboarding has an adaptive ankle that can be used and that allows more movement in all directions then a typical ankle[33] (**Fig. 12**). Most of the literature in para skiing, both alpine and nordic, focus on injury rates and have traditionally shown higher injury at winter Olympics (strains, fractures, lacerations). Once para snowboarding was added officially to the Paralympic Games, it had higher acute injury rates, including lower limb, head/neck/face injuries.[39,42] In the 2018 Winter Paralympic Games, of the 100 injuries reported, 50 of them and a majority were in athletes with LL/LD.[42]

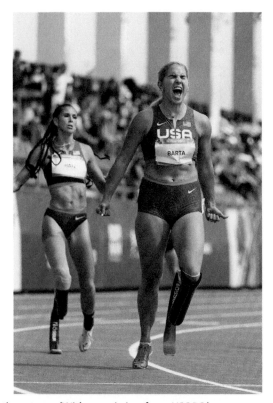

Fig. 5. Para athletics runner. (With permission from USOPC.)

Para Swimming

Para swimming includes the following events: backstroke, freestyle, butterfly, breast-stroke, medley, and relay events. It has 3 overall classifications: physical, vision, and intellectual. Persons with LL/LD are in the physical class. In general, para swimming follows the same rules as Olympic swimming[43] and no prosthesis is allowed for us in competition. Current research in para swimming includes mental health, injury

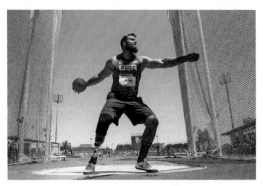

Fig. 6. Para athletics discus. (With permission from USOPC.)

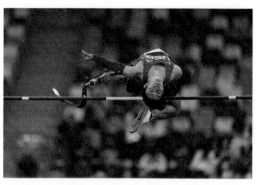

Fig. 7. Para athletics high jump. (With permission from USOPC.)

prevention programs, as well as critiquing classification methods for athletes with LL/LD to make groups more equal.[44–46] Para swimming has a high percentage of athletes competing at Paralympic Games, but with a significant lower injury rate reported compared to other summer para sports.[47] There is equipment to help with adaptive swimming outside of formal competition, such as a swim fin that can be attached to a socket. There are specific waterproof knee and ankle components designed for swimming. An ankle can be switched from walking to swimming position and can be versatile for someone walking on a pool deck or shore that can lock and unlock in position (**Figs. 13** and **14**).

Para Triathlon

Para triathlon has events in which athletes race in 3 disciplines: 750 m of swimming, followed by 20 km of cycling, and 5 km of running. Athletes may use a hand cycle, tandem bicycle, or bicycle in the cycling portion with or without a prosthesis, and wheelchairs are permitted on the running portion of the course. Classes are para triathlon wheelchair (PTWC) 1 to 2: athletes with limitations in lower limbs (PTWC2) and upper limbs (PTWC1) using a handcycle for the cycling segment and a racing chair for the running segment. Para triathlon standing 2 to 5: athletes with limitations in lower and/or upper limbs (lower class number means there are more limitations) who compete in bicycling and running. Assistive devices such as prosthetic limbs and/or bike modifications are regulated by the international federation of para triathlon. Para triathlon visual

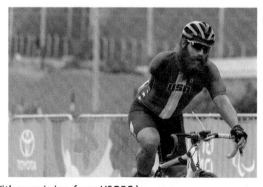

Fig. 8. Cycling. (With permission from USOPC.)

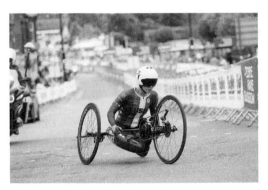

Fig. 9. Hand cycling. (With permission from USOPC.)

impairment (PTVI) 1 to 3: athletes with vision impairment, subdivided in 3 classes by severity of vision loss (visual acuity and/or visual field). Athletes in the PTWC and PTVI classes compete in combined events, with an interval start system per sport class.[48] Para triathlon pushes the endurance of participants and thermoregulation has been studied in competition, highlighting risk factors such as lack of capacity for evaporative heat loss, or augmented metabolic heat production, or lack of pace awareness, increasing thermoregulatory strain.[18]

Seated Volleyball

Seated volleyball is played on a smaller court and with a lower net. All athletes must keep contact of their pelvis with the ground while playing. There are only 2 sports classes and athletes can be capable of standing when off the court (eg, using prosthetic limb or may use arm crutches).[49] There are limited studies in seated volleyball, some suggesting high injury rates diffusely to the musculoskeletal system; while a recent study reported in athletes with LL/LD, shoulder, elbow, and finger injuries had higher incidence, including significant dominant versus nondominant shoulder asymmetry that can contribute to injury[50,51] (**Fig. 15**).

Wheelchair Basketball

In wheelchair basketball, 2 teams of 5 players compete in 4 periods of 10 minutes. The player class is assessed based on capacity to complete skills on the court and they are

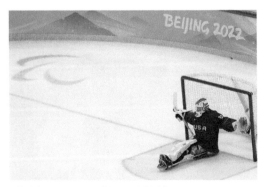

Fig. 10. Sled hockey. (With permission from USOPC.)

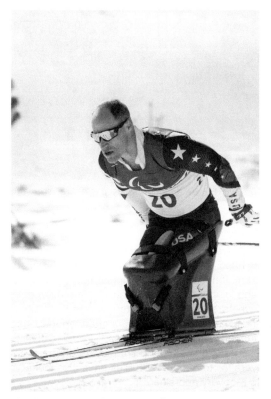

Fig. 11. Para skiing. (With permission from USOPC.)

given an assigned number of points based on these skills combined. Points assigned can never total more than 14 on the court at once for the team.[52] Wheelchair basketball has a significant body of literature compared to other adaptive sports, including community and Paralympic programs. Literature suggests that shoulder and upper limbs are most injured, followed by head/face and then trunk. Lower limb injury is less likely. Injuries are more likely overuse versus acute, historically[40,53] (**Fig. 16**).

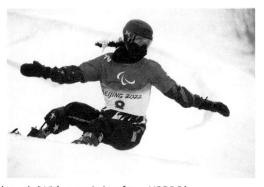

Fig. 12. Para snowboard. (With permission from USOPC.)

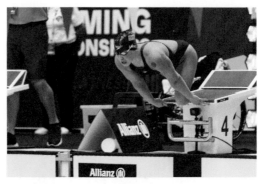

Fig. 13. Para swimming. (With permission from USOPC.)

Wheelchair Rugby

In wheelchair rugby, players play in specialized manual wheelchairs, offensive or defensive. Each team has 5 players, and their players are classified via a point system based on arm and trunk functions and wheelchair use.[54] Wheelchair rugby research focuses on injuries and injury prevention. Shoulders are the most commonly injured; additionally elbows, wrists, and hands are often reported.[35,40] Shoulder impingement, biceps tendinosis, and rotator cuff disorders are often reported, as are mononeuropathies, that is, carpal tunnel, in wheelchair athletes.[35] Patterns of falls have been studied to understand injuries; for example, low point players often fall to elbows/shoulders, while high point players fall to hands.[55] Studies have also looked at the sport's relationship to heart rate recovery and sleep[56,57] **(Fig. 17).**

Wheelchair Tennis

Wheelchair tennis is like able-bodied tennis, but a double bounce is permitted. There are 2 athlete groups, the open class (one or both legs impaired) and the quad class (includes limited arm function as well).[58] Athletes may use a sports or daily use wheelchair. Equipment can be modified, including taping racquets to the player's arm/hand in the quad group. Balls can also be adapted depending on the court or altitude.[35] Research shows that wheelchair tennis has lower injury risk compared to cycling, basketball, and rugby. Shoulder and soft tissue injuries are the highest reported injuries.[35,59]

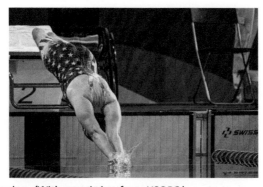

Fig. 14. Para swimming. (With permission from USOPC.)

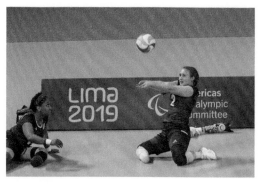

Fig. 15. Seated volleyball. (With permission from USOPC.)

EMERGING SPORTS
Adaptive Surfing

There are 3 para surfing stand classes, 1 kneeling, 1 sit, 2 prone, and 2 vision. People with LL/LD can compete in para surf stand, kneel, sit, or prone depending on the level of amputation and location. For example, in para surfing kneel, the athlete must have a below-the-knee LD/LD or both lower limb LD/LL.[60]

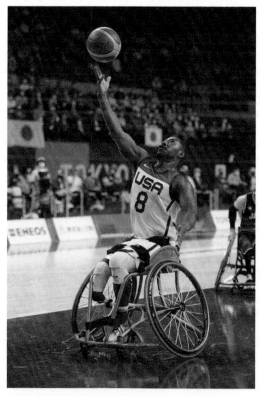

Fig. 16. Wheelchair basketball. (With permission from USOPC.)

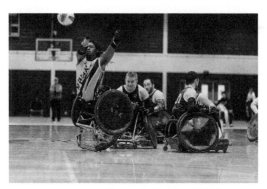

Fig. 17. Wheelchair rugby. (Credit: Sydney Verlinde, University of Michigan Adaptive Sports & Fitness. Photo taken at the 2023 Coupie Classic Wheelchair Rugby Tournament hosted by University of Michigan Adaptive Sports & Fitness.)

Para Dance Sport

This sport was formerly known as wheelchair dance sport and rebranded in 2016. Although well established in other countries, it is a new and growing adaptive sport in the United States.

There are 2 sport classes: 1 for less impaired and 1 for more impaired. Dancers compete in standard, latin, singles, and freestyle categories. The inclusivity of this sport makes it unique with categories of 1 standing dancer and 1 using a wheelchair (combi) or 2 dancers using wheelchairs (duo)[61] (**Fig. 18**).

Para Standing Tennis

Para standing tennis is tennis for those with ambulatory disabilities who play without the use of a wheelchair. The court is a full-size regulation court across all categories. Rules are similar to able-bodied tennis. Classifications for lower impairments are defined as PST1, a person with unilateral upper LL/LD or similar impairment, and PST2 is a person with a unilateral below-knee LL/LD, mild cerebral palsy, or similar impairment, and both get one bounce. PST3 is a person with above-knee, or bilateral below-knee LL/LD, bilateral arm impairment, moderate-to-severe cerebral palsy, or similar impairment, and PST4 is a person with short stature or similar impairment, and both get 2 bounces.[62]

Stand-up Basketball

Stand-up basketball allows for LL/LD athletes to play the game of basketball using prosthetic devices (for lower limb) rather than playing wheelchair basketball. Individuals can compete if they have at least one amputation. The sport is inclusive of both upper and lower LL/LD.[63]

ADAPTIVE ACTIVITY

There are many adaptive activities for exercise or recreation that are not specifically for sports competition. Clinicians often recommend adaptive exercise as a progression from basic locomotion, to aid in long-term mobility. Running and cycling will be reviewed as they are common adaptive activities reviewed in current research.

Adaptive Running

A person may pursue running after progressing in activity with their daily use prosthesis. They may have goals to run for exercise or running may be a requirement as

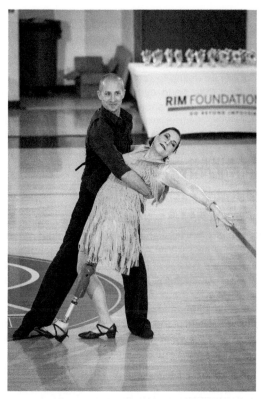

Fig. 18. Para dance sport. (With permission from Dance Mobility.)

part of a specific sport. Low-to-moderate running/jogging for short periods can be performed utilizing a dynamic response prosthetic foot. If a person wants to run with improved performance for increased distance or speed, then a running-specific prosthesis (RSP) will be needed. Understanding running biomechanics can help in RSP selection.[64] Running requires higher impact compared to what a daily use prostheses can provide. Understanding loading of the prosthesis and force are important considerations for RSP prescription.[65] Another variable to consider is prosthetic stiffness. The exact stiffness of the running blade is not always known. The less stiff a prosthesis is, the more muscle activation is needed in the residual limb for stability, which leads to greater metabolic demand.[65] Currently, selection of a prosthetic running foot or running blade begins with the person being assigned a stiffness category that is based on expected activity level and body mass. Alignment can also affect stiffness of the RSP during running[66] and should be taken into account when selecting a running blade. Considerations for persons with transfemoral amputation include determining which knee components may suit the runner best if they choose to utilize an articulated prosthesis versus non-articulated for running. Gait training with an RSP is also important to avoid injury and optimize running biomechanics.[67] Overall a person using an RSP is able to achieve similar speed and aerobic capacity similar to able-bodied runners, showing no physiologic advantage.[68] In comparison to the use of a daily use prosthesis for running, an RSP can reduce the energy cost,[68] which is why an RSP should be carefully considered when addressing the activity needs of a person with LL/LD.

Adaptive Cycling

The biomechanics of cycling requires increased flexion of the joints in the lower extremities compared to walking.[69] Specifically with reduced knee range of motion, a hinged crank arm can be utilized. In a scoping review on bicycling participation in people with LL, a stiffer foot or adjusting the crank length can reduce pedaling asymmetry in high-intensity bicycling.[69] In hand cycling, factors such as body measurement, comfort, range of motion, and pace should be used to facilitate crank length selection.[70] These considerations illustrate where the combination of evaluation of athlete, the ASP, and cycle all are working in concert for optimal function. Other adaptations to facilitate cycling include magnetic clips for pedals, sling-back pedals, or electric motors.

ACTIVITY-SPECIFIC PROSTHESES AND EQUIPMENT

Optimizing a daily use prosthesis may be enough for participation in activities including sports. Clinical discussion with the patient and their prosthetist helps determine need and appropriateness for an ASP. The limb prescription may not require a full ASP but utilize a person's socket and change the foot or terminal device required for a particular sport.[35] Knowing what ASP components are available and working with a knowledgeable prosthetist is important when prescribing these components and determining further rehabilitation needs beyond basic locomotion. In many cases, insurance does not cover ASPs or adaptive sports equipment that may limit the clinician's experience with ASP prescription. With legislation changing from state to state that expands insurance coverage for ASPs and other adaptive sports equipment for physical activity, this knowledge is critical for providers.[71]

PROSTHESIS PRESCRIPTION CONSIDERATIONS

When prescribing an ASP, evaluating the physical capabilities of the participant and the condition of the residual limb are first. In combination, the biomechanics of the sport should be considered in relation to the participant and access to appropriate training and coaching for a particular sport or activity. Additional rehabilitation may be needed to adjust to use of an ASP. When working with a prosthetist, discussion regarding several elements that are unique to the demands of a particular sport in relation to what the prosthesis can provide is critical.

Bench alignment accounts for a person's thigh orientation and hip mobility. There is limited evidence in the literature for alignment recommendations for running prosthetic feet or running blades requiring providers to rely on manufacturer guidelines.[72] Although standard bench alignment may be adequate for moderate physical activity, it is difficult to attain dynamic alignment, in relation to equipment use, like a cycle or a snowboard. This would necessitate aligning the prosthesis with the adaptive sports equipment with which it will be used **Fig. 19**.

Due to increased forces in sports, higher energy return in a prosthetic foot is required. This may be adequate with a dynamic response foot, but as speed/performance requirements are needed, a running blade can be selected. For activities that require more jumping, dynamic loading should be taken into account[65] and shock absorption is needed to help disperse forces that then translate to the residual limb. This can be accomplished through a prosthetic knee that provides hydraulic dampening or a prosthetic foot with built-in shock absorption or adding a vertical shock-absorbing pylon. Understanding joint loading informs prosthetic prescription and how an athlete might train with that prosthesis.[73] If an activity requires rotation, this

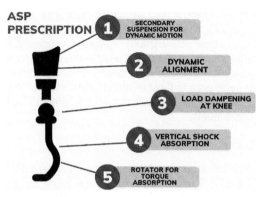

Fig. 19. ASP prescription considerations.

can put stress on the residual limb. In order to reduce this type of stress, it can be accomplished with a torsion adaptor or rotator that can provide torque absorption. Suspension of the socket in an ASP is critical in very dynamic activity for safety and security and an athlete may require auxiliary suspension, such as a suspension sleeve or dual suspension pin lock.

For the person with upper LL/LD, research is limited for the design and use of ASPs. A terminal device can be interchangeable based on the sport, such as cycling or skiing. Energy expenditure, in regard to upper extremity prosthesis use, is unknown, but based on limited prototype testing for a cycling prosthesis, weight is a factor for ease of use.[74]

There is limited research looking at the pros and cons of ASPs for recreational users and no studies focusing on children.[75] Current models intended for the design of sports technology or the creation of assistive technology lack the detail and application to the design of prosthetic limbs required for competitive sport, although there is one proposed framework for the development of ASPs at the elite level.[76]

Although we have discussed a few common wheelchair sports, we will not be discussing wheelchair prescription as this has its own extensive body of research. General considerations apply to any adaptive sports equipment. It is important to have a good fit with reduction in pressure and friction, similar to a prosthesis. Customization to the individual is best when prescribing a sports wheelchair, sit ski, hockey sled, or adaptive cycle.

PARTICIPANT CONSIDERATIONS

Participation in adaptive sports for the individual with LL/LD requires some key areas for consideration. Several physical characteristics include a requisite amount of upper, lower,[77] and core body strength[78] along with the ability to rapidly generate force, adequate range of motion of the spine, upper and lower body joints, muscular endurance (especially for muscle groups that may not be typically used for extended periods of time), cardiovascular endurance,[79] and a potential of increased energy need based on the demands of the sport[80] and use of adaptive equipment. It is also important to note that asymmetries,[77] for those with unilateral limb difference, most likely exist when comparing sides. These requirements differ depending on the sport. The ability to withstand increased forces of stress, torque, and friction on the skin is also required. For sports with prostheses and socket usage, the residual limb must be able to build up tolerance to prevent skin breakdown and discomfort.[33,81] In addition to physical considerations, there is also emotional readiness. Participants in adaptive sport will engage in activities that will challenge them, maybe at levels not encountered before, and may require closer assessment to ensure participant success. There are events that will include spectators and thus require the participant to be emotionally ready.[82] While these identified areas are important for participation, it is important to keep in mind that each area is flexible and adjustable; the adaptive sport should be modified to allow maximum participation from the athlete, especially at the introductory and recreational levels.

SAFETY CONSIDERATIONS

Inherent to any sports participation, safety concerns must be taken into account.[83,84] In adaptive sports literature, it is difficult to determine injury and illnesses in only athletes with LL/LD. Paralympic literature is helpful, and constantly improving with lead from the International Paralympic Committee (IPC).[85] Para athletes did have higher illness and injury rates compared to their Olympic counterparts.[86]

Injuries

Injuries in limb-deficient athletes have been reported to be most common in the shoulder or lumbar region.[87,88] Most injuries are first time, with less being recurrence or exacerbation. However, those with quadruple LL/LD had 2 times the number of recurrent injuries versus those with single or double limb amputations.[88] In the Tokyo Summer Games, taekwondo and judo had higher rates of injury then other sports, and similar to other studies, acute injuries were highest in shoulder, followed by hand/fingers.[89] Athletes with LL/LD in 2016 Tokyo Summer Games had the highest number of injuries compared to other impairments; the number one injury was again upper extremity.[47] In 2018 Winter Games, para snowboard had a high incidence of lower limb injuries, but across all winter para sports, acutely and consistent with Summer Games, the shoulder was again the most common.[42] In general, with wheelchair sports, shoulder is the most commonly reported injury as well.[90]

Illnesses

The medical team must also monitor mental health, medical illnesses, and support nutrition. Mental health should be monitored routinely with wellness surveys, particularly anxiety and depression that are common before and during games.[8] Further in adaptive athletes, one must consider the effect of altitude, cold or heat conditions, and travel fatigue. Medical teams must be prepared to treat environmental impacts.[91] Illnesses must also be considered and time loss, which can vary to involve any organ/system. Adaptive athletes may have other medical history that makes them at high risk for respiratory illness and time loss from sport. Tokyo 2020 reported that dermatologic and respiratory illnesses were most common illnesses.[89]

CLINICAL OUTCOMES

Participating in adaptive sports allows for individuals with LL/LD a method to improve functional fitness, overall health, body image, as well as improved mood and quality of life.[92–95] Multiple studies across adaptive sports have demonstrated the positive impact that adaptive sports has had on the athlete's sense of self and belonging in a community.[96] In addition, the improvements in physical characteristics such as strength, endurance, and balance result in participants having greater self-confidence and self-esteem leading to improved engagement in work and leisure activities and overall improvement in quality of life.[77,82,97–100] There is also evidence that participation in adaptive team sports and the social skills required to navigate this environment also provides improvements in emotional and social well-being as the athlete develops a larger sense of belonging.[97,101]

DISCUSSION

Utilizing the framework that considers the participant, demands of the sport, and the ASP/equipment required leads to successful participation in adaptive sports.

Further, this framework takes an interdisciplinary approach with everyone working in concert with the athlete, including the clinical provider, certified prosthetist, physical or occupational therapist, coach, and athletic trainer. This points to the multitude of aspects of adaptive sports that could be studied.

The campaign, "So Every BODY Can Move," spearheaded by the American Orthotics and Prosthetics Association, is lobbying state by state to improve insurance coverage for ASPs and other adaptive sports equipment.[71] Physical activity inequities have been studied, but as insurance coverage is changing, more access leads to more participation, leading to more data. This can push innovation in ASP limb design, if more people are utilizing them. Research on different adaptive sports not in current literature, can inform design of programs and equipment for that sport and safety recommendations. There is a lack of research in persons with LD compared to those with LL. If access to ASPs improves in childhood, this can help facilitate the high levels of activity expected of children with LD compared to their peers. This work is fundamental to sustaining mobility and improving physical activity and health outcomes for persons with LL/LD.

CLINICS CARE POINTS

- To facilitate adaptive sports participation, one must consider the characteristics of the athlete, the demands of the sport, and the design of the ASP or equipment.
- Knowing what ASP components are available and working with a knowledgeable prosthetist is important when prescribing these components and determining further rehabilitation needs beyond basic locomotion.
- Consideration should be given for additional rehabilitation to adjust to use of an ASP and access to appropriate training and coaching for a particular sport or activity.
- In general, the upper extremity is the most injured area in adaptive athletes, typically from overuse. In high-velocity sports, acute injuries like fractures can occur more often. Unique to adaptive athletes, skin breakdown is frequent.
- Participation in adaptive sport for people with LL/LD improves an athlete's fitness, overall health, body image, mood, quality of life, and sense of self and belonging and accountability in a community.

DISCLOSURES

E.M. Lamberg is the current President of the American Amputee Soccer Association.

REFERENCES

1. Ziegler-Graham K, MacKenzie EJ, Ephraim PL, et al. Estimating the prevalence of limb loss in the United States: 2005 to 2050. Arch Phys Med Rehabil 2008; 89(3):422–9.

2. Heavey E. The multiple meanings of "disability" in interviews with amputees. Commun Med 2013;10(2):129–39.

3. de Hollander EL, Proper KI. Physical activity levels of adults with various physical disabilities. Prev Med Rep 2018;10:370–6.

4. CDC. Disability and Health Data System (DHDS) | CDC. Centers for Disease Control and Prevention. 2023. Available at: https://www.cdc.gov/ncbddd/disability andhealth/dhds/index.html. [Accessed 24 November 2023].

5. Arem H, Moore SC, Patel A, et al. Leisure time physical activity and mortality: a detailed pooled analysis of the dose-response relationship. JAMA Intern Med 2015;175(6):959–67.

6. Ekelund U, Tarp J, Steene-Johannessen J, et al. Dose-response associations between accelerometry measured physical activity and sedentary time and all cause mortality: systematic review and harmonised meta-analysis. The BMJ 2019;366:l4570.

7. Puce L, Okwen PM, Yuh MN, et al. Well-being and quality of life in people with disabilities practicing sports, athletes with disabilities, and para-athletes: Insights from a critical review of the literature. Front Psychol 2023;14:1071656.

8. Rodríguez Macías M, Giménez Fuentes-Guerra FJ, Abad Robles MT. The sport training process of para-athletes: a systematic review. Int J Environ Res Public Health 2022;19(12):7242.

9. Bentzen M, Kenttä G, Karls T, et al. Monitoring mental distress in Para athletes in preparation, during and after the Beijing Paralympic Games 2022: A 22 week prospective mixed-method study. Front Sports Act Living 2022;4:945073.

10. IPC Classification - Paralympic Categories & How to Qualify. International Paralympic Committee. Available at: https://www.paralympic.org/classification. [Accessed 12 December 2023].

11. Tweedy SM, Beckman EM, Connick MJ. Paralympic classification: conceptual basis, current methods, and research update. Pharm Manag PM R 2014;6(8 Suppl):S11–7.

12. IPC. Paralympic Sports List - Summer & Winter Paralympic Sports. International Paralympic Committee. 2023. Available at: https://www.paralympic.org/sports. [Accessed 23 November 2023].

13. Overview - World Abilitysport. 2020. Available at: https://worldabilitysport.org/world-abilitysport-games/overview/. [Accessed 12 December 2023].

14. Invictus Games. Invictus Games. Available at: https://www.invictusgames foundation.org/hosting-invictus-games. [Accessed 12 December 2023].

15. Affairs D of V. VA National Veterans Sports Programs. 2022. Available at: https://department.va.gov/veteran-sports/. [Accessed 12 December 2023].

16. Sanctioned Competitions. Move United. Available at: https://moveunitedsport.org/events/sanctioned-competitions/. [Accessed 12 December 2023].

17. Move United. Move United. Available at: https://moveunitedsport.org/. [Accessed 11 December 2023].

18. Stephenson BT, Hoekstra SP, Tolfrey K, et al. High thermoregulatory strain during competitive paratriathlon racing in the heat. Int J Sports Physiol Perform 2020;15(2):231–7.

19. NAGA Home. National Amputee Golf Association. Available at: http://www.nagagolf.org/. [Accessed 30 November 2023].

20. Golf. Move United. Available at: https://moveunitedsport.org/sport/golf/. [Accessed 30 November 2023].

21. Parziale JR, De Luigi AJ. Golf in the paralympic games. Am J Phys Med Rehabil 2023;102(11):1040–1.

22. Sidiropoulos AN, Nelson LM, Pruziner AL, et al. Evaluation of weight shift and x-factor during golf swing of veterans with lower limb loss. Am J Phys Med Rehabil 2023;102(1):85–91.

23. Heasley V, Meyer D, Foster T, et al. A model of collaboration can expand the opportunities in adaptive sports equipment. Am J Phys Med Rehabil 2022; 101(8):798.

24. Adaptive Sport | U.S. Amputee Soccer Team. U.S. Amputee Soccer. Available at: https://www.usampsoccer.org. [Accessed 12 December 2023].

25. Maehana H, Miyamoto A, Koshiyama K, et al. Profile of match performance and heart rate response in Japanese amputee soccer players. J Sports Med Phys Fitness 2018;58(6):816–24.

26. Nowak A. Match performance in Polish amputee soccer Extra Ligue – a pilot study. Adv Rehabil 2020;34(2):16–25.

27. Lamberg E, Pierre-Glaude J. Athletic ability in the sport of amputee soccer. Soccer Soc 2022;23(1):1–7.

28. Esatbeyoglu F, Hazir T, İsler AK. Match characteristics of professional outfield amputee soccer players during official amputee soccer matches. Spor Hekim DergisiTurkish J Sports Med 2022;57(4):189–95.

29. Aytar A, Pekyavas NO, Ergun N, et al. Is there a relationship between core stability, balance and strength in amputee soccer players? A pilot study. Prosthet Orthot Int 2012;36(3):332–8.

30. About Para Track & Field. Available at: https://www.usparatf.org/about-para-track-and-field. [Accessed 1 December 2023].

31. Grobler L, Derman W, Racinais S, et al. Illness at a Para Athletics Track and Field World Championships under Hot and Humid Ambient Conditions. PM&R 2019; 11(9):919–25.

32. UCI. Para-cycling. 2023. Available at: https://www.uci.org/discipline/para-cycling/24eju96onGN1Fo94jnlhZK. [Accessed 24 November 2023].

33. Bragaru M, Dekker R, Geertzen JH. Sport prostheses and prosthetic adaptations for the upper and lower limb amputees: an overview of peer reviewed literature. Prosthet Orthot Int 2012;36(3):290–6.

34. De Luigi AJ. Adaptive sports medicine: a clinical guide. springer international publishing AG. 2017. Available at: http://ebookcentral.proquest.com/lib/umichigan/detail.action?docID=5050100. [Accessed 30 November 2023].

35. De Luigi AJ, editor. Adaptive sports medicine: a clinical guide. Springer International Publishing; 2018. https://doi.org/10.1007/978-3-319-56568-2.

36. World Para Ice Hockey/IPC. Para Ice Hockey - About the Sport. International Paralympic Committee. 2023. Available at: https://www.paralympic.org/ice-hockey/about. [Accessed 24 November 2023].

37. Webborn N, Emery C. Descriptive epidemiology of paralympic sports injuries. PM&R 2014;6(8S):S18–22.

38. Blauwet C, Willick SE. The paralympic movement: using sports to promote health, disability rights, and social integration for athletes with disabilities. PM&R 2012;4(11):851–6.

39. Wu F, Liu Y, Zhuang M. Lessons from the Winter Paralympic Games disclosing the epidemiology of winter sports injury in paralytic athletes: a meta-analysis. BMC Sports Sci Med Rehabil 2022;14(1):1–8.

40. Soo Hoo JA, Latzka E, Harrast MA. A descriptive study of self-reported injury in non-elite adaptive athletes. PM&R 2019;11(1):25–32.

41. IPC. Para alpine skiing rules & classification. International Paralympic Committee. 2023. Available at: https://www.paralympic.org/alpine-skiing/classification. [Accessed 24 November 2023].

42. Derman W, Runciman P, Jordaan E, et al. High incidence of injuries at the Pyeongchang 2018 Paralympic Winter Games: a prospective cohort study of 6804 athlete days. Br J Sports Med 2020;54(1):38–43.

43. IPC. World Para Swimming Classification & Categories - SB9, SM8. International Paralympic Committee. 2023. Available at: https://www.paralympic.org/swimming/classification. [Accessed 24 November 2023].

44. Hogarth L, Payton C, Van de Vliet P, et al. A novel method to guide classification of para swimmers with limb deficiency. Scand J Med Sci Sports 2018;28(11):2397–406.

45. Hogarth L, Payton C, Van De Vliet P, et al. The impact of limb deficiency impairment on Para swimming performance. J Sports Sci 2020;38(8):839–47.

46. Salerno J, Tow S, Regan E, et al. Injury and injury prevention in United States para swimming: a mixed-methods approach. Int J Sports Phys Ther 2022;17(2):293–306.

47. Derman W, Runciman P, Schwellnus M, et al. High precompetition injury rate dominates the injury profile at the Rio 2016 Summer Paralympic Games: a prospective cohort study of 51 198 athlete days. Br J Sports Med 2018;52(1):24–31.

48. Para Triathlon Classification & Categories. International Paralympic Committee. Available at: https://www.paralympic.org/triathlon/classification. [Accessed 1 December 2023].

49. IPC. Sitting Volleyball Classification & Categories. International Paralympic Committee. 2023. Available at: https://www.paralympic.org/sitting-volleyball/classification. [Accessed 24 November 2023].

50. Ahmadi S, Gutierrez GL, Uchida MC. Asymmetry in glenohumeral muscle strength of sitting volleyball players: an isokinetic profile of shoulder rotations strength. J Sports Med Phys Fitness 2020;60(3):395–401.

51. Zwierzchowska A, Gaweł E, Gómez MA, et al. Prediction of injuries, traumas and musculoskeletal pain in elite Olympic and Paralympic volleyball players. Sci Rep 2023;13:11064.

52. IWBF. Classification Wheelchair Basketball. IWBF - International Wheelchair Basketball Federation. 2018. Available at: https://iwbf.org/the-game/classification/. [Accessed 24 November 2023].

53. Sá K, Costa e Silva A, Gorla J, et al. Injuries in wheelchair basketball players: a systematic review. Int J Environ Res Public Health 2022;19(10):5869.

54. IPC. Wheelchair rugby Classification & Categories. International Paralympic Committee. 2023. Available at: https://www.paralympic.org/wheelchair-rugby/classification. [Accessed 24 November 2023].

55. Tashiro T, Maeda N, Sasadai J, et al. Characteristics of Falls Among Men's Wheelchair Rugby Players in the Rio 2016 and Tokyo 2020 Summer Paralympic Games: A Video Analysis. J Hum Kinet 2022;84:233–7.

56. Heart rate response and recovery in wheelchair tetraplegic rugby athletes: a pilot study. J Sports Med Phys Fit 2018;58(9):1349–53. Available at: https://www.minervamedica.it/en/journals/sports-med-physical-fitness/article.php?cod=R40Y2018N09A1349. [Accessed 13 December 2023].

57. Murphy CJ, Hartescu I, Roberts IE, et al. Sleep characteristics of highly trained wheelchair rugby athletes with and without a cervical spinal cord injury during the competitive season. Front Sports Act Living 2021;3:643233.

58. Wheelchair Tennis Classification & Categories. International Paralympic Committee. Available at: https://www.paralympic.org/wheelchair-tennis/classification. [Accessed 7 December 2023].

59. Ultrasonographic evaluation of the shoulder in elite wheelchair tennis players. J Sport Rehabi 2010;19(2). Available at: https://journals-humankinetics-com.proxy.lib.umich.edu/view/journals/jsr/19/2/article-p161.xml. [Accessed 13 December 2023].

60. ISAsurf. ISA Para Surfing Classification. International Surfing Association. 2023. Available at: https://isasurf.org/learning/para-surfing/isa-para-surfing-classification/. [Accessed 24 November 2023].

61. Para dance sport - Fast Facts. International Paralympic Committee. Available at: https://www.paralympic.org/dance-sport-fast-facts. [Accessed 1 December 2023].

62. Para-Standing Tennis. Para-Standing Tennis. Available at: https://www.parastandingtennis.com. [Accessed 13 December 2023].

63. Ability J. AMP1: Newest Addition to 360 Sports. Ability360 | Phoenix, AZ. 2018. Available at: https://ability360.org/livability/amp1-newest-addition-360-sports/. [Accessed 13 December 2023].

64. Hobara H, Sakata H, Amma R, et al. Loading rates in unilateral transfemoral amputees with running-specific prostheses across a range of speeds. Clin Biomech Bristol Avon 2020;75:104999.

65. Agnew S, Geil MD, Gharai MH. Dynamic stiffness of pediatric prostheses during rapid loading. J Prosthet Orthot 2020;32(4):245–50.

66. Groothuis A, Houdijk H. The effect of prosthetic alignment on prosthetic and total leg stiffness while running with simulated running-specific prostheses. Front Sports Act Living 2019;1. https://doi.org/10.3389/fspor.2019.00016.

67. Santer J, MacDonald S, Rizzone K, et al. Strategies for gait retraining in a collegiate runner with transfemoral amputation: a case report. Int J Sports Phys Ther 2021;16(3):862–9.

68. Brown MB, Millard-Stafford ML, Allison AR. Running-specific prostheses permit energy cost similar to nonamputees. Med Sci Sports Exerc 2009;41(5):1080.

69. Poonsiri J, Dekker R, Dijkstra PU, et al. Bicycling participation in people with a lower limb amputation: A scoping review. BMC Musculoskelet Disord 2018;19(1).

70. Mason BS, Stone B, Warner MB, et al. Crank length alters kinematics and kinetics, yet not the economy of recumbent handcyclists at constant handgrip speeds. Scand J Med Sci Sports 2021;31(2):388–97.

71. So Every BODY Can Move | AOPA – AMERICAN ORTHOTIC & PROSTHETIC ASSOCIATION. Available at: https://aopanet.org/so-kids-can-move/. [Accessed 13 December 2023].

72. Migliore GL, Petrone N, Hobara H, et al. Innovative alignment of sprinting prostheses for persons with transfemoral amputation: Exploratory study on a gold medal Paralympic athlete. Prosthet Orthot Int 2021;45(1):46.

73. Funken J, Willwacher S, Heinrich K, et al. Three-dimensional takeoff step kinetics of long jumpers with and without a transtibial amputation. Med Sci Sports Exerc 2019;51(4):716.

74. Tiele A, Soni-Sadar S, Rowbottom J, et al. Design and development of a novel upper-limb cycling prosthesis. Bioengineering 2017;4(4).

75. Hadj-Moussa F, Ngan CC, Andrysek J. Biomechanical factors affecting individuals with lower limb amputations running using running-specific prostheses: A systematic review. Gait Posture 2022;92:83–95.

76. Dyer B. Development of high performance parasport prosthetic limbs: A proposed framework and case study. Assist Technol 2020;32(4):214–21.

77. Nolan L. Lower limb strength in sports-active transtibial amputees. Prosthet Orthot Int 2009;33(3):230–41.

78. Cavedon V, Brugnoli C, Sandri M, et al. Physique and performance in male sitting volleyball players: implications for classification and training. PeerJ 2022;10:e14013.

79. Chin T, Sawamura S, Fujita H, et al. Physical fitness of lower limb amputees. Am J Phys Med Rehabil 2002;81(5):321.

80. Innocencio da Silva Gomes A, Gonçalves Ribeiro B, de Abreu Soares E. Nutritional profile of the Brazilian Amputee Soccer Team during the precompetition period for the world championship. Nutr Burbank Los Angel Cty Calif. 2006; 22(10):989–95.

81. Wang YN, Sanders JE. How does skin adapt to repetitive mechanical stress to become load tolerant? Med Hypotheses 2003;61(1):29–35.

82. Bragaru M, van Wilgen CP, Geertzen JHB, et al. Barriers and facilitators of participation in sports: a qualitative study on dutch individuals with lower limb amputation. PLoS One 2013;8(3):e59881.

83. Klenck C, Gebke K. Practical management: common medical problems in disabled athletes. Clin J Sport Med 2007;17(1):55.

84. Ferrara MS, Peterson CL. Injuries to athletes with disabilities: identifying injury patterns. Sports Med Auckl NZ 2000;30(2):137–43.

85. Thompson WR, Vanlandewijck YC. Perspectives on research conducted at the Paralympic Games. Disabil Rehabil 2021;43(24):3503–14.

86. Anderson T, Cali MG, Clark SC, et al. Team USA injury and illness incidence at the 2022 Beijing Winter Olympic and Paralympic Games. Br J Sports Med 2023. https://doi.org/10.1136/bjsports-2023-107185.

87. Heneghan NR, Heathcote L, Martin P, et al. Injury surveillance in elite Paralympic athletes with limb deficiency: a retrospective analysis of upper quadrant injuries. BMC Sports Sci Med Rehabil 2020;12:36.

88. Heneghan NR, Collacott E, Martin P, et al. Lumbosacral injuries in elite Paralympic athletes with limb deficiency: a retrospective analysis of patient records. BMJ Open Sport Exerc Med 2021;7(1):e001001.

89. Derman W, Runciman P, Eken M, et al. Incidence and burden of illness at the Tokyo 2020 Paralympic Games held during the COVID-19 pandemic: a prospective cohort study of 66 045 athlete days. Br J Sports Med 2023;57(1): 55–62.

90. Weith M, Junge A, Rolvien T, et al. Epidemiology of injuries and illnesses in elite wheelchair basketball players over a whole season - a prospective cohort study. BMC Sports Sci Med Rehabil 2023;15(1):84.

91. Fagher K, Baumgart JK, Solli GS, et al. Preparing for snow-sport events at the Paralympic Games in Beijing in 2022: recommendations and remaining questions. BMJ Open Sport Exerc Med 2022;8(1):e001294.

92. Deans SA, McFadyen AK, Rowe PJ. Physical activity and quality of life: A study of a lower-limb amputee population. Prosthet Orthot Int 2008;32(2):186–200.

93. da Silva R, Rizzo JG, Gutierres Filho PJB, et al. Physical activity and quality of life of amputees in southern Brazil. Prosthet Orthot Int 2011;35(4):432–8.

94. Wetterhahn KA, Hanson C, Levy CE. Effect of participation in physical activity on body image of amputees. Am J Phys Med Rehabil 2002;81(3):194.

95. Christensen J, Ipsen T, Doherty P, et al. Physical and social factors determining quality of life for veterans with lower-limb amputation(s): a systematic review. Disabil Rehabil 2016;38(24):2345–53.
96. Jaarsma EA, Dijkstra PU, Geertzen JHB, et al. Barriers to and facilitators of sports participation for people with physical disabilities: A systematic review. Scand J Med Sci Sports 2014;24(6):871–81.
97. Auricchio JR, Bernardes N, Moreno MA. Study of the quality of life in amputee soccer players. Man Ther Posturology Rehabil J 2017;1–5.
98. Yazicioglu K, Taskaynatan MA, Guzelkucuk U, et al. Effect of playing football (soccer) on balance, strength, and quality of life in unilateral below-knee amputees. Am J Phys Med Rehabil 2007;86(10):800–5.
99. Adamsen L, Andersen C, Midtgaard J, et al. Struggling with cancer and treatment: young athletes recapture body control and identity through exercise: qualitative findings from a supervised group exercise program in cancer patients of mixed gender undergoing chemotherapy. Scand J Med Sci Sports 2009;19(1):55–66.
100. Sporner ML, Fitzgerald SG, Dicianno BE, et al. Psychosocial impact of participation in the National Veterans Wheelchair Games and Winter Sports Clinic. Disabil Rehabil 2009;31(5):410–8.
101. Monteiro R, Pfeifer L, Santos A, et al. Soccer practice and functional and social performance of men with lower limb amputations. J Hum Kinet 2014;43:33–41.

Prosthetic Componentry in Lower Limb Prosthetic Restoration

Rebecca A. Speckman, MD, PhD[a],*, Wayne T. Biggs, BS, CPO[a]

KEYWORDS

- Socket • Prosthetic suspension • Transtibial prosthesis • Transfemoral prosthesis
- Prosthetic knee

KEY POINTS

- Some historical prosthetic componentry such as the thigh corset and side joints are still used in modern practice for specific clinical scenarios.
- Ischial containment transfemoral prosthesis sockets are designed to promote anatomic femur adduction.
- Most prosthetic knees utilize passive control mechanisms such as brakes or hydraulic dampening, and do not actively generate power.
- Most prosthetic knees designed for low-mobility users provide very little resistance if the knee is flexed.

INTRODUCTION

This article presents a framework for understanding the role and indications for different lower limb prosthesis designs and components.

The prosthetic *socket* is the load-bearing part of the prosthesis. It acts as a connector between the prosthesis user and the prosthesis.

The *suspension system* of a prosthesis is the mechanism by which the prosthesis is secured on the prosthesis user.

The *interface* is material between the socket and the residual limb. (Terminology can sometimes overlap—the socket is an interface between the residual limb and the rest of the prosthesis.)

The overall structure of a lower limb prosthesis can be of endoskeletal or exoskeletal design.

The prosthetic *knee* and *foot* are components designed to simulate some of the function of the anatomic knee or foot and ankle, respectively.

[a] Regional Amputation Center, Rehabilitation Care Services, VA Puget Sound Health Care System, 1660 South Columbian Way, Seattle, WA 98108, USA
* Corresponding author. 1660 South Columbian Way, Seattle, WA 98108.
E-mail address: Rebecca.Speckman@va.gov

Phys Med Rehabil Clin N Am 35 (2024) 795–815
https://doi.org/10.1016/j.pmr.2024.06.010
1047-9651/24/Published by Elsevier Inc.

SOCKETS

Pressures experienced by the residual limb within the socket impact patient comfort, prosthesis use, and residual limb health.[1] Specific designs may vary by how much and where the socket contacts the residual limb, socket contours, areas of relief, socket brim height, and other variables.

Historical Perspective

Through the first half of the twentieth century, standard lower limb sockets were carved from wood and were open at the distal end of the residual limb. Loadbearing through the socket and lack of contact at the distal limb created risk for distal skin breakdown, edema, and verrucous hyperplasia.[2]

Proximal structures were used to help bear some of the user's weight or to stabilize the knee or hip. These structures were bulky and limited movement.

In the *total contact socket* approach, the entire socket is in contact with the residual limb, reducing factors that lead to tissue complications with wooden sockets. This design evolved when plastic laminates became available.[3] Standard-of-care transtibial and transfemoral socket designs in modern practice are total contact.

Transtibial Sockets

Early to mid-twentieth CE transtibial prostheses usually had a *thigh corset with side joints,* a leather corset laced tightly around the thigh and attached to the socket by steel struts with hinge joints (**Fig. 1**). The objective of the thigh corset was to

- Reduce motion about the knee

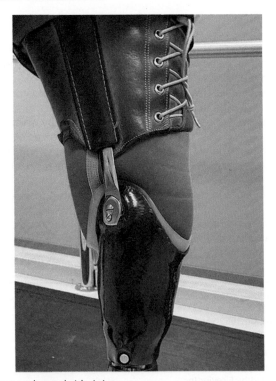

Fig. 1. Thigh corset and metal side joints.

- Share load with the limb–socket interface

The thigh corset sometimes served as the suspension mechanism for the prosthesis and sometimes was used with a waist belt and forked strap.

Patellar tendon-bearing socket

The patellar tendon-bearing (PTB) socket, developed in the 1950s to 1960s, was a total contact socket designed to preferentially load and offload areas of the residual limb.[4,5]

- *Pressure tolerant areas*: Patellar tendon, muscular compartments (anterior compartment, posterior compartment, [a]popliteal fossa), and flatter surfaces of bones (medial tibial flare, medial and lateral aspects of the tibial crest, fibular shaft).
- *Pressure sensitive areas*: Bony prominences (tibial tubercle, tibial crest, fibular head, distal tibia, and fibula), fibular nerve, hamstring tendons.

The PTB design allowed many users to bear their full weight through the prosthesis, reducing the need for use of a thigh corset.[3]

Supracondylar and supracondylar/suprapatellar sockets

The PTB supracondylar (SC) socket's medial and lateral brims come in over the condyles, increasing mediolateral stability.[6] This design can also create *anatomic* suspension. The supracondylar-suprapatellar (SC-SP) socket's anterior brim comes in over the patella, preventing knee hyperextension (**Fig. 2**).

Total surface-bearing socket

The total surface-bearing (TSB) socket came into widespread use in the 1990s. The TSB socket was designed to distribute pressures uniformly over the residual limb and to be used with suction suspension.[7] Traditional TSB sockets were sometimes used with no interface between the hard socket and the residual limb, and sometimes with a liner or insert of a softer material such as foam.

Hydrostatic sockets (a TSB variation) are fabricated using a pressure chamber around the residual limb to apply uniform pressure during casting.[8]

Transtibial Socket Selection

Most transtibial sockets are a hybrid between the traditional PTB socket and the TSB socket, and the TSB is the "go-to" design if suction or vacuum suspension is being used.[9] Practice patterns vary. The contours of a PTB socket can reduce socket rotation. SC and SCSP sockets are still used at times to stabilize the knee (eg, a short residual limb), and sometimes for suspension.

Transfemoral

Standard transfemoral prostheses in the first half of the twentieth century had a metal hip joint and pelvic band for suspension.[10] The invention of a good expulsion valve in the 1940s led to the development of above-knee suction sockets that achieved more secure suspension.[11]

Quadrilateral socket

The classic *quadrilateral* socket was originally made from wood and later with plastic laminates. Characteristics included

---

[a] The proximal gastrocnemius is sometimes considered part of the popliteal fossa.

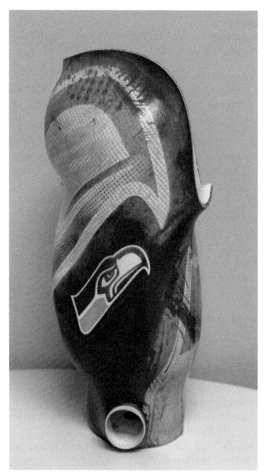

Fig. 2. SC/SP transtibial socket.

- Weight-bearing through an ischial seat
- Narrow dimension in the anteroposterior plane and focused pressure over Scarpa's triangle to keep the ischium seated (**Fig. 3**)
- Mediolateral dimension similar to that of the residual limb
- Brim *channels* for prominent musculature and tendons

This socket was designed to create some suction. It allowed many users to utilize a waist belt or Silesian bandage for suspension rather than the conventional hip joint and pelvic band.[10]

With this design, contraction of the hip abductors in stance phase led to lateral shift of the socket and significant distal lateral limb pressure. A wide-based gait and lateral trunk lean were compensatory strategies.[12]

Ischial containment socket
The *ischial containment* socket (ICS) was designed to promote normal adduction of the femur in stance phase and reduce lateral socket movement, distal lateral limb pressure.[13] The ICS's characteristics include

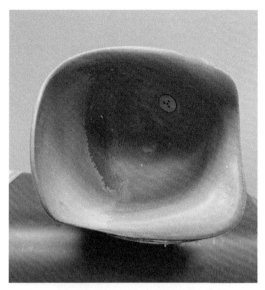

Fig. 3. Quadrilateral socket, axial view.

- Brim lies medial to the ischial ramus.
- The socket is narrower than the quadrilateral socket in the coronal plane (**Figs. 4** and **5**).
- The medial and lateral brim are intended to create a "bony lock" for coronal plane control.

Other names for this socket design include *ischial ramus containment* prosthesis, or the *normal shape normal alignment* socket.[14]

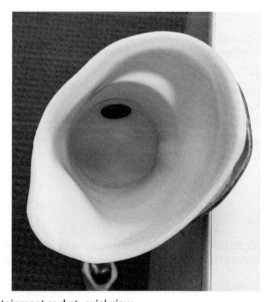

Fig. 4. Ischial containment socket, axial view.

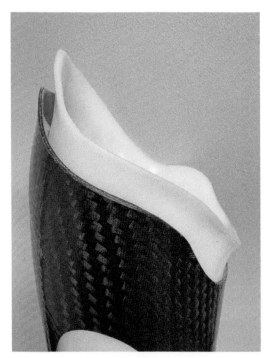

Fig. 5. Ischial containment socket, anterior view.

While there are mixed opinions as to the importance of capturing the ischium to mediolateral stability, as well as to how often the ischial ramus is truly captured on a case-by-case basis, the ICS is the predominant transfemoral socket design in modern practice. It is typically used with a flexible inner socket, allowing a flexible medial brim.

Subischial socket

Subischial sockets paired with vacuum-assisted suction may improve comfort compared to the ICS without sacrificing prosthesis control and stability.[15,16]

Inner flexible sockets

The inner flexible socket is a thermoplastic inner socket that is more flexible than the laminated hard socket (**Fig. 6**). This can be used to

- Create a more comfortable socket brim
- Add options for relief over bony prominences
- As part of an adjustable volume system with cables

Inner flexible sockets add bulk and weight, and friction with the prosthetic liner may impede donning.

SKELETAL STRUCTURE

After the advent of plastic laminates, lower limb prostheses used *exoskeletal* structure, which have a hard outer shell and a hard inner socket (**Fig. 7**). This was needed for structural stability.

In *endoskeletal* prostheses, the socket is connected directly to distal prosthetic componentry (see **Fig. 6**). Due to the evolution of sturdier materials, most lower

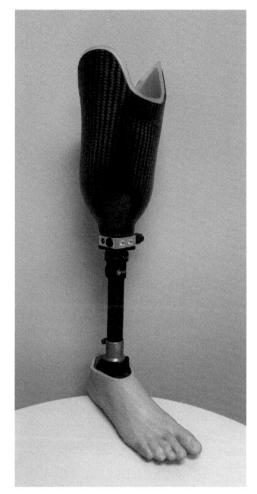

Fig. 6. Endoskeletal transtibial prosthesis with inner flexible socket.

limb prostheses in modern practice are endoskeletal. It is much easier to perform alignment changes with endoskeletal prosthesis.

The *shank* is the structure between the knee and the foot and is also called the *pylon* for endoskeletal prostheses.

LINERS: INTERFACES BETWEEN SOCKET AND RESIDUAL LIMB
Closed-Cell Foam Inserts

Socket inserts (also called "liners") crafted from heat-pliable closed-cell foam were a mainstay in lower limb prosthetics for decades, used with residual limb socks (**Fig. 8**). In modern practice, potential indications are

- The patient cannot tolerate viscoelastic prosthetic liners.
- Skin/soft tissue or hygiene concerns warrant using socks against the skin.
- As part of a historical system (eg, if thigh corset is used to stabilize and offload short transtibial residual limb).

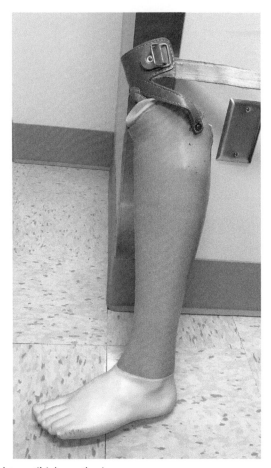

Fig. 7. Exoskeletal transtibial prosthesis.

Prosthetic Liners

Modern prosthetic liners are made from viscoelastic materials: thermoplastic elastomers (TPEs), silicones, and polyurethanes (**Fig. 9**, modern prosthetic liner with pin). Silicone and polyurethane liners are stiffer than TPE liners.[17] Prosthetic liners are rolled onto the residual limb and secured by friction. Prosthetic liners tend to improve load distribution and comfort in comparison to traditional foam interfaces.[1] Liners can vary by shape, thickness, and special features.

Prosthetic Socks

In modern practice, prosthetic socks are usually worn over the prosthetic liner. Socks of different thicknesses (ply) are used to accommodate residual limb volume changes.

SUSPENSION SYSTEMS
Traditional Suspension Systems

Traditional suspension systems are sometimes used in modern practice as auxiliary (secondary) or primary suspension in special situations.

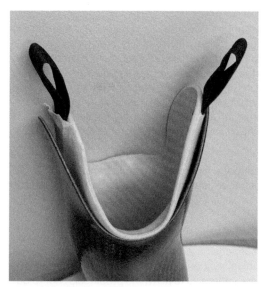

Fig. 8. Transtibial socket with closed cell foam insert.

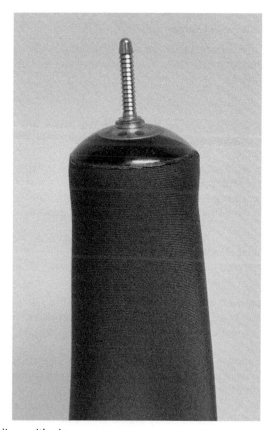

Fig. 9. Prosthetic liner with pin.

Transtibial

SC cuffs (cuff straps) create purchase proximal to the femoral condyles. Cuff straps are still sometimes used for very low-mobility prosthesis.

The *waist belt with forked strap* is sometimes used in modern practice when a thigh corset is used for stability or offloading—thigh corsets can sometimes provide suspension, but occasionally a separate dedicated suspension mechanism is needed (forked strap and waist belt, pin-lock suspension).

Neoprene *sleeves* were used as primary suspension.

SC sockets were historically used more frequently for suspension.

Transfemoral

The traditional transfemoral hip joint and pelvic band are rarely used in modern practice. The Silesian bandage is sometimes used as primary suspension for longtime prosthesis users or as auxiliary suspension.

Socket-Based Anatomic Suspension

With socket-based suspension (sometimes called "anatomic suspension"), the socket itself creates mechanical suspension. Doors, windows, clamshell designs, removable brims, and wedges are strategies to allow the prosthesis user to don and doff the prosthesis (**Fig. 10**). In the *stovepipe* design, a foam insert is used to achieve close anatomic fit, and the hard socket is more cylindrical.

Negative Pressure Differential Suspension

Suction suspension utilizes a negative pressure differential. To achieve negative pressure, 2 things are needed: a way for air to leave but not reenter and a sealing strategy to create a closed system.

Sealing strategies

- *Suction with sealing sleeve.* A nonpermeable TPE sleeve around the socket creates a seal with proximal skin or a reflected prosthetic liner. (This is not traditional sleeve suspension.)
- *Seal-in suction.* A prosthetic liner with flexible ring(s) creates a barometric seal with the interior of the socket.
- *Skin-fit suction.* The residual limb creates a seal with the inner surface of the socket. There is no soft interface between the skin and the socket.

Passive suction

In passive suction suspension, air is expelled through an expulsion valve (a 1 way valve) when the prosthesis is donned (**Fig. 11**). Alternatively, air can escape around the residual limb during donning.

- Passive suction with sealing sleeve and a cushion gel liner is a common combination for transtibial prostheses as it provides good suspension, residual limb protection, and the ability to use prosthetic socks for volume control.
- Passive seal-in suction can work well for transfemoral prosthesis users with fairly stable limb volume. It can be more difficult to maintain the integrity of the seal for transtibial prosthesis users.
- Skin fit suction is most often used for transfemoral prosthesis users with healthy skin and soft tissue, fairly stable limb volume, and good neuromuscular control.

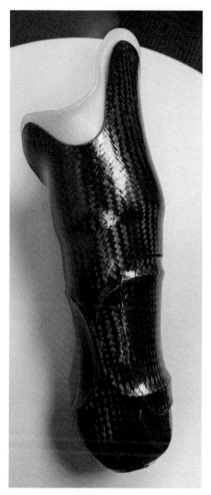

Fig. 10. Knee disarticulation socket that utilizes anatomic suspension.

Vacuum-assisted suction

In vacuum-assisted suction (VAS), sometimes called "elevated vacuum," a motorized or mechanical pump elevates and maintains a greater pressure differential compared to passive suction. A sealing sleeve or seal-in prosthetic liner can be used. VAS suspension can stabilize limb volume and improve the pressure distribution during ambulation.[1] Subject matter experts suggest that correct use of a VAS system may demand more skill and attention on the part of the prosthesis user, as skin blisters or other complications can result from improper use.[18]

VAS permits less pistoning (vertical movement within the socket during the gait cycle) in comparison to passive suction, which permits less pistoning than locking liner-based mechanical suspension.[1] All permit less pistoning than traditional suspension methods.[19,20]

Mechanical Attachment of Prosthetic Liner

Prosthetic *locking liners* have a distal umbrella that accepts a metal pin or lanyard strap (see **Fig. 9**). Prosthetic socks with distal holes can be used.

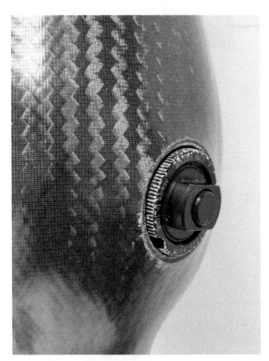

Fig. 11. 1 way expulsion valve.

In *pin-lock suspension*, a pin engages with a shuttle lock fabricated into the socket. Ridged pins can give the prosthesis user auditory and tactile feedback that the pin is engaged in the lock. The number of clicks and speed of clicks can guide sock ply management. Pin-lock is a common suspension method for transtibial prostheses and can be used for transfemoral prosthesis users with sufficient dexterity.

In *lanyard suspension*, a lanyard strap secured to the liner is secured on the outside of the socket. Lanyard suspension is often appropriate for transfemoral prosthesis users with poor hand dexterity and neuromuscular control, who might have difficulty lining up the pin correctly. Furthermore, the lanyard can be threaded through the transfemoral socket while the user is seated, allowing the prosthesis user to partially don the socket in a secure manner before standing.

Auxiliary Suspension

Auxiliary suspension is a secondary suspension mechanism used to improve the security of suspension or to control movement of the prosthesis. For example, a total elastic suspension belt could be used as auxiliary suspension for an active transfemoral prosthesis user who uses skin fit suction but occasionally has had complete loss of suspension due to hyperhidrosis.

KNEES

Prosthetic knees are designed to flex in the sagittal plane. Like the anatomic knee, a prosthetic knee can collapse ("buckle") into flexion if weight is put through it without a counteracting force but cannot collapse into extension. The art of using an above-knee prosthesis includes allowing the knee to bend when desired (eg, swing phase, when sitting down) without accidentally putting weight through a flexed knee, which may result in the knee buckling if the user cannot compensate with voluntary hip extension.

Prosthetic knees can be classified by 3 core attributes: the mechanism that prevents the knee from collapsing during stance phase (*stance control,* or *stance stability mechanism*), the mechanism for control of knee flexion during swing phase (*swing control*), and the type of center of rotation at the joint that allows knee flexion.[10,21]

Core Attributes of Prosthetic Knees

Axis

Monocentric (often called "*single axis*") knees have a simple hinge joint (**Fig. 12**), the bolt of the hinge is the center-of-rotation. Some monocentric knees are very simple and lightweight, and some are heavier and more complex.

Polycentric knees (**Fig. 13**) have an instantaneous center-of-rotation that varies with degree of flexion.[22] The polycentric knee's complex movement is created by bars and linkages that change relative position as the knee flexes, similar to the anterior cruciate ligament (ACL) and posterior cruciate ligament (PCL's) positioning during anatomic knee flexion. Polycentric knees may allow the distal knee to tuck under the proximal knee, which can effectively shorten the knee when it is flexed.

Swing phase control
Free swing. Some prosthetic knees do not have a dedicated mechanism to control knee movement during swing phase.

Constant friction. A constant amount of friction at the knee joint slows rise of the heel during entry to swing phase and slows forward momentum of the shank during swing.

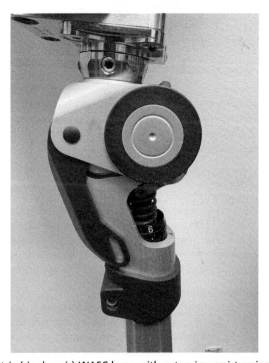

Fig. 12. Monocentric (single axis) WASC knee with extension assist spring.

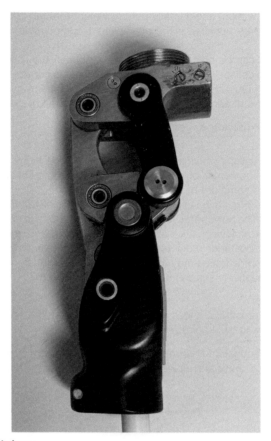

Fig. 13. Polycentric knee.

This is appropriate for single-speed ambulators, as changing the cadence can result in the knee being flexed on entry to stance phase, causing risk of buckling.

The term *constant friction knee* sometimes refers to a single-axis knee with constant friction swing control, and *no* dedicated stance control mechanism. This type of knee is rarely used in modern practice.[21]

Hydraulic or pneumatic. Fluid-controlled dampening of swing phase is responsive to changes in cadence and offers closer to normal swing phase movement.[21]

Extension assist. Extension assist is a spring or spring-like mechanism that stores energy when the knee is flexed and then returns some energy to promote extension (see **Fig. 11**). This can aid the user in achieving full knee extension by terminal swing and can also control heel rise in terminal stance phase. Extension assist mechanisms can be found in conjunction with friction or pneumatic swing control mechanisms.

Stance phase control (stance stability)
In normal gait, eccentric contraction of the quadriceps in early stance phase allows controlled yielding (controlled progressive knee flexion under a load), then isometric contraction of the quadriceps prevents further flexion (ie, prevents buckling of the knee).[23] The primary role of prosthetic knee stance control is to prevent the knee from buckling during stance phase, and some have more sophisticated capabilities.

Prosthetic knee alignment is always considered. Ground reaction force vector (GRFV) behind the knee creates a flexion moment, and GRFV in front of the knee creates an extension moment (stabilizing). The prosthetist aims for dynamic alignment that promotes stability in stance phase and does not impede the prosthesis user from breaking into swing.

Non-articulated prosthesis. Some prostheses for persons with amputations at the knee, transfemoral, or at the hip do *not* have a prosthetic knee. A non-articulated prosthesis could be used in low mobility or early mobility situations where stability is paramount (eg, early prosthesis training for a person with bilateral transfemoral amputations), for activities involving uneven terrain (eg, panning for gold), or for high-level activities.

Polycentric knee. The typical 4 bar polycentric knee's instantaneous center-of-rotation in full flexion is high and posterior relative to the physical center of the knee, which lessens knee flexion moment or creates a knee extension moment in early stance. Polycentric knees may have additional stance stability mechanisms such as hydraulic stance control.

Locking knee. A manual locking knee has a mechanism that locks the knee when the knee is unweighted and in extension and does not disengage and flex until the knee has been fully offloaded and the user generates a knee flexion moment. Because gait deviations caused by a fixed knee are very difficult to unlearn, this is only used for very unstable prosthesis users. Manual locks are also available in some prosthetic knees appropriate for more active persons, who may benefit from an optional lock for activities requiring extra stability or still standing.

Weight-activated stance control knee. The weight-activated stance control (WASC) knee's friction brake engages when an axial load is put through the knee in full extension[23] (see **Fig. 11**). WASC knees are usually single axis with constant friction swing control and may be appropriate for household or low-level community ambulators.[b]

Hydraulic stance control. Unlike the other stance control mechanisms, hydraulic resistance can allow controlled yielding under high loads (often called *stance flexion yielding*). High stance-yielding resistance coupled with a larger range of motion of resistance has potential benefits:[23,24]

1. Controlled knee flexion in early stance phase, a characteristic of normal gait.
2. Weight-bearing through a flexed knee while descending slopes or stairs.
3. *Stumble recovery*: Strong yielding resistance that allows the user enough time to catch themselves if they suddenly put weight through a bent knee.

Mechanical hydraulic swing and stance control knees are suitable for users with good range of motion and neuromuscular control.

Pneumatic fluid control is not suitable for stance control due to the much higher amount of resistance required.

Stance flexion. Stance flexion is any mechanism that allows controlled knee flexion as the knee is loaded in early stance phase. This can be achieved by hydraulic dampening or an elastomeric bumper.

---

[b] Synonyms: *safety knee," load-activated brake.*

Microprocessor knees

Microprocessor-controlled knees have computers that analyze information from sensors monitoring the user's gait and then adjust the knee's resistance in real time to match the perceived situation (such as faster walking speed). Most microprocessor knees (MPKs) are single-axis knee with fluid-controlled stance and swing phase. Adaptive control of resistance has the potential to improve theoretic benefits of fluid-controlled knees.

MPKs differ in characteristics such as

- Types and frequency of sensor inputs
- Default resistance—stance versus swing
- Adaptive control of swing and stance, versus stance only
- Range of motion with effective resistance for different activities

Some MPKs are designed to support higher level activities (eg, step-over-step stair descent, walking backward), while some have features focused on lower mobility community ambulators. In higher level community ambulators, MPKs can improve users' ability to walk on even and uneven terrain,[25] slopes and stairs,[26] stumble recovery, and balance.[25] In limited community ambulators, MPKs reduce incidence of falls, fear of falling, and risk of falling, while leading to improved mobility, self-selected walking speed, and patient-reported ambulation.[27]

MPKs are heavier and more expensive than mechanical knees. The effectiveness of specific MPKs for activities varies for specific situations. For example, some MPKs' resistance qualities impact their effectiveness for stumble recovery.[28]

Externally powered knees. Externally powered knees (EPKs), also called *active knees* or *propulsive* knees, are microprocessor-controlled knees with powered knee extension. Early research suggested EPKs may lessen power required by the contralateral knee during sit-to-stand transfers and stair ascent for some users.[29,30] EPKs might impede mobility in older persons.

EPKs have significantly heavier batteries and shorter battery life than fluid-controlled MPKs and generate noise during use. Performance of specific EPKs can vary due to qualities of the knee and patient factors. Currently available EPKs are not well suited to lower mobility prosthesis users and are not available for most users.[31]

FEET AND ANKLES
Elements of Prosthetic Feet and Ankles

The objectives of the prosthetic foot (or foot–ankle) include[32]

- Energy absorption during early stance
- Achieve stable foot position following initial contact
- Provide close-to-normal center-of-pressure progression (shank kinematics, or *rollover*)
- Contribute to push-off in late stance phase and transition into swing.

The *keel* of a prosthetic foot is the longitudinal portion that parallels the midfoot and forefoot and creates an anterior lever arm.[33]

Solid ankle cushioned heel foot

The solid ankle cushioned heel (SACH) foot is a non-articulated prosthetic foot—"solid ankle" means "no ankle joint"—with a rigid wooden keel and a compressible cushion heel. The heel absorbs energy and allows progression forward in early stance phase.[34]

Single-axis foot

The traditional single-axis foot's mechanical joint allows some plantarflexion and dorsiflexion.[35] In comparison to the SACH foot, the single-axis foot achieves a faster foot flat in stance phase. This swings the center-of-pressure and thus GRFV forward earlier, which lessens knee flexion moment in early stance. This could be considered for patients with lower mobility at risk of knee collapse, such as elderly persons with transfemoral amputation. Elastomeric bumpers control motion.

Flexible keel foot

A flexible keel foot has a keel made from a flexible material such as plastic or carbon fiber. This allows smoother rollover through stance phase and is suitable for a low-mobility community ambulator.

Multi-axis foot

A multi-axis foot has a mechanical joint that allows some movement in the sagittal plane, the mediolateral plane, and sometimes the transverse plane (rotation). Multi-axis feet are appropriate for a community ambulator who encounters uneven terrain, as the increased motion can accommodate the terrain. However, some limited community ambulators may feel more stable with a foot that has less inherent motion. Prosthetic feet and ankles can achieve multiaxial movement by means other than a mechanical joint.

Energy storing-and-return or dynamic response

An *energy storing-and-return* (ESAR) *foot* is a spring design made with carbon fiber, fiberglass, or composite materials (see **Fig. 13**). The spring design stores energy as it compresses and returns that energy in transition to swing phase (push-off).[36] Some ESAR feet have a split keel to allow more multiaxial movement. ESAR feet with an integrated shank can reduce weight of the prosthesis and sometimes can provide more spring. ESARs began as a continuum with what are now called flexible keel feet.

Hydraulic ankles

Hydraulic foot–ankle systems use a hydraulic ankle to control the sagittal plane. This allows for increased range of motion while walking on uneven surfaces like hills, ramps, and traversing over obstacles. In comparison to feet with similar features but a fixed ankle, hydraulic ankles have a smoother forward progression of center of pressure[37] and may permit higher walking speeds,[38,39] better mimic ankle resistance moments,[40] and decrease the energy cost of ambulation.[41] The ankle plantarflexion and dorsiflexion resistance can be adjusted.

Microprocessor-controlled ankles. Microprocessor-controlled ankles may improve knee stability on slopes compared to mechanical hydraulic ankles.[42,43] A microprocessor ankle with "standing support" may reduce kinematic compensations during still standing.[44]

Externally powered ankles The first commercially available externally powered foot–ankle system uses electronic motors and mechanical springs to create push-off.[45] Externally powered foot–ankles may improve peak push-off and external knee moments on the contralateral limb, but findings have been inconsistent.[32] Such devices have heavy batteries and generate noise during active use.

CONSIDERATIONS

When taken together, the characteristics of transfemoral and transtibial prosthetic componentry have key implications about prosthesis use and candidacy.

Sit-to-Stand Transfers

The ability to transition from the seated position to the standing position (sit-to-stand transfer) and vice versa (stand-to-sit transfer), is fundamental building blocks for any activities that involve standing or walking. Put simply—if one cannot safely and independently perform standing-up and sitting-down transfers throughout the day, one cannot safely stand or walk in real-world settings.

Let us consider forces through the knees during sit-to-stand. In healthy adults, both lower limbs bear weight as they stand up, with the dominant limb tending to experience slightly higher loads.[46] Unilateral transtibial prosthesis users have less weight-bearing symmetry and tend to put more weight through the non-amputated limb but still bear a considerable proportion of their weight through the prosthesis.[47] In contrast, unilateral transfemoral prosthesis users bear only a negligible amount of weight through the prosthesis during sit-to-stand transfers.[48]

Why? As we discussed earlier, prosthetic knees' main objectives are to use resistance to prevent knee flexion—they are not designed to create active knee extension torque sufficient to lift body weight. Furthermore, all prosthetic knees buckle if a load is put through them when significantly bent (and some when bent more than a few degrees).

So, a transfemoral prosthesis does not help a person stand up, nor does it help them perform squat-pivot transfers (transitioning from one seated position to another with the knees bent).

Implications for Transfemoral Prosthesis Candidacy

A person with a transfemoral amputation would not be able to functionally benefit from a prosthesis *unless*, at a bare minimum:

- They can easily perform sit-to-stand and stand-to-sit transfers using only their contralateral lower limb, upper extremities, and real-world supports and assistive devices. (One cannot pull oneself up to the parallel bars in normal day-to-day circumstances!) They must be capable of doing this many times throughout the day.
- They can maintain a standing position on the contralateral lower limb for at least 5 to 10 minutes, with good balance. (This is required for prosthesis fitting.)

Good dynamic balance on the contralateral lower limb is also required for transfemoral prosthesis donning.

DISCUSSION

There are numerous considerations and options for lower limb prosthesis componentry, and there is no one "best" approach. However, one does not have to know a lot of details about prosthetic componentry to add valuable perspective for patients and other members of the clinical team! Understanding some of the major components of the prosthesis and being able to communicate how these components can be helpful—or not helpful—goes a long way.

CLINICS CARE POINTS

- For patients with a high likelihood of residual limb volume changes day-to-day or overtime, consider a prosthesis suspension method that allows the use of prosthetic socks for volume accommodation.

- Suction and vacuum suspension are very secure when there is a good socket fit and the sealing method is intact.

- Pin-lock and lanyard suspension allow the use of prosthetic socks and can make it easier for some users to know when their limb is seated and secured in the socket.

- SC and SC/SP transtibial sockets can be used to stabilize the knee.

- A transtibial prosthesis thigh corset with side joints can be used to partially offload or stabilize the knee and residual limb. Additional suspension may be needed.

- IC design is the standard of care for transfemoral sockets. It is difficult to don this type of socket when seated, and the brim is uncomfortable and can lead to skin breakdown.

- Most prosthetic knees, including computer-controlled knees, are passive devices and do not actively create forces to support and lift the user when going from sitting to standing or walking up hills or stairs.

- Transfemoral prosthesis fitting and use require a much higher threshold of physical function and neuromuscular control than transtibial prosthesis use.

DISCLOSURE

None of the authors have any commercial or financial conflicts of interest and any funding sources.

REFERENCES

1. Stevens PM, Depalma RR, Wurdeman SR. Transtibial socket design, interface, and suspension: A clinical practice guideline. J Prosthet Orthot 2019;31(3): 172–8.
2. Thompson RG. The patellar tendon bearing total contact prosthesis for below-knee amputees. Orthot Pros 1962;16:238–44.
3. Foort J. The patellar-tendon-bearing prosthesis for below-knee amputees, a review of technique and criteria. Artif Limbs 1965;9(1):4–13.
4. Radcliffe CW, Foort J. The Patellar-Tendon-Bearing below-Knee Prosthesis. Biomechanics Laboratory. Berkeley: University of California; 1961.
5. Fergason J, Smith DG. Socket considerations for the patient with a transtibial amputation. Clin Orthop Relat Res 1999;361:76–84.
6. Kapp S. Suspension systems for prostheses. Clin Orthop Relat Res 1999;361: 55–62.
7. Staats TB, Lundt J. The UCLA total surface bearing suction below-knee prosthesis. Clinical Prosthetics and Orthotics 1987;11(3):118–30.
8. Kahle JT. Conventional and hydrostatic transtibial interface comparison. J Prosthet Orthot 1999;11(4):85–91.
9. Childers WL, Wurdeman SR. Transtibial amputation: prosthetic management. In: Krajbich JI, Pinzur MS, Potter BK, et al, editors. Atlas of amputations and limb deficiencies surgical, prosthetic, and rehabilitation principles. 5th edition. Rosemont, IL: American Academy of Orthopaedic Surgeons; 2023. p. 1648–701.
10. Wilson EB. Recent Advances in Above Knee Prosthetics. Artif Limbs 1968; 12(2):1–27.
11. von Werssowetz OF. Above-the-knee Suction-socket. J Bone Joint Surg 1952; 34(3):731–9.
12. Radcliffe CW. Functional Considerations in the Fitting of Above-Knee Prostheses. Artif Limbs 1955;2(1):35–60.

13. Long IA. Normal shape-normal alignment (NSNA) above-knee prosthesis. Clinical Prosthetics & Orthotics 1985;9(4):9–14.

14. Redhead RG. Total surface bearing self suspending above-knee sockets. Prosthet Orthot Int 1979;3(3):126–36.

15. Fatone S, Caldwell R. Northwestern University Flexible Subischial Vacuum Socket for persons with transfemoral amputation-Part 1: Description of technique. Prosthet Orthot Int 2017;41(3):237–45.

16. Kahle JT, Highsmith MJ. Transfemoral sockets with vacuum-assisted suspension comparison of hip kinematics, socket position, contact pressure, and preference: Ischial containment versus brimless. J Rehabil Res Dev 2013;50(9):1241–52.

17. Cagle JC, Hafner BJ, Taflin N, et al. Characterization of prosthetic liner products for people with transtibial amputation. J Prosthet Orthot 2018;30(4):187–99.

18. Gholizadeh H, Lemaire ED, Eshraghi A. The evidence-base for elevated vacuum in lower limb prosthetics: Literature review and professional feedback. Clin Bio-Mech 2016;37:108–16.

19. Highsmith MJ, Kahle JT, Miro RM, et al. Prosthetic interventions for people with transtibial amputation: Systematic review and meta-analysis of high-quality prospective literature and systematic reviews. J Rehabil Res Dev 2016;53(2):157–83.

20. Safari MR, Meier MR. Systematic review of effects of current transtibial prosthetic socket designs—Part 2: Quantitative outcomes. J Rehabil Res Dev 2015;52(5):509–26.

21. Michael JW. Modern prosthetic knee mechanisms. Clin Orthop Relat Res 1999;361:39–47.

22. Radcliffe CW. Four-bar linkage prosthetic knee mechanisms: kinematics, alignment and prescription criteria. Prosthet Orthot Int 1994;18(3):159–73.

23. Stewart RE, Staros A. Selection and application of knee mechanisms. Bull Prosthet Res 1972;9:90–158.

24. Mauch HA. Stance control for above-knee artificial legs – design considerations in the S-N-S knee. Bull Prosthet Res 1968;5(2):61–72.

25. Kaufman KR, Levine JA, Brey RH, et al. Gait and balance of transfemoral amputees using passive mechanical and microprocessor-controlled prosthetic knees. Gait Posture 2007;26(4):489–93.

26. Bellmann M, Schmalz T, Blumentritt S. Comparative biomechanical analysis of current microprocessor-controlled prosthetic knee joints. Arch Phys Med Rehabil 2010;91(4):644–52.

27. Hahn A, Bueschges S, Prager M, et al. The effect of microprocessor controlled exo-prosthetic knees on limited community ambulators: systematic review and meta-analysis. Disabil Rehabil 2022;44(24):7349–67.

28. Ernst M, Altenburg B, Schmalz T, et al. Benefits of a microprocessor-controlled prosthetic foot for ascending and descending slopes. J NeuroEng Rehabil 2022;19(1):9.

29. Wolf EJ, Everding VQ, Linberg AA, et al. Comparison of the Power Knee and C-Leg during step-up and sit-to-stand tasks. Gait Posture 2013;38(3):397–402.

30. Wolf EJ, Everding VQ, Linberg AL, et al. Assessment of transfemoral amputees using C-Leg and Power Knee for ascending and descending inclines and steps. J Rehabil Res Dev 2012;49(6):831–42.

31. Hafner BJ, Askew RL. Physical performance and self-report outcomes associated with use of passive, adaptive, and active prosthetic knees in persons with unilateral, transfemoral amputation: Randomized crossover trial. J Rehabil Res Dev 2015;52(6):677–700.

32. Major MJ, Stevens PM. Prosthetic foot and ankle mechanisms. In: Krajbich JI, Pinzur MS, Potter BK, et al, editors. Atlas of amputations and limb deficiencies surgical, prosthetic, and rehabilitation principles. 5th edition. Rosemont, IL: American Academy of Orthopaedic Surgeons; 2023. p. 1399–451.

33. Versluys R, Beyl P, Van Damme M, et al. Prosthetic feet: state-of-the-art review and the importance of mimicking human ankle-foot biomechanics. Disabil Rehabil Assist Technol 2009;4(2):65–75.

34. Carroll K, Rheinstein J, Pollard E. Understanding prossthetic feet. In: Chui K, Yen S, Jorge M, Lusardi M, editors. Orthotics & prosthetics in rehabilitation. 4th edition. St. Louis, MO: Elsevier; 2020. p. 566–76.

35. Hafner BJ. Clinical prescription and use of prosthetic foot and ankle mechanisms: a review of the literature. Journal of Prosthetics and Orthotics 2005;17(4):S5–11.

36. Michael J. Energy storing feet: A clinical comparison. Clinical Prosthetics and Orthotics 1987;11(3):154–68.

37. De Asha AR, Johnson L, Munjal R, et al. Attenuation of centre-of-pressure trajectory fluctuations under the prosthetic foot when using an articulating hydraulic ankle attachment compared to fixed attachment. Clin BioMech 2013;28(2):218–24.

38. Moore R. Effect on stance phase timing asymmetry in individuals with amputation using hydraulic ankle units. J Prosthet Orthot 2016;28(1):44–8.

39. Barnett CT, Brown OH, Bisele M, et al. Individuals with Unilateral Transtibial Amputation and Lower Activity Levels Walk More Quickly when Using a Hydraulically Articulating Versus Rigidly Attached Prosthetic Ankle-Foot Device. J Prosthet Orthot 2018;30(3):158–64.

40. Bai X, Ewins D, Crocombe AD, et al. Kinematic and biomimetic assessment of a hydraulic ankle/foot in level ground and camberwalking. PLoS One 2017;12(7):e0180836.

41. Askew GN, McFarlane LA, Minetti AE, et al. Energy cost of ambulation in transtibial amputees using a dynamic-response foot with hydraulic versus rigid "ankle": Insights from body centre of mass dynamics. J NeuroEng Rehabil 2019;16(1):39.

42. Struchkov V, Buckley JG. Biomechanics of ramp descent in unilateral trans-tibial amputees: Comparison of a microprocessor controlled foot with conventional ankle-foot mechanisms. Clin BioMech 2016;32:164–70.

43. McGrath M, Laszczak P, Zahedi S, et al. The influence of a microprocessor-controlled hydraulic ankle on the kinetic symmetry of trans-tibial amputees during ramp walking: A case series. J Rehabil Assist Technol Eng 2018;5. 2055668318790650.

44. Davies KC, Laszczak P, Rek B, et al. The influence of hydraulic ankles and microprocessor-control on the biomechanics of trans-tibial amputees during quiet standing on a 5° slope. Canadian Prosthetics and Orthotics Journal 2019;2(2):33517.

45. Herr HM, Grabowski AM. Bionic ankle-foot prosthesis normalizes walking gait for persons with leg amputation. Proc Biol Sci 2012;279(1728):457–64.

46. Schofield JS, Parent EC, Lewicke J, et al. Characterizing asymmetry across the whole sit to stand movement in healthy participants. J Biomech 2013;46(15):2730–5.

47. Ozyurek S, Demirbuken I, Angin S. Altered movement strategies in sit-to-stand task in persons with transtibial amputation. Prosthet Orthot Int 2014;38(4):303–9.

48. Burger H, Kuzelicki J, Marincek C. Transition from sitting to standing after trans-femoral amputation. Prosthet Orthot Int 2005;29(2):139–51.

Prosthetic Componentry in Upper Limb Prosthetic Restoration

Rebecca A. Speckman, MD, PhD[a,b,*], Wayne T. Biggs, BS, CPO[a]

KEYWORDS

- Body-powered prostheses • Externally powered prostheses • Myoelectric
- Transradial prosthesis • Transhumeral prosthesis • Terminal device

KEY POINTS

- In comparison to externally powered prostheses, upper limb body-powered prostheses are lighter, more durable, easier to repair, and more forgiving of residual limb volume and shape changes.
- Upper limb body-powered devices are considered intuitive to operate, with precise prehensile (grasping) ability.
- Externally powered upper limb devices can allow a user to have multiple grasping pattern options and operate in a larger functional work envelope.
- Externally powered control mechanisms for upper limb prostheses often utilize input from surface myoelectric sensors but sometimes utilize other input devices such as a linear transducer or a switch.

INTRODUCTION
Upper Limb Kinesiology

Upper limb prosthetic components are often characterized by the *degrees of freedom* (DOFs), or different planes of movement, that they allow.[1] For example, the elbow has 1 key DOF (flexion/extension), and the wrist has 3 DOFs (flexion/extension, supination/pronation, and radial/ulnar deviation). The goal of prosthetic design is not always to include all "normal" DOFs, as adding DOFs can increase the cost, weight, and fragility of a device. Instead, focus is often on prioritization of DOFs for practical use. Movement patterns such as specific grasps can involve multiple DOFs simultaneously.

There are different types or classes of upper limb activities. *Prehension* is the grasping and releasing of objects.[2] Nonprehensile activities do not include grasping

---

[a] Regional Amputation Center, VA Puget Sound Health Care System, 1660 South Columbian Way, Seattle, WA 98108, USA; [b] Department of Rehabilitation Medicine, University of Washington, 325 Ninth Avenue, Box 359612, Seattle, WA 98104, USA
* Corresponding author. 1660 South Columbian Way, Seattle, WA 98108.
E-mail address: Rebecca.Speckman@va.gov

Phys Med Rehabil Clin N Am 35 (2024) 817–831
https://doi.org/10.1016/j.pmr.2024.06.011
1047-9651/24/Published by Elsevier Inc.

or seizing. Nonprehensile activities could include specific finger actions (eg, depressing a piano key) or the hand (eg, pushing a shopping cart). Human hands are important for gestures and have social and cultural significance.[3]

Napier proposed that most prehensile movements could be classified as *precision grips*, in which an object is pinched between the distal aspects of the opposing thumb and finger(s), and *power grips*, in which an object is held "as in a clamp between the flexed fingers and the palm," with counter pressure from the palmar surface of the thumb.[4] Taylor and Schwarz further classified prehension patterns into 3 precision grasps (tip pinch, palmar pinch, and lateral pinch) and 3 power grasps (spherical, cylindrical, and hook).[5] There are many taxonomies of hand prehension or grasping patterns, some with a great variety of patterns.[6,7]

Frameworks for Describing Upper Limb Prostheses

Upper limb prostheses are often categorized by their overall type of *control mechanism*, or the method by which prosthesis movement is controlled or created.

- Body-powered (BP) devices have elements that actively move in real time under the direct control of volitional body movement.
- Externally powered (EP) devices have an electric motor that generates movement in response to input from the prosthesis user. Input may be from surface electrodes picking up muscle contraction signals (*myoelectric control*) or other methods such as a switch.
- A *hybrid* prosthesis has BP and EP elements.
- *Passive* devices are stationary within the device itself. The overall prosthesis can still change position as the user changes position, and some passive devices can be repositioned (eg, wrist rotated, hand opened or closed) using the contralateral limb or other means.

An upper limb prosthesis can be described using a similar framework to that presented for lower limb prostheses, with a few adjustments:

- The *control* mechanism
- The prosthetic *socket* is a connector between the user and the rest of the prosthesis. It transmits movements and forces and may have other functions such as suspension or housing electrical components.
- The structural type of the prosthesis could be *exoskeletal,* with a hard external shell-like structure creating structural integrity, or *endoskeletal*, with an internal support structure (usually components linked directly together).
- The prosthesis *suspension system* is the mechanism by which the prosthesis is secured on the user.
- There may be an *interface* between the prosthetic socket and the user's residual limb or other body parts in contact with the socket, such as the torso.
- An upper limb prosthesis could have elements designed to simulate some function of the anatomic shoulder, elbow, wrist, or hand.
- An element designed to simulate some function of the anatomic hand is usually called a *(prosthetic) hand* if its appearance is similar to an anatomic hand, and a *terminal device* if its appearance is not similar to an anatomic hand.

CONTROL MECHANISMS
Body-Powered Control

BP upper limb prostheses as used in modern practice remain similar to their development in the 1950s, during the push for advancements in prostheses after World War

II.[8] In BP control, volitional movement of the proximal upper extremity and shoulder girdle is used to exert force and create linear movement (called *excursion*) of cable(s) that operate the terminal device (TD) or elbow.[9] Proper fitment of the prosthesis and positioning of the cable(s) are needed to optimize translation of volitional movement into TD or elbow control.

The *work envelope*, or *functional work envelope*, is the area in which the prosthesis user can operate the TD.[9]

- The working envelope for a BP TD is usually somewhere in front of the torso, below the shoulders, above the waist, and between shoulder width.
- Ability of the user to use glenohumeral flexion and scapular protraction together or isolated can expand the functional envelope. For example, isolated scapular protraction could allow TD control closer to the body.
- A cable that is too long might require the user to utilize full glenohumeral flexion and biscapular protraction to achieve sufficient excursion for TD control, which would move the functional envelope further away from the front of the body. (A cable could even be loose enough to make it impossible for the user to create sufficient excursion to control the TD in any position.)
- Specific componentry such as type of wrist can affect the work envelope.

Comparison to lower limb prosthesis terminology

For lower limb prosthetics, the term BP is sometimes used in a broader sense to describe a prosthesis or element whose movement is controlled in real time by body movement.[10] However, in modern practice for lower limb prosthetics, there are not direct analogs to upper limb BP cable control. A historical example of lower limb BP movement more analogous to cable control is the use of straps from the torso to the shank to actively translate trunk extension into prosthetic knee extension (TFA).

Transradial Body-Powered Prostheses

Control sequence

In a traditional transradial BP prosthesis, the control cable operates a TD. Glenohumeral flexion and biscapular abduction (also called scapular protraction) are used to activate a single-cable control system. Glenohumeral flexion is able to create a larger excursion than biscapular abduction.

Harnesses

Figure-of-eight harness: suspension and cable anchor. The figure-of-eight harness functions as both an anchor for the control cable and as a suspension mechanism. The *axillary loop* goes around the contralateral shoulder, creating an anchor. The cable is attached to the lower posterior strap of the harness on the ipsilateral side of the prosthesis and then begins its course at the posterior upper arm, typically to a *triceps cuff*. An ipsilateral anterior strap (sometimes called an inverted Y suspensor strap) attaches directly to the prosthesis to create suspension.

Figure-of-nine harness: cable anchor. If a suspension system other than a harness is used, for example, self-suspension, the figure-of-eight harness's suspension strap is not necessary. The figure-of-nine harness's contralateral axillary loop (**Fig. 1**) has a posterior strap that attaches to the control cable and serves solely as an anchor for the cable.

Chest strap and shoulder saddle. The shoulder saddle is an alternative harness that utilizes a pad on the shoulder of the amputation side as the point of origination of cable(s), with a chest strap (a strap around the thorax) for stabilization. This could be

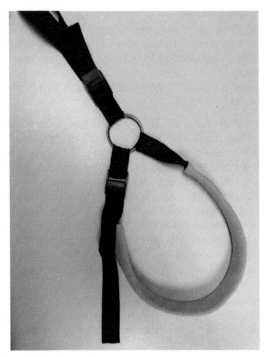

Fig. 1. Figure-of-nine axillary loop.

used if the figure-of-eight harness has caused complications at the contralateral axilla and may be easier to don.[11]

Terminal devices

The TD of an upper limb prosthesis is the most distal element of the prosthesis and the prehensile (grasping) element. Traditional BP TDs are usually a *hook* or a *hand*, with the latter term used to denote any TD with its appearance made to look like an anatomic hand.

Voluntary opening hook. The classic BP upper limb prosthesis TD is a voluntary opening (VO) hook (**Fig. 2**), sometimes called a "split-hook" as the design has 2 tines that meet side by side to create grasping ability. Specialized rubber bands hold the tines closed at rest, and the user creates excursion on the control cable to separate the tines (**Fig. 3**). One rubber band creates about 1.5 pounds of grip force. Rubber bands can be added or removed by the patient or prosthetist. The prosthesis user must create force greater than the maximum grip force of the TD to open the hook. This design allows for precise grasping. VO hooks can vary, for example, by the cant (slant), shape of the tines, width of opening, or gripping surface. VO hooks are considered very functional, and appropriate for settings including hard labor or outdoors. Some persons may not prefer the esthetic of hooks.

Advantages of VO hooks:[11]

- Lightweight
- Easy to see the object to be grasped
- Work well for heavy-duty activities
- Can be used in adverse weather conditions

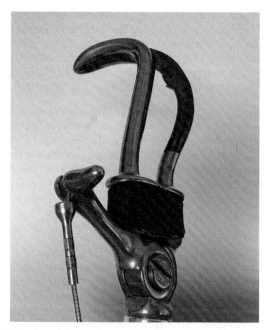

Fig. 2. VO hook BP TD, closed (in resting position).

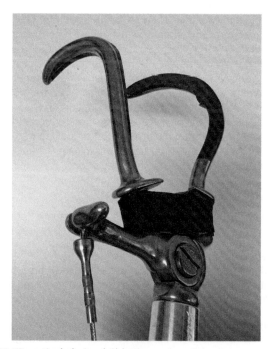

Fig. 3. VO hook BP TD, actively being held open.

Voluntary opening hand. There are BP VO hands available, which usually utilize a 3 jaw chuck grip pattern (the thumb opposes the index and middle fingers). VO hands are considered to be less functional than VO hooks as VO hands are heavier, it is more difficult to see objects, and precise actions such as manipulating clothing fasteners are more difficult. Furthermore, VO hands tend to deliver lower pinch forces than VO hooks.[12] Some users may prefer the cosmesis of a mechanical hand.

Voluntary closing hook. Voluntary closing (VC) hooks are open at rest, and excursion of the control cable closes the hook. The user can control the speed of closure and the grip force. This design allows varied grip force and opens more easily than a VO hook. This may be advantageous for activities in which a quick release may be preferred for safety reasons, for example, a power tool, or for activities that require a gentler grasp, such as cooking. VC hooks are generally less preferred than VO hooks as VC hooks require the user to maintain the grip force for the entire time they are grasping an item, and the open position of a VC at rest can be unwieldy.

Wrists

Prosthetic wrists are the point of attachment of the TD and allow repositioning of the TD.[9] The 3 DOFs of the anatomic wrist are flexion/extension, ulnar and radial deviation, and supination/pronation (often called "rotation").[13] Some prosthetic wrists allow movement in one plane, while others allow positioning in multiple planes. Some wrists are passive, and some have elements operated by a control cable. Wrists may be held in position by friction or locking mechanisms. Quick-disconnect wrists allow users to easily switch between TDs, or to rotate the TD and "lock" it in a secure position. When switching between TDs, it is possible to "stow" the cable so that a passive TD can be attached.

Friction wrists have sufficient friction to prevent rotation of the device (and thus the TD) under a given amount of loading. The position of a friction wrist can be changed using the contralateral upper limb, by striking the TD against another surface, or by grasping a stationary item with the TD and rotating about the TD.

A wrist with flexion feature can better allow the user to reach midline, which is helpful for many activities of daily living. This is especially important for a bilateral upper limb prosthesis user. Flexion elements are often spring-loaded, locking into place once flexed. Wrists with flexion capability tend to be heavier and larger, and flexion units can break down. Wrists with spring-loaded pronation can be locked in supination, and release of the lock allows spring-assisted pronation. In BP wrists, the user can control a lock or positioning of the wrist using a control cable. Some wrists have more complex capabilities such as multiple DOFs, or locking into different positions in one plane. Low-profile wrists can be used to minimize added length for persons with wrist disarticulation or long transradial amputations.

Transhumeral Body-Powered Prostheses

Classic transhumeral BP prostheses utilize a 2 cable system to control a mechanical locking elbow and a VO hook TD.

Body-powered elbows

The traditional style of mechanical prosthetic elbow allows flexion and extension (1 DOF) and locks into place. Elbows may have other features such as spring-assisted flexion, or capability of rotation. Some elbows utilize friction to hold position.[14]

Transhumeral body-powered prosthesis cables and functions

Control cable. The transhumeral (TH) prosthesis control cable (**Fig. 4**), also called the dual control cable, opens the TD or flexes the elbow and has similar placement to the

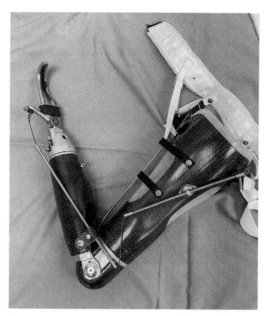

Fig. 4. Transhumeral BP prosthesis with dual control cable and elbow locking cable.

transradial (TR) control cable. The TH control cable originates from a posterior strap of a figure-of-eight harness, and excursion and force are generated by glenohumeral flexion or biscapular abduction. Split housing of the cable allows excursion and force generation to preferentially act at the elbow, creating elbow flexion, when the elbow is unlocked. When the elbow is locked, excursion of the cable opens the TD.

Elbow locking cable. A second cable locks and unlocks the elbow. The elbow lock cable originates at the anterior shoulder, such as on the anterior strap of a figure-of-eight harness, and runs anterior to the upper arm in the deltoid pectoral groove to connect to the elbow's locking mechanism. Excursion on the elbow lock cable is generated by glenohumeral extension, abduction, and depression of the shoulder.[14]

Control sequence
Starting with the elbow unlocked, 3 separate actions are needed to position and operate the TD of a transhumeral BP prosthesis.[9]

1. Elbow is moved to the desired amount of flexion. (TH control cable; excursion and force are generated by glenohumeral flexion and biscapular abduction.)
2. Locking of the elbow. (Elbow locking cable; tension to operate the lock is created by glenohumeral extension and abduction, shoulder depression.)
3. Operation of the TD (TH control cable).

Advantages and Disadvantages of Body-Powered Control

Advantages
BP upper limb prostheses have multiple advantages:[15]

- Lower weight, lower cost compared to externally powered devices
- Durable
- Sensory feedback via cable tension and force
- Good prehensile function

Disadvantages

- Harness can lead to discomfort or nerve compression at contralateral axilla.[15]
- Some prosthesis users may have difficulty generating sufficient excursion or force to operate a BP device.
- The functional envelope of operation of the TD can be limited.

EXTERNALLY POWERED CONTROL

EP devices contain electric motor(s) that actively generate movement. *Myoelectric* EP components receive input from surface myoelectric signals.

Myoelectric Control

In myoelectric control, electrical signals from muscle contraction are amplified and translated into powered movement of a prosthetic component.[16] Traditional myoelectric control utilizes input from surface electrodes. Most modern myoelectric components have programmable microprocessors (onboard computers) that allow more sophisticated and adjustable signal interpretation and control.[17] Programmable microprocessors can add or improve features, for example, customizable grip patterns, switching between proportional and nonproportional control, increasing the user-adjustability.

Direct control

In *direct control* myoelectric components, activation from a muscle is translated directly into a single movement or movement within a single degree of freedom.[18] (This direct translation might occur for multiple different functions, but only one function operates at a time.) In direct control, muscles typically are mapped to the movement that best parallels their innate function, for example, wrist extensors would be used to control hand opening. Most modern myoelectric components have *proportional control*, meaning that a stronger muscle contraction translates into faster movement or higher grip force.

In *dual*, or *2 channel control*, myoelectric signals are picked up from 2 muscles in the residual limb, usually an agonist/antagonist pair such as wrist flexors and extensors, or elbow flexors and extensors.[16] The prosthetist works with the prosthesis user to determine a muscle signal for switching between different grips or movements. Co-contraction of the muscle pair is commonly used; other options are the use of a long "open" or long "closed" muscle contraction signal to switch between different DOFs, which might be different functions of the same joint/section (eg, different prehension patterns), or movement at different joints. *Single-site* or *single-channel* control is possible if there is only 1 useable muscle site but is generally considered unwieldy. There are numerous single-site control strategies, and proportional control is possible.[18]

Conventional dual-channel control myoelectric components do not allow simultaneous myoelectric control of more than 1 DOF. *Sequential control* means that the user can only operate grip pattern or other movement at a time and must switch through a sequence of movements to operate a different movement.

Pattern recognition

In *pattern recognition* myoelectric control, patterns of muscle activation (rather than single muscle site activation) are used to control different DOFs.[19] An array of electrodes over 1 or more muscles picks up numerous myoelectric signals, which are processed and classified (translated) by an on-board microprocessor into control signals.[16] Specific muscle activation patterns are designated to control specific grip patterns or other movements during prosthesis fitting and training.

Pattern recognition myoelectric control has several potential advantages over direct control: (1) users can go from one grip pattern or movement to another without the separate switch step (muscle co-contraction, etc.); (2) independent muscle signals free of cross-talk are *not* required; and (3) users may find the control to be more intuitive.[20] Furthermore, pattern recognition has the potential to allow simultaneous control of multiple DOF or movements, which is especially advantageous in the setting of additional powered joints (eg, simultaneously closing the hand while extending the elbow).[21] Potential drawbacks of pattern recognition include a patient may not have sufficient area for the electrode array in the prosthetic design, and accuracy in classification of muscle activation patterns varies.[22,23]

Other Externally Powered Control Mechanisms

Although the term "myoelectric" is sometimes used to refer broadly to powered upper limb components, not all EP components are controlled by myoelectric input. In fact, some components that use myoelectric control also have other input pathways. Other potential mechanisms of input include hardware switches (eg, manual bump switches or cable-pull mechanical switches), buttons, linear potentiometers, movement detection, and force sensing resistors.[18] Utilizing an alternate control mechanism alongside myoelectric control is a potential strategy to allow simultaneous operation in multiple DOF.

Linear potentiometers translate linear movements, such as generated by a control cable from a BP prosthesis, into electrical signal. This can allow proportional control. One centimeter of excursion is considered sufficient for a prosthesis user to utilize this type of control.

Externally Powered Components

Myoelectric hands vary in DOF, number of actuators (effectors of movement), grip (prehension) patterns, maximum grip force and carry load, size, weight, compatibility with other devices, and other characteristics.[1,24–26] Some myoelectric hands have multiple fingers controlled by an actuator, some have actuators for flexion/extension of each finger and for thumb opposition (or more), while some require passive thumb movement.[24,27] There is a wide range of variation in grasp force and carry load among commercial myoelectric components, which is at least partially attributable to differences in materials.[24–26] Preprogrammed grip patterns in commercial myoelectric hands range from 3 to more than 10. Some commercial hands have *adaptive grip,* in which the grip conforms to the shape of different objects.

There are also several myoelectric TDs designed to have a single grasping function, similar to a BP split-hook TD.[27] Some myoelectric hands or upper limb units have integrated powered wrists with at least 1 DOF, while some incorporate passive wrist movement.[24] There are several myoelectric elbows, as well as EP elbows controlled by mechanical switch, which may weigh less than available myoelectric components.

Additional considerations in component selection

While it might be assumed that more grip patterns or DOF are better, the practicality and ease of use of available movements and the ease of switching between movements are more important than the designed capabilities of a component. Furthermore, increase in intended features may be accompanied by an increase in component weight, for example, if the number of actuators is increased.[27]

Comparison of myoelectric control with body-powered control

The decision on using EP (usually myoelectric) components or BP can be impacted by a number of considerations, and there is insufficient evidence to recommend for or against specific control strategies.[28–30]

- The operation of BP prostheses is intuitive and generally requires less training than myoelectric systems.
- BP prostheses generally require less adjustments and are less sensitive to changes in fit compared to myoelectric prostheses.
- BP prostheses are easier to clean, more durable, and more suitable for use in rougher environments or heavy-duty activities than myoelectric prostheses.
- BP prostheses have sensory feedback for grip force and proprioception, while myoelectric prostheses historically have not provided sensory feedback. (However, some modern myoelectric components have incorporated sensory feedback features.)
- BP prostheses may have a faster time from prescription to fitting and readiness for use due to the combination of being potentially easier to fit and less expensive, which in turn may influence success and adoption of prosthesis use.
- Switching between TDs may be more difficult with BP prostheses as the control cable must be disconnected and reconnected.
- BP hooks (not hands) have excellent prehension abilities.
- Myoelectric prostheses are often considered to have better cosmesis than BP prostheses.
- Subject-matter expertise of the interdisciplinary team may be particularly important for myoelectric prostheses. The prosthetist and occupational therapist may need to spend a large amount of time training or collaborating with device specialists.

HYBRID CONTROL

A hybrid-controlled prosthesis has BP and EP elements.[11] Hybrid control is typically seen with transhumeral prostheses, for example, with a BP elbow and a myoelectric hand. Hybrid prostheses could have several advantages compared to a dual-cable control full BP system or all EP control:[29]

- A hybrid prosthesis typically weighs less than most EP elbow and TD combinations.
- With a hybrid BP elbow and myoelectric TD, the user does not need to lock the elbow to operate the TD. Furthermore, the excursion requirement to move the elbow is lessened.
- Can permit simultaneous control (performing simultaneous functions, such as elbow flexion and grasp).

Ability to create excursion to operate a BP joint and candidate sites for myoelectric pickup are factors in determining if a hybrid control system would be suitable.

SOCKETS, SUSPENSION, AND INTERFACE

Design priorities for socket, suspension, and interface of upper limb prostheses include comfortable load forces, stabilization of the prosthesis, utilizing available range of motion, and secure suspension of the prosthesis.[31–33] Maintaining consistent residual limb contact with electrodes is essential for myoelectric prostheses, and many socket designs have been developed with an eye toward this goal.[34]

Prosthetic sockets

Sockets for upper limb prostheses are often *double walled*, with an inner socket that surrounds the residual limb closely and an outer wall with profile similar to an anatomic limb. (This is exoskeletal design, but the term "double-walled" is often used when referring to upper limb prostheses.) Double-walled (exoskeletal) design was originally used to improve the durability of prostheses in the early era of fabrication using laminates. While durability of single-walled sockets is less of a concern with newer materials, double-walled sockets are often used in upper limb prostheses for improved cosmesis and to house elements of powered control systems.

Self-suspending sockets utilize anatomic structure to create suspension, thus obviating the need for a harness or other suspension method. A socket that can "grab the boney structures" well can provide good stability and control.[34] For BP or hybrid upper limb prostheses, this could allow the use of a figure-of-nine harness, which is solely a control cable anchor, rather than a figure-of-eight, which provides both prosthesis suspension and anchoring of cables.

Thermoplastic inner flexible sockets are often used for myoelectric upper limb prostheses. The flexible inner allows for placement of surface electrodes, is a suitable surface for skin-fit suction, and may add some ability to accommodate for volume changes. However, inner flexible sockets add bulk and weight to the prosthesis.

Transradial sockets

The Muenster socket was designed to provide self-suspension (socket-based suspension) for persons with short transradial limbs, aiming to create stability by anteroposterior compression in the cubital fold.[31,35] The Northwestern socket, or Northwestern University Supracondylar Suspension Technique, was designed to provide self-suspension for longer residual limbs.[31,35] The Northwestern design created mediolateral compression proximal to the humeral condyles. The features of these sockets that were intended to create self-suspension also limited range of motion at the elbow and made donning and doffing the prosthesis more difficult.[32] There are numerous newer strategies for transradial self-suspension that may alleviate these concerns, such as the window over the posterior elbow seen with the three-fourth transradial socket.[35]

Transhumeral sockets

The soft tissue envelope and lack of distal bony structure to act as an anchor can make it challenging to achieve good socket stability and control.[34] Strategies to achieve better socket control and reduction of rotation include the use of harness-based suspension, the use of a socket design with trimlines that extend to the anterior and posterior shoulder, and others.[31,34]

Wrist disarticulation and elbow disarticulation sockets

Self-suspending sockets are often used for wrist disarticulation and elbow disarticulation levels of amputation, as close fit of the socket and interface about the distal bony structure can create secure suspension and control of rotation. This may allow trimlines of the socket and interface to be brought down (or made more distal), potentially allowing more motion at proximal joints.[36]

Compression/release stabilized sockets

The compression-stabilized interface (socket) design, also called the high-fidelity socket, is intended to stabilize the longitudinal axis by creating longitudinal alternating compression and release.[32] This socket design is thought to be particularly helpful in the setting of transhumeral amputation, where the soft tissue envelopes create a challenging environment for achieving good socket stability and control, and for myoelectric limbs, where socket stability and consistent residual limb contact are paramount.[32]

Suspension and Interface

As described in other sections, there are upper limb prosthetic harnesses that function as both suspension mechanism and cable anchors. Self-suspension is still employed, especially for the wrist or elbow disarticulation levels. Harnesses are sometimes used as adjunct or additional suspension, or to help reduce socket rotation.[34] At the transradial level, suspension is typically anatomic or harness. At the transfemoral level, suspension is typically with suction, harness, or pin-lock.

Traditionally, socks were often the only interface between the hard socket and the residual limb, and this is still seen with socket-based suspension or harness-based suspension. Elastomer prosthetic liners are used for pin-lock suspension.

SUMMARY

In this article, the authors introduced the basics of BP and EP control for upper limb prostheses, and other features of upper limb prosthetics design. Upper limb prosthetics is considered to be a very specialized area of clinical care.[37] With some basic understanding of the concepts presented in this article, non-prosthetist team members can better communicate and collaborate with prosthetists in the care of patients with upper limb amputation.

CLINICS CARE POINTS

- VO hooks are generally preferred to hand-shaped TDs as they are lightweight, allow good visualization of the object to be grasped, and work well for heavy-duty activities. Grip force is controlled by rubber bands.

- In comparison to VO hooks, VC hooks allow variable grip force. VC hooks require continuous effort and cable tension to maintain grasp and may obstruct visualization of objects.

- The movements used to operate the TD of a BP device are glenohumeral flexion and biscapular protraction (abduction).

- For upper limb prostheses, harnesses are sometimes used for suspension alone, sometimes used for both suspension and cable anchoring (BP devices), and sometimes used only for anchoring (BP devices).

- BP upper limb prostheses are low weight and durable, provide sensory feedback, and have very good prehensile function. BP systems may be more robust to socket fit changes than EP devices.

- In comparison to BP devices, upper limb EP devices are heavy and less durable. EP devices can allow users to operate a TD in a larger area and utilize different grasps. EP devices may have a preferable cosmetic appearance to some users.

DISCLOSURES

None of the authors have any commercial or financial conflicts of interest and any funding sources.

REFERENCES

1. Vujaklija I, Farina D. Mechatronic Design of Functional Prosthetic Systems. In: Aszmann OC, Oskar CA, Farina D, Dario F, editors. Bionic limb reconstruction. Cham: Springer; 2021. p. 77–93.
2. Light TR. Kinesiology of the upper limb. In: Krajbich JI, Pinzur MS, Potter BK, editors. Atlas of amputations and limb deficiencies: surgical, prosthetic, and rehabilitation principles, vol. 1. Rosemont, IL: American Academy of Orthopaedic Surgeons; 2023. p. 222–55.
3. Alpenfels EJ. The anthropology and social significance of the human hand. Artif Limbs 1955;2(2):4–21.
4. Napier JR. The prehensile movements of the human hand. J Bone Joint Surg Br 1956;38-B(4):902–13.
5. Taylor CL, Schwarz RJ. The anatomy and mechanics of the human hand. Artif Limbs 1955;2(2):22–35.
6. Kamakura N, Matsuo M, Ishii H, et al. Patterns of static prehension in normal hands. Am J Occup Ther 1980;34(7):437–45.
7. Casanova JS, Grunert BK. Adult prehension: Patterns and nomenclature for pinches. J Hand Ther 1989;2(4):231–44.
8. Hashim NA, Abd Razak NA, Abu Osman NA, et al. Improvement on upper limb body-powered prostheses (1921–2016): A systematic review. Proc Inst Mech Eng H 2018;232(1):3–11.
9. Rotter D. Harnessing and controls for upper limb body-powered prostheses. In: Krajbich JI, Pinzur MS, Potter BK, editors. Atlas of amputations and limb deficiencies: surgical, prosthetic, and rehabilitation principles, vol. 2. Rosemont, IL: American Academy of Orthopaedic Surgeons; 2023. p. 506–69.
10. Michael JW, Stevens PM. Lower limb prosthetic components: updated classification and passive, body-powered components. In: Krajbich JI, Pinzure MS, Potter BK, editors. Atlas of amputations and limb deficiencies, vol. 3, 4th edition. Rosemont, IL: American Academy of Orthopaedic Surgeons; 2016. p. 429–44.
11. Uellendahl J. Body-powered prosthetic systems. In: Aszmann OC, Farina D, editors. Bionic limb reconstruction. Cham, Switzerland: Springer International Publishing; 2021. p. 56–75.
12. Smit G, Bongers RM, Van der Sluis CK, et al. Efficiency of voluntary opening hand and hook prosthetic devices: 24 years of development? J Rehabil Res Dev 2012; 49(4):523–34.
13. Bajaj NM, Spiers AJ, Dollar AM. State of the Art in Artificial Wrists: A Review of Prosthetic and Robotic Wrist Design. IEEE Trans Robot 2019;35(1).
14. Stark G, Gerald S, LeBlanc M, et al. Overview of body-powered upper extremity prostheses. In: Meier RH, Robert H, Atkins DJ, et al, editors. Functional restoration of adults and children with upper extremity amputation. New York: Demos Medical Pub; 2004. p. 175–86.
15. Hess A. Upper limb body-powered components. In: Krajbich JI, Pinzur MS, Potter BK, et al, editors. Atlas of amputations and limb deficiencies: surgical, prosthetic, and rehabilitation principles. 5th edition. Rosemont, IL: American Academy of Orthopaedic Surgeons; 2023. p. 424–506.
16. Hahne J, Janne H, Prahm C, Cosima P, Vujaklija I, Ivan V, Farina D, Dario F. Control Strategies for Functional Upper Limb Prostheses. In: Aszmann OC, Oskar CA, Farina D, Dario F, editors. Bionic limb reconstruction. Cham: Springer; 2021. p. 285–308.

17. Lake C, Miguelez JM. Comparative analysis of microprocessors in upper limb prosthetics. J Prosthet Orthot 2003;15(2):48–63.
18. Hosie RS, Lock BA. Control options for upper limb externally powered components. In: Krajbich JI, Pinzur MS, Potter BK, et al, editors. Atlas of amputations and limb deficiencies: surgical, prosthetic, and rehabilitation principles. Rosemont, IL: American Academy of Orthopaedic Surgeons; 2023. p. 637–62.
19. Scheme E, Englehart K. Electromyogram pattern recognition for control of powered upper-limb prostheses: State of the art and challenges for clinical use. J Rehabil Res Dev 2011;48(6):643.
20. Zhang W, White M, Zahabi M, et al. Cognitive workload in conventional direct control vs. pattern recognition control of an upper-limb prosthesis. In: 2016 IEEE International Conference on Systems, Man, and Cybernetics. October 9 - 12, 2016. Budapest, Hungary. SMC 2016 - Conference Proceedings. 2017.
21. Young AJ, Smith LH, Rouse EJ, et al. A comparison of the real-time controllability of pattern recognition to conventional myoelectric control for discrete and simultaneous movements. J NeuroEng Rehabil 2014;11(1).
22. Van Der Niet Otr O, Reinders-Messelink HA, Bongers RM, et al. The i-LIMB hand and the DMC plus hand compared: A case report. Prosthet Orthot Int 2010;34(2): 216–20.
23. Roche AD, Rehbaum H, Farina D, et al. Prosthetic myoelectric control strategies: a clinical perspective. Curr Surg Rep 2014;2(3).
24. Calado A, Soares F, Matos D. A review on commercially available anthropomorphic myoelectric prosthetic hands, pattern-recognition-based microcontrollers and sEMG Sensors used for Prosthetic Control. In: 19th IEEE International Conference on Autonomous Robot Systems and Competitions April 24-26, 2019. Porto, Portugal, ICARSC. 2019.
25. Belter JT, Segil JL, Dollar AM, et al. Mechanical design and performance specifications of anthropomorphic prosthetic hands: A review. J Rehabil Res Dev 2013; 50(5):599–618.
26. Belter JT, Dollar AM. Performance characteristics of anthropomorphic prosthetic hands. In: IEEE International Conference on Rehabilitation Robotics June 29 - July 1, 2011. Zurich, Switzerland. 2011.
27. Damerla R, Qiu Y, Sun TM, et al. A Review of the Performance of Extrinsically Powered Prosthetic Hands. IEEE Trans Med Robot Bionics 2021;3(3).
28. Carey SL, Lura DJ, Highsmith MJ. Differences in myoelectric and body-powered upper-limb prostheses: Systematic literature review. J Rehabil Res Dev 2015; 52(3):247–62.
29. Uellendahl J. Myoelectric versus body-powered upper-limb prostheses: a clinical perspective. J Prosthet Orthot 2017;29(4):25–9.
30. Crunkhorn A, Andrews E, Fantini C, et al. Management of upper limb amputation rehabilitation. Am J Phys Med Rehabil 2023;102(3):245–53.
31. Lake C. The evolution of upper limb prosthetic socket design. J Prosthet Orthot 2008;20(3):85–92.
32. Alley RD, Williams TW, Albuquerque MJ, et al. Prosthetic sockets stabilized by alternating areas of tissue compression and release. J Rehabil Res Dev 2011; 48(6):669–96.
33. Stark G, Fantini C. Elbow disarticulation and transhumeral amputation. In: Krajbich JI, Pinzur MS, Potter BK, editors. Atlas of amputations and limb deficiencies: surgical, prosthetic, and rehabilitation principles, vol. 2. Rosemont, IL: American Academy of Orthopaedic Surgeons; 2023. p. 837–89.

34. Andrew JT. Transhumeral and elbow disarticulation anatomically contoured socket considerations. J Prosthet Orthot 2008;20(3):107–17.
35. Sang Y, Li X, Luo Y. Biomechanical design considerations for transradial prosthetic interface: A review. Proc Inst Mech Eng H 2016;230(3).
36. Fantini C, Stark GE. Wrist disarticulation and transradial amputation. In: Krajbich JI, Pinzur MS, Potter BK, editors. Atlas of amputations and limb deficiencies: surgical, prosthetic, and rehabilitation principles, vol. 2. Rosemont, IL: American Academy of Orthopaedic Surgeons; 2023. p. 759–811.
37. Lake C, Dodson R. Progressive upper limb prosthetics. Phys Med Rehabil Clin N Am 2006;17(1).

Predicting Functional Outcomes Following Dysvascular Lower Limb Amputation

An Evidence Review of Personalizing Patient Outcomes

Daniel C. Norvell, PhD[a],*, Alison W. Henderson, PhD[b],
Elizabeth G. Halsne, PhD, CPO[a], David C. Morgenroth, MD[a]

KEYWORDS

- Amputation • Prosthetics • Predicting outcomes • Decision support tools

KEY POINTS

- Amputation-level and prosthesis prescription decisions are complex and can significantly impact future functional outcomes and quality of life for people with limb loss.
- The ability to predict individualized functional outcomes following amputation is a key element in providing personalized rehabilitation.
- Decision support tools and patient decision aids used for shared decision-making can reduce decisional conflict between providers and patients, leading to greater decisional satisfaction and quality of life.

INTRODUCTION

More than 1 million individuals live with a major lower limb amputation (LLA) in the United States.[1] Annually, over 150,000 individuals in the United States undergo LLAs (including partial foot) related to peripheral artery disease (PAD) or diabetes.[2] Due to increasing rates of dysvascular disease, including PAD and diabetes, it is predicted that the population with LLA will double by 2050,[1] giving rise to an increasing overall health care burden.[3]

[a] VA Center for Limb Loss and Mobility (CLiMB), VA Puget Sound Health Care System, 1660 South Columbian Way, MS 151-R, Seattle, WA 98108, USA; [b] Department of Rehabilitation Medicine, University of Washington, 325 Ninth Avenue, Box 359612, Seattle, WA 98104, USA
* Corresponding author. 1660 South Columbian Way, Seattle, WA 98108.
E-mail address: daniel.norvell@va.gov

Phys Med Rehabil Clin N Am 35 (2024) 833–850
https://doi.org/10.1016/j.pmr.2024.06.005   **pmr.theclinics.com**
1047-9651/24/© 2024 Elsevier Inc. All rights are reserved, including those for text and data mining, AI training, and similar technologies.

LLA due to dysvascular disease can be performed at different levels. Many factors influence the choice of amputation level, including limb perfusion, the presence of comorbidities, prior mobility status, social support system availability, surgeons' clinical experience, individual prioritization of each outcome, and knowledge of the existing evidence. The most common major amputation levels are across the middle portion of the foot (transmetatarsal [TM]), between the knee and the ankle (transtibial [TT]) and between the hip and the knee (transfemoral [TF]). There is no clear evidence in favor of one amputation level over another in the setting of dysvascular disease,[4,5] and thus, there is uncertainty as to which level will result in the best patient outcomes. Further, several studies have indicated that clinician knowledge of factors contributing to poor outcomes is lacking.[6,7] Similarly, while appropriate prosthesis prescription is critical in the successful rehabilitation of those with LLA, predicting a patient's probable level of prosthesis mobility to aid in matching an appropriate prosthesis and rehabilitation plan lacks guiding evidence[8] and is challenging.[9] The purpose of this review is to provide an evidence-based discussion of the impact that amputation level, prosthesis provision, and patient-specific factors have on future patient functional outcomes. In addition, considering how patient-specific factors may predict future function (ie, personalized rehabilitation) will lead to improved outcomes in key domains. We have thus organized this review by discussing (1) the impact that amputation level and prosthesis prescription have on key outcomes; (2) the importance of how predicting outcomes may help facilitate deciding on the optimal amputation level (when a decision is possible) and prosthesis prescription; (3) predicting outcomes and personalized rehabilitation; (4) existing published prediction models; and (5) how prediction models can be leveraged to develop decision support tools to facilitate provider/patient shared decision-making (SDM) to ensure decisions consider each individual patient's priorities and preferences.

LOWER LIMB AMPUTATION LEVELS EFFECT ON OUTCOMES

Among those able to walk prior to their amputation surgery, individuals with TF amputations are significantly less likely to return to ambulation than those with TT amputations,[10] rendering a more distal amputation potentially more functionally advantageous. However, the potential mobility benefits of a more distal amputation may not be realized because of the increased risk of delayed or compromised healing, especially at the TM level.[11] Failure of healing results in the need for ongoing wound care and potential reamputation at a more proximal level, which may result in a loss of functional mobility that exceeds that which would have occurred if the amputation was performed at a more proximal level initially.[12,13] An additional critical factor in the decision process is mortality risk; amputation secondary to dysvascular disease results in a higher mortality risk than in the majority of cancer diagnoses,[14] with average 1 and 5 year mortality risks as high as 44% and 77%, respectively.[15] The limited survival period creates an imperative to make decisions that will best ensure patients' remaining life years are lived consistent with their priorities and preferences. The challenge is that each patient is unique; therefore, relying on population averages when counseling an individual patient often falls short of helping providers and patients make informed decisions that are specific to the individual patient's attributes and goals.

PREDICTING FUNCTIONAL OUTCOMES TO AID IN AMPUTATION-LEVEL DECISIONS

In some cases, especially in emergencies, there are limited amputation-level options (ie, an obvious level is warranted, or there is no time to consider options). However, in many dysvascular amputations, more than one amputation-level option is viable, and the decision involves weighing multiple risks and benefits for each level (eg, more distal amputation levels may lead to better mobility outcomes but may increase the risk of poor healing, sometimes necessitating reamputation at a more proximal level). Poor amputation-level decisions can have a significant negative impact on quality of life (QoL) and likewise can prove costly to the health care system.[16,17] An evidence-based approach to predicting functional outcomes will facilitate better amputation-level decision-making. A recent systematic review concluded that surgeons are generally good at predicting perioperative risk but are poor at predicting longer term outcomes.[18] Predicting future functional outcomes will not only facilitate improved transparency regarding surgical implications, but greater knowledge of a future outcome often leads to greater decisional satisfaction and decreased decisional conflict.[19,20] Physician decisional conflict has been associated with decreased well-being, poor work satisfaction,[21] poor patient compliance,[22] and poorer quality of care,[23] all of which lead to poor patient outcomes. Among patients living with diabetes, there is a positive relationship between decisional conflict and distress,[24] and several studies have found that diabetes-related distress is associated with reduced QoL and poor psychological well-being.[25,26] Therefore, the ability to predict functional outcomes based on the choice of amputation level will better inform providers and patients so they can make decisions that align most with each patient's priorities and preferences, which will play a prominent role in reducing decisional conflict and improve QoL for patients and providers alike.

PATIENT INVOLVEMENT IN AMPUTATION-LEVEL DECISIONS

Patient involvement in amputation-level decision-making is often limited. In a recent qualitative study, 22 patients and 21 providers were interviewed regarding amputation-level decisions among patients with dysvascular disease. Four themes were identified: (1) providers recognized the importance of incorporating patient preferences into amputation-level decisions and strived to do so; (2) patients did not perceive that they are included as equal partners in decisions around amputation or amputation level; (3) providers perceived several obstacles to including patients in amputation-level decisions; and (4) patients described facilitators to their involvement including presentation of clear, concise information, and the importance of communicating concern during the discussion.[27]

PREDICTING FUNCTIONAL OUTCOMES TO AID IN PROSTHESIS PRESCRIPTION

For patients whose amputations heal and who are candidates to walk again, restoring mobility through rehabilitation and lower limb prosthesis (LLP) fitting is associated with improved QoL.[28,29] Increased prosthesis use has been associated with higher levels of independence and function through improved self-care and mobility,[30] employment success,[31] and improved perceived QoL.[32–34] Successful prosthesis provision is, therefore, integral to the rehabilitation of those with LLA. However, predicting a patient's probable level of prosthesis mobility to aid in matching an appropriate prosthesis and rehabilitation plan is challenging. LLP prescription includes a multitude of choices including socket design, socket interface, suspension system, prosthetic feet, and prosthetic knees in the case of TF amputation.

There are myriad choices for prosthetic feet and knee components, which vary immensely in their cost and design characteristics. Prosthesis prescription typically includes a comprehensive history and physical examination, often including an estimation of that patient's likely mobility potential. The Centers for Medicare and Medicaid Services developed a 5 level mobility classification system (Medicare Functional Classification Levels [MFCL] or "K-levels"), which is used in the civilian sector to determine approval of prosthesis type and cost for individual patients based upon their actual or potential for ambulation. Although the MFCL classification system has never been validated and its predictive validity is uncertain, it has been widely adopted and used as a national guideline matching functional mobility descriptors with the prescription of prosthetic devices.[35–37] Furthermore, prescribing clinicians do not have confidence in the accuracy or utility of the K-level system. In a survey of US prosthesis prescribers, 67% of respondents did not believe that the K-level system accurately assigns a level of rehabilitation potential.[9]

The language in each K-level descriptor includes the "potential to ambulate," which is used to determine the medical necessity for certain prosthetic components or additional features. Given the importance that "potential" mobility has on prosthetic component provision, it is vital to predict future mobility as accurately as possible. However, there is a lack of evidence to guide prosthesis prescription as reported in a prior Cochrane review[8] and illustrated practically in a qualitative study including 23 experienced rehabilitation clinicians,[38] which highlighted the difficulties clinicians experience in estimating outcomes and suggested inequity of prosthesis provision and variation in the provision of high-cost items because of these challenges. The primary challenge is predicting an individual patient's future mobility, thereby making it difficult to prescribe a prosthetic limb to match that mobility. This results in significant concerns of providing a prosthetic limb that will be inadequate for optimally restoring mobility or potentially exposing patients to the risk of injury related to falls and a potential loss of functional life years.[39]

PREDICTING OUTCOMES FOR PERSONALIZED REHABILITATION

In addition to the importance of predicting mobility outcomes in general, considering each patient's unique characteristics and goals is vital. Personalized medicine (also known as precision medicine) shifts away from traditional "one-size-fits-all" approaches to patient care, which have often been deemed ineffective, inefficient, and not driven by patient values.[40] Personalized medicine is accomplished by predicting patients' specific risks for key outcomes so that interventions can be delivered at the right time, place, and setting to improve overall outcomes.[41,42] As computing power increases, the ability to use advanced machine learning techniques to identify and quantify personalized risk has improved.[43] Personalized medicine is well underway in many medical disciplines, including genetics and oncology; however, the power of personalized medicine in rehabilitation is emerging (ie, personalized rehabilitation).[40] Predicting functional outcomes is essential to achieve personalized rehabilitation through prediction modeling. Prediction models enable the determination of how individual patient characteristics lead to probable outcomes.[40,44–46] The implementation of these models needs to be done with careful thought and planning to include experienced teams with diverse scientific and clinical backgrounds to ensure maximum accuracy and utility.[45,47,48] In order to enhance the likelihood of clinical translation of prediction models, it is important to include predictors that are easy to collect[40] and that do not add significant clinician time.[49]

PREDICTION MODELS FOR PEOPLE WITH LOWER LIMB AMPUTATION

Since personalized medicine is dependent on prediction models, knowing what is available in the literature concerning prediction models in people with LLA is important. A recently published systematic review identified and evaluated the performance characteristics of post-LLA outcome prediction models.[50] This systematic search of decades of literature identified 12 studies describing 13 prediction models. Among the 13 models (one predicting two outcomes), 9 predicted mortality,[51–59] 2 predicted postoperative morbidity,[51,58] 2 predicted mobility,[60,61] and 1 predicted reamputation.[62] Among the 9 mortality prediction models, 8 models predicted short-term risk (30 days or in hospital) and only 1 predicted 12 month risk.[59] The 2 mobility prediction models predicted 12 month mobility, one assessed predictors at the time of prosthesis prescription[60] and the other predicted mobility prior to amputation in patients undergoing an incident TM, TT, and TF amputation.[61] The latter model does not require a prosthesis prescription and can be used alongside the comparable mortality and reamputation risk models at the time of the amputation-level decision.[59,62] Only 4 studies exclusively included patients undergoing an incident (ie, first) amputation.[58,59,61,62] The remaining studies included a mixture of incident and reamputations. Such heterogeneous populations that do not separate or isolate first from repeat amputations can confound the functional outcome predictions, thus rendering it unclear whether it was the sequelae of prior surgeries versus other factors contributing to the predicted risks. Clinical translation for individual patients can be more challenging when using data from more heterogenous samples.

Two recent models that predict mobility have been published since the aforementioned systematic review. One predicts 12 month post-prescription mobility at the time of prosthesis prescription[63] and the other predicts 6 month mobility after discharge from rehabilitation (mixture of inpatient and outpatient) with a prosthesis.[64] Finally, one model that predicts reamputation was developed based on predictors available in the preamputation period and predicts reamputation to the same or higher level within 12 months of incident amputation.[62] **Table 1** lists each of these models and summarizes the final predictors included in the model.

A major challenge in the utility of prediction models is their ease of clinical application. While the dissemination of prediction models through publication is an important first step, it falls short of translating science into tools readily available at the point of care. Clinical translation requires converting these models into point-of-care tools that can predict future outcomes as part of the clinical workflow. Progress in technology and available data create unprecedented opportunities for prediction models to inform, personalize, and improve care by developing decision support tools,[65] as described further later.

DECISION SUPPORT TOOLS FACILITATE THE CLINICAL TRANSLATION OF PREDICTION MODELS

Prediction models that are converted to point-of-care decision support tools have the greatest potential to be implemented clinically and thereby positively impact patient care and outcomes. However, despite the existence of the 13 prediction models discussed earlier, few have been converted into decision support tools. Evidence-based decision support tools, which often come in the form of a risk calculator, have been shown to be more effective at estimating future outcomes than clinical "gestalt," which is subject to potential biases.[18] Three of the published prediction models described earlier[59,61,62] have been translated into a point-of-care decision support tool to aid in amputation-level decision-making known as the AMPREDICT decision support tool (www.ampredict.org; **Fig. 1**).[49] The single tool predicts 12 month postamputation mortality, reamputation, and mobility at the TM, TT, and TF levels based on the 3 validated models. It has been used by over 3500 providers from 66 countries. It has a parallel set of patient-facing tools known as the AMPDECIDE patient decision aids (PtDAs) to aid in the TM versus TT and TT versus TF decisions (www.ampdecide.org/decison-making; **Fig. 2**). A separate PtDA has been developed to assist in the

Table 1
Studies reporting on risk prediction models and factors involved in risk prediction*

Study	Tool Used	Predicted Outcomes	Predictors Included in Risk Tool
Feinglass et al,[53] 2001	Novel tool (un-named)	30 d mortality	TT 30 d mortality: *Comorbidities:* Current smoker, dyspnea at rest, totally dependent functional health status, COPD, previous revascularization/amputation, gangrene, hepatomegaly, HTN (requiring treatment), dialysis, CVA with no neurologic deficit, impaired sensorium, disseminated cancer, ASA IV or V *Labs:* Albumin TF 30 d mortality: *Demographics:* Age, DNR status, Emergency operation *Comorbidities:* Current pneumonia, ventilator dependent, HTN (requiring treatment), disseminated cancer, ASA IV *Labs:* Bilirubin, K, Urea, WCC
Tang et al,[57] 2009	Novel modified "VBHOM"	30 d mortality	*Demographics:* Age, gender, mode of admission *Investigations:* Hb, WCC, urea, creatinine, Na, K
Nelson et al,[55] 2012	Novel tool (un-named)	30 d mortality	*Demographics:* Age *Comorbidities:* Dependent functional status, dialysis, steroid use, preoperative sepsis, impaired sensorium (confusion/delirium), DNR status *Labs:* Thrombocytopenia, increased INR, and azotemia
Patterson et al,[56] 2012	VBHOM and a novel modified VBHOM	30 d mortality	*Demographics:* Age *Labs:* Na, K, creatinine, albumin
Easterlin et al,[52] 2013	Novel tool (un-named)	30 d mortality	*Demographics:* Age *Comorbidities:* CHF, COPD, major cardiac surgery, steroid use, dependent functional status, dyspnea, dialysis, impaired sensorium, preoperative sepsis
Wied et al,[58] 2016	Surgical Apgar score	30 d mortality and major morbidity	*Operative factors:* Estimated blood loss, intraoperative lowest mean arterial pressure, intraoperative lowest heart rate

Study	Tool	Outcome	Variables
Czerniecki et al,[61] 2017	Novel "AMPREDICT-mobility"	1 year ambulation	*Demographics:* Age, BMI, race, married/partnered *Comorbidities:* DM, dialysis, COPD, treatment of anxiety/depression, self-rated health *Operative factors:* Amputation level
Norvell et al,[59] 2019	Novel "AMPREDICT-mortality"	1 year mortality	*Demographics:* Age, BMI, race *Comorbidities:* Functional status, CHF, dialysis *Labs:* Urea, WCC, and platelet count *Operative factors:* Amputation level
Jolissaint et al,[54] 2019	Novel tool (un-named)	30 d mortality	*Demographics:* Age, DNR status *Comorbidities:* CKD, COPD, CHF, CAD, dependent living status *Operative factors:* Amputation level (TF)
Czerniecki et al,[62] 2019	Novel "AMPREDICT-reamputation"	1 year reamputation	*Demographics:* Sex *Comorbidities:* Current smoker, alcohol abuse, rest pain/gangrene, anticoagulant therapy, DM, COPD, CKD, previous revascularization *Labs:* WCC *Operative factors:* Amputation level
Bowrey et al,[60] 2019	Novel "BLARt" score	1 year ambulation	*Demographics:* Age, gender, BMI *Comorbidities:* Cause of amputations (trauma, congenital, orthopedic, cancer, vascular), cognitive capacity, preamputation mobility, severe respiratory disease, dialysis, CVA/neurologic disease, recent MI/Angina, contralateral limb problem *Operative factors:* Amputation level
Ambler et al,[51] 2020	Novel "UKAmpRisk"	In-hospital mortality and major morbidity	*Demographics:* Age, emergency admission, weight *Comorbidities:* Abnormal ECG, albumin, ASA grade *Labs:* Creatinine, WCC, previous ipsilateral intervention *Operative factors:* Bilateral/unilateral operation, amputation level

(continued on next page)

Table 1
(continued)

Study	Tool Used	Predicted Outcomes	Predictors Included in Risk Tool
Norvell et al,[63] 2023	Novel "AMPREDICT PROsthetics"	1 year mobility	*Demographics:* Age, BMI, marital Status *Comorbidities:* DM, dialysis, PAD, CAD, COPD, CHF, depression, anxiety, PTSD, schizophrenia, smoking, alcohol-use disorder, cocaine-use disorder, opioid-use disorder *Operative factors:* Amputation level, days to prosthetic prescription, history of revascularization
Wafi et al,[64] 2023	Novel tool (unnamed)	6 mo mobility	*Demographics:* Age, sex *Comorbidities:* Active malignancy, cerebrovascular disease, end-stage renal disease, cognitive impairment *Operative factors:* Amputation level

Abbreviations: ASA, American Society of Anesthesiologists; BLARt, Blatchford Allman Russell tool; BMI, body mass index; CAD, coronary artery disease; CHF, congestive heart failure; COPD, chronic obstructive pulmonary disease; CVA, cerebrovascular accident; DM, diabetes mellitus; DNR, do not attempt resuscitation order; Hb, hemoglobin; HTN, hypertension; INR, International normalized ratio; K, serum potassium; MI, myocardial infarction; Na, serum sodium; TF, transfemoral; VBHOM, vascular biochemistry and hematology outcome models; WCC, white cell count.
*Wied et al model predicts two outcomes.

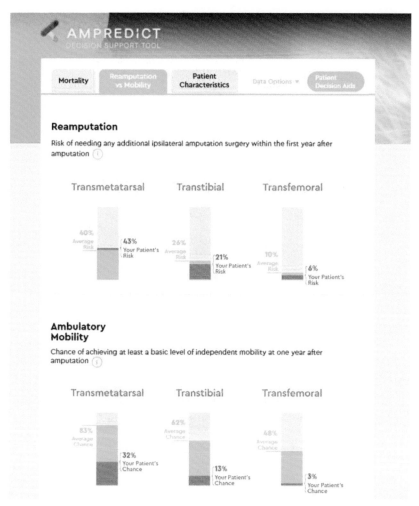

Fig. 1. Example from the AMPREDICT decision support tool. (With permission from AMPREDICT.)

partial foot versus TT amputation-level decision (www.amputationdecisionaid.com; **Fig. 3**).[66] The content available within these decision aid Web sites provides a plethora of high-quality information that emphasizes the critical importance of patients participating in the amputation-level decision consistent with their priorities and preferences. All these decision aids were developed using the International Patient Decision Aid Standards. In addition to the amputation-level decision support tools, the AMPREDICT PROsthetics prediction model[63] is currently being translated into an online point-of-care decision support tool to aid in prosthesis prescription and rehabilitation planning and will be available in the near future. Ultimately, being able to predict functional outcomes has the potential to lead to improved clinical outcomes, especially if there are tools available at the point of care; however, this is best accomplished when the risks generated from these tools are shared with the patient to empower them to participate in such critical decisions that will have a major impact on their remaining functional life years. A barrier to this process is inconsistent or poor provider

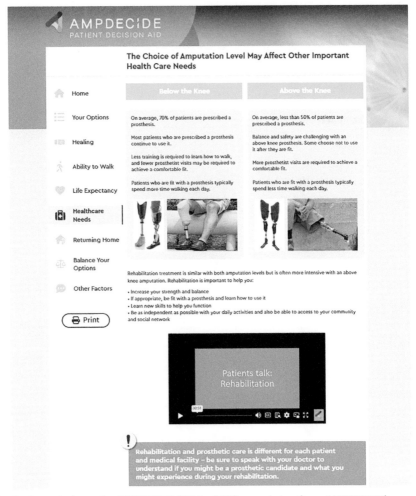

Fig. 2. Example from the AMPDECIDE PtDAs. (With permission from AMPREDICT.)

communication about treatment options and predicted outcomes.[67] Evidence-based clinical decision support tools, such as the PtDAs referenced earlier, help mitigate some of these barriers, acting as a supplement to important patient–provider conversations around treatment options to aid in SDM.[68]

USING DECISION SUPPORT TOOLS FOR SHARED DECISION-MAKING

Decision support tools, in the form of probability/risk calculators or PtDAs, are vital tools to facilitate SDM. SDM is "the process by which a health care provider communicates information about options, outcomes, probabilities, and scientific uncertainties of available treatment options, and the patient communicates his or her values and the relative importance he or she places on benefits and harms."[69] It occurs when an *informed clinician* involves an *informed patient* as a partner in treatment decisions, balancing the risks and benefits of different care options with the patient's priorities and preferences.[69] In SDM, the assumption that the health care provider is

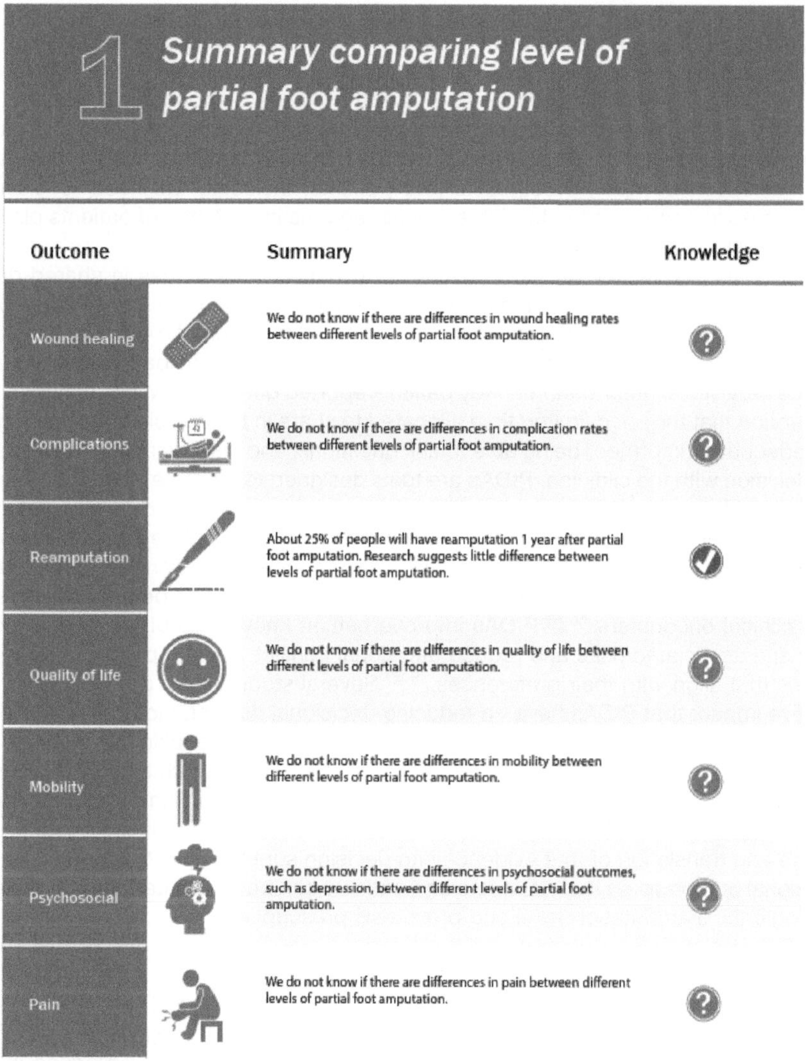

	Summary comparing level of partial foot amputation	
Outcome	**Summary**	**Knowledge**
Wound healing	We do not know if there are differences in wound healing rates between different levels of partial foot amputation.	?
Complications	We do not know if there are differences in complication rates between different levels of partial foot amputation.	?
Reamputation	About 25% of people will have reamputation 1 year after partial foot amputation. Research suggests little difference between levels of partial foot amputation.	✓
Quality of life	We do not know if there are differences in quality of life between different levels of partial foot amputation.	?
Mobility	We do not know if there are differences in mobility between different levels of partial foot amputation.	?
Psychosocial	We do not know if there are differences in psychosocial outcomes, such as depression, between different levels of partial foot amputation.	?
Pain	We do not know if there are differences in pain between different levels of partial foot amputation.	?

Fig. 3. Example from the amputation decision aid. (Dillon MP, Fatone S, Quigley M. (2017) A decision aid for people facing partial foot amputation due to peripheral arterial disease. http://amputationdecisionaid.com Accessed Dec 2023.)

the only party who needs to access evidence in decision-making is discarded.[70] It allows patients to play a part in, and be willing to commit to, potential outcomes when they are involved in the decision.[70] To help them cope, patients report wanting and needing more information about what to expect physically, functionally, and psychologically.[71,72]

Qualitative studies have identified important patient perceptions of rehabilitation after amputation with respect to a desire to be more informed.[73,74] In a study of patients who had undergone an LLA due to vascular disease and were about to undergo prosthesis rehabilitation, participants described having vague expectations secondary to being inadequately informed, which then led to passive participation in the rehabilitation process.[73] Primary recommendations from this study included the importance of clinicians having clear discussions with patients before and during prosthesis rehabilitation to help shape realistic expectations about future outcomes so they can take a more active, informed role in the process. Another qualitative study aimed to identify common interactions between individuals with LLA and prosthetists from the patient's point of view.[74] The results emphasized the need for improved communication between prosthetists and patients, including the need to discuss the process in a more understandable manner and the importance of patients playing a larger role in the decision-making.

In an extensive systematic review evaluating patient preferences in shared decisions, 71% of studies indicated that patients want to be active partners with their providers in making their health care decisions.[75] Another systematic review evaluating patient barriers to SDM indicated that the greatest barrier to participation was an inadequate provision of information.[76] Key patient-reported barriers identified included the perception that they had limited time allocated to share in the decision, including getting adequately informed, being able to ask questions, and discussing the tradeoffs of the decision with the clinician. PtDAs are tools designed to facilitate patient participation in health care decisions by describing the available options and helping patients determine their priorities and preferences around these options. They have been identified as an important tool to enhance the SDM process by serving as catalysts to engage patients in decision-making processes and can be used before, during, and after clinical encounters.[77,78] PtDAs improve patient knowledge of the possible options and associated risks and reduce decisional conflict, helping patients make decisions that align with their preferences.[79,80] Several studies have demonstrated the positive impact that PtDAs have on reducing decisional conflict, including in patients with cancer,[81] diabetes,[82] and osteoarthritis.[83] PtDAs have also been found to improve decisional knowledge and decisional satisfaction,[84] which are key outcomes noted earlier to positively influence quality of care, patient compliance, psychological well-being, and QoL. The critical element that ties this all together is the need for evidence and translation of that evidence into decision support tools that predict future functional outcomes so that providers and patients can be adequately informed when making critical amputation-level and prosthesis prescription decisions.

DISCUSSION

This evidence review aimed to provide an evidence-based discussion about the importance of predicting functional outcomes after LLA. More specifically, the authors covered applications in 2 key areas that impact future functional outcomes — amputation-level decision-making and prosthesis prescription. The focus was on the critical role that predicting future functional outcomes has in ensuring that decision-making in these areas is informed by the evidence of patient-specific factors. Clinical "gestalt," which is commonly used to make decisions, is often not sufficiently evidence-based and can lead to decisional conflict, leading to further downstream consequences and adverse effects on the QoL of patients and providers.

While traditional studies often report averages across population samples, personalized rehabilitation approaches to decision-making after LLA enable a more patient-centered method of accounting for different patients' unique characteristics and goals. Amputation level and prosthesis prescription are complex decisions that both benefit from being able to predict future function at the time of the decision, with corresponding tools to help facilitate communication and SDM between the provider and the patient. Prediction models are a key first step, but these models need to be translated into point-of-care tools (eg, provider-facing risk calculators and patient-facing decision aids) to facilitate clinical use and positive impacts on patient care. The AMPREDICT decision support tool for amputation-level decision-making,[49] its parallel AMPDECIDE PtDAs (www.ampdecide.org), as well as the Amputation Decision Aid (www.amputationdecisionaid.com)66 are useful examples of this translation and are being used by thousands of providers in dozens of countries. The next step in this translational evolution is the integration of decision support tools into the electronic health record for easy point-of-care access.

SUMMARY

Predicting functional outcomes in patients undergoing a dysvascular LLA is a critical step in personalizing both amputation level selection and prosthesis prescription, ensuring that these decisions align with individual patients' priorities and preferences. As we move into an era of personalized rehabilitation, prediction models are the first step. However, these models will only have an impact if they are translated into point-of-care decision support tools and PtDAs.

CLINICS CARE POINTS

- Personalized rehabilitation should be the goal when considering amputation-level and prosthesis prescription decisions in patients undergoing LLA for dysvascular disease.
- The ability to predict individualized functional outcomes following amputation is a key element in providing personalized rehabilitation.
- Decision support tools available at the point of care can ensure that patients receive the best evidence-based data regarding their future outcomes and will better allow them to participate in these critical decisions. Such tools are available and can be accessed at www.ampdecide.org and www.amputationdecisionaid.com.

DISCLOSURE

No authors have any commercial or financial conflicts of interest nor any funding sources to report at the time of this submission.

REFERENCES

1. Ziegler-Graham K, MacKenzie EJ, Ephraim PL, et al. Estimating the prevalence of limb loss in the United States: 2005 to 2050. Arch Phys Med Rehabil 2008;89(3): 422–9.
2. Dillingham TR, Pezzin LE, Shore AD. Reamputation, mortality, and health care costs among persons with dysvascular lower-limb amputations. Arch Phys Med Rehabil 2005;86(3):480–6.
3. Dillingham TR, Pezzin LE, MacKenzie EJ. Limb amputation and limb deficiency: epidemiology and recent trends in the United States. South Med J 2002;95(8): 875–83.
4. Heyns A, Jacobs S, Negrini S, et al. Systematic review of clinical practice guidelines for individuals with amputation: Identification of best evidence for rehabilitation to develop the WHO's package of interventions for rehabilitation. Arch Phys Med Rehabil 2021;102(6):1191–7.

5. Webster JB, Crunkhorn A, Sall J, et al. Clinical practice guidelines for the rehabilitation of lower limb amputation: an update from the Department of Veterans Affairs and Department of defense. Am J Phys Med Rehab 2019;98(9):820–9.

6. Klaphake S, de Leur K, Mulder PG, et al. Mortality after major amputation in elderly patients with critical limb ischemia. Clin Interv Aging 2017;12:1985–92.

7. van Netten JJ, Fortington LV, Hinchliffe RJ, et al. Early Post-operative Mortality After Major Lower Limb Amputation: A Systematic Review of Population and Regional Based Studies. Eur J Vasc Endovasc Surg 2016;51(2):248–57.

8. Hofstad C, Linde H, Limbeek J, et al. Prescription of prosthetic ankle-foot mechanisms after lower limb amputation. Cochrane Database Syst Rev 2004;2004(1): Cd003978.

9. Borrenpohl D, Kaluf B, Major MJ. Survey of U.S. Practitioners on the Validity of the Medicare Functional Classification Level System and Utility of Clinical Outcome Measures for Aiding K-Level Assignment. Arch Phys Med Rehabil 2016;97(7): 1053–63.

10. Cruz CP, Eidt JF, Capps C, et al. Major lower extremity amputations at a Veterans Affairs hospital. Am J Surg 2003;186(5):449–54.

11. Daniel CN, Czerniecki JM. Risks and risk factors for ipsilateral reamputation in the first year following first major unilateral dysvascular amputation. Euro J Vasc Endovasc Surg 2020;60(4):614–21.

12. O'Brien PJ, Cox MW, Shortell CK, et al. Risk factors for early failure of surgical amputations: an analysis of 8,878 isolated lower extremity amputation procedures. J Am Coll Surg 2013;216(4):836–42 [discussion 842-4].

13. Phair J, DeCarlo C, Scher L, et al. Risk factors for unplanned readmission and stump complications after major lower extremity amputation. J Vasc Surg 2018; 67(3):848–56.

14. Armstrong DG, Wrobel J, Robbins JM. Guest Editorial: are diabetes-related wounds and amputations worse than cancer? Int Wound J 2007;4(4):286–7.

15. Fortington LV, Geertzen JH, van Netten JJ, et al. Short and long term mortality rates after a lower limb amputation. Eur J Vasc Endovasc Surg 2013;46(1): 124–31.

16. Columbo JA, Davies L, Kang R, et al. Patient experience of recovery after major leg amputation for arterial disease. Vasc Endovasc Surg 2018;52(4):262–8.

17. Franklin H, Rajan M, Tseng CL, et al. Cost of lower-limb amputation in U.S. veterans with diabetes using health services data in fiscal years 2004 and 2010. J Rehabil Res Dev 2014;51(8):1325–30.

18. Dilaver NM, Gwilym BL, Preece R, et al. Systematic review and narrative synthesis of surgeons' perception of postoperative outcomes and risk. BJS Open 2020; 4(1):16–26.

19. Légaré F, Adekpedjou R, Stacey D, et al. Interventions for increasing the use of shared decision making by healthcare professionals. Cochrane Database Syst Rev 2018;(7).

20. Orom H, Biddle C, Underwood IIIW, et al. What is a "good" treatment decision? Decisional control, knowledge, treatment decision making, and quality of life in men with clinically localized prostate cancer. Med Decis Making 2016;36(6): 714–25.

21. Mishel MH, Germino BB, Lin L, et al. Managing uncertainty about treatment decision making in early stage prostate cancer: a randomized clinical trial. Patient Educ Counsel 2009;77(3):349–59. Epub 2009 Oct 9.

22. Meeuwesen L, van den Brink-Muinen A, Hofstede G. Can dimensions of national culture predict cross-national differences in medical communication? Patient Educ Counsel 2009;75(1):58–66. Epub 2008 Nov 13.

23. Mazzi MA, Rimondini M, Deveugele M, et al. What do people appreciate in physicians' communication? An international study with focus groups using video-taped medical consultations. Health Expect 2015;18(5):1215–26.

24. Bruno BA, Choi D, Thorpe KE, et al. Relationship among diabetes distress, decisional conflict, quality of life, and patient perception of chronic illness care in a cohort of patients with type 2 diabetes and other comorbidities. Diabetes Care 2019;42(7):1170–7. Epub 2019 May 2.

25. Glasgow RE, Ruggiero L, Eakin EG, et al. Quality of life and associated characteristics in a large national sample of adults with diabetes. Diabetes Care 1997; 20(4):562–7.

26. Jannoo Z, Wah YB, Lazim AM, et al. Examining diabetes distress, medication adherence, diabetes self-care activities, diabetes-specific quality of life and health-related quality of life among type 2 diabetes mellitus patients. J Clin Transl Endocrinol 2017;9:48–54.

27. Leonard C, Sayre G, Williams S, et al. Perceived shared decision-making among patients undergoing lower-limb amputation and their care teams: a qualitative study. Prosthet Orthot Int 2023;47(4):379–86.

28. Columbo JA, Nolan BW, Stucke RS, et al. Below-knee amputation failure and poor functional outcomes are higher than predicted in contemporary practice. Vasc Endovasc Surg 2016;50(8):554–8.

29. Suckow BD, Goodney PP, Nolan BW, et al. Domains that determine quality of life in vascular amputees. Ann Vasc Surg 2015;29(4):722–30.

30. Chan KM, Tan ES. Use of lower limb prosthesis among elderly amputees. Ann Acad Med Singapore 1990;19(6):811–6.

31. Whyte AS, Carroll LJ. A preliminary examination of the relationship between employment, pain and disability in an amputee population. Disabil Rehabil 2002;24(9):462–70.

32. Asano M, Rushton P, Miller WC, et al. Predictors of quality of life among individuals who have a lower limb amputation. Prosthet Orthot Int 2008;32(2):231–43.

33. Schaffalitzky E, Gallagher P, Maclachlan M, et al. Understanding the benefits of prosthetic prescription: exploring the experiences of practitioners and lower limb prosthetic users. Disabil Rehabil 2011;33(15–16):1314–23.

34. Singh R, Ripley D, Pentland B, et al. Depression and anxiety symptoms after lower limb amputation: the rise and fall. Clin Rehabil 2009;23(3):281–6.

35. Tricare. Durable Medical Equipment, Prosthetics, Orthotics, and Supplies (DME-POS). 2011. Available at: http://www.tricare.mil/DMEPOS/. [Accessed 1 February 2011].

36. Anthem Blue Cross Blue Shield. Lower Limb Prosthesis. 1/2/11. 2011. Available at: http://www.anthem.com/medicalpolicies/guidelines/gl_pw_a053639.htm.

37. Blue Cross Blue Shield of Florida. Medical Policies (Medical Coverage Guidelines) Prosthetics. Available at: https://mcgs.bcbsfl.com/MCG?activity=openSearchedDocMcg&imgId=76AA2MDI165FKA4KZA1. (Accessed 11 March 2011), 2011.

38. Sansam K, O'Connor RJ, Neumann V, et al. Clinicians' perspectives on decision making in lower limb amputee rehabilitation. J Rehabil Med 2014;46(5):447–53.

39. Sansam K, Neumann V, O'Connor R, et al. Predicting walking ability following lower limb amputation: a systematic review of the literature. J Rehabil Med 2009;41(8):593–603.

40. French MA, Roemmich RT, Daley K, et al. Precision rehabilitation: optimizing function, adding value to health care. Arch Phys Med Rehabil 2022. https://doi.org/10.1016/j.apmr.2022.01.154.

41. National Research Council. Toward precision medicine: building a knowledge network for biomedical research and a new taxonomy of disease. Washington, DC: National Academies Press; 2011.

42. Edwards AG, Naik G, Ahmed H, et al. Personalised risk communication for informed decision making about taking screening tests. Cochrane Database Syst Rev 2013;(2).

43. Ankolekar A, Dekker A, Fijten R, et al. The benefits and challenges of using patient decision aids to support shared decision making in health care. JCO clinical cancer informatics 2018;2:1–10.

44. Lo A, Chernoff H, Zheng T, et al. Why significant variables aren't automatically good predictors. Proc Natl Acad Sci U S A 2015;112(45):13892–7.

45. Poldrack RA, Huckins G, Varoquaux G. Establishment of best practices for evidence for prediction: a review. JAMA Psychiatr 2020;77(5):534–40.

46. Varga TV, Niss K, Estampador AC, et al. Association is not prediction: a landscape of confused reporting in diabetes - A systematic review. Diabetes Res Clin Pract 2020;170:108497.

47. Ngiam KY, Khor IW. Big data and machine learning algorithms for health-care delivery. Lancet Oncol 2019;20(5):e262–73.

48. Obermeyer Z, Emanuel EJ. Predicting the future - big data, machine learning, and clinical medicine. N Engl J Med 29 2016;375(13):1216–9.

49. Norvell DC, Henderson A, Sukow B, et al. The development and usability of the AMPREDICT decision support tool: translating research to shared decision making for veterans facing lower limb amputation. Eur J Vasc Endovasc Surg 2021. https://doi.org/10.1016/j.ejvs.2021.03.031.

50. Preece RA, Dilaver N, Waldron CA, et al. A systematic review and narrative synthesis of risk prediction tools used to estimate mortality, morbidity, and other outcomes following major lower limb amputation. Eur J Vasc Endovasc Surg 2021; 62(1):127–35.

51. Ambler GK, Thomas-Jones E, Edwards AGK, et al. Prognostic risk modelling for patients undergoing major lower limb amputation: an analysis of the UK national vascular registry. Eur J Vasc Endovasc Surg 2020;59(4):606–13.

52. Easterlin MC, Chang DC, Wilson SE. A practical index to predict 30-day mortality after major amputation. Ann Vasc Surg 2013;27(7):909–17.

53. Feinglass J, Pearce WH, Martin GJ, et al. Postoperative and late survival outcomes after major amputation: findings from the Department of Veterans Affairs National Surgical Quality Improvement Program. Surgery 2001;130(1):21–9.

54. Jolissaint JS, Shah SK, Martin MC, et al. Risk prediction of 30-day mortality after lower extremity major amputation. J Vasc Surg 2019;70(6):1868–76.

55. Nelson MT, Greenblatt DY, Soma G, et al. Preoperative factors predict mortality after major lower-extremity amputation. Surgery 2012;152(4):685–94 [discussion 694-6].

56. Patterson AJ, Degnan AJ, Walsh SR, et al. Efficacy of VBHOM to predict outcome following major lower limb amputation. Vasc Endovasc Surg 2012;46(5):369–73.

57. Tang TY, Prytherch DR, Walsh SR, et al. The development of a VBHOM-based outcome model for lower limb amputation performed for critical ischaemia. Eur J Vasc Endovasc Surg 2009;37(1):62–6.

58. Wied C, Foss NB, Kristensen MT, et al. Surgical apgar score predicts early complication in transfemoral amputees: Retrospective study of 170 major amputations. World J Orthop 2016;7(12):832–8.

59. Norvell DC, Thompson ML, Boyko EJ, et al. Mortality prediction following non-traumatic amputation of the lower extremity. Br J Surg 2019;106(7):879–88.

60. Bowrey S, Naylor H, Russell P, et al. Development of a scoring tool (BLARt score) to predict functional outcome in lower limb amputees. Disabil Rehabil 2019; 41(19):2324–32.

61. Czerniecki JM, Turner AP, Williams RM, et al. The development and validation of the AMPREDICT model for predicting mobility outcome after dysvascular lower extremity amputation. J Vasc Surg 2017;65(1):162–71.

62. Czerniecki JM, Thompson ML, Littman AJ, et al. Predicting reamputation risk in patients undergoing lower extremity amputation due to the complications of peripheral artery disease and/or diabetes. Br J Surg 2019;106(8):1026–34.

63. Norvell DC, Thompson ML, Baraff A, et al. AMPREDICT PROsthetics-predicting prosthesis mobility to aid in prosthetic prescription and rehabilitation planning. Arch Phys Med Rehabil 2023;104(4):523–32.

64. Wafi A, Ribeiro L, Kolli V, et al. Predicting prosthetic mobility at discharge from rehabilitation following major amputation in vascular surgery. Eur J Vasc Endovasc Surg 2023. https://doi.org/10.1016/j.ejvs.2023.09.034.

65. Pencina MJ, Goldstein BA, D'Agostino RB. Prediction models - development, evaluation, and clinical application. N Engl J Med 2020;382(17):1583–6.

66. Quigley M, Dillon MP, Fatone S. Development of shared decision-making resources to help inform difficult healthcare decisions: An example focused on dysvascular partial foot and transtibial amputations. Prosthet Orthot Int 2018;42(4): 378–86.

67. Covvey JR, Kamal KM, Gorse EE, et al. Barriers and facilitators to shared decision-making in oncology: a systematic review of the literature. Support Care Cancer 2019;27:1613–37.

68. O'Connor AM, Llewellyn-Thomas HA, Flood AB. Modifying unwarranted variations in health care: shared decision making using patient decision aids: a review of the evidence base for shared decision making. Health Aff 2004;23(Suppl2). VAR-63-VAR-72.

69. Consortium NL. Shared Decision Making (Fact Sheet). 2013.

70. Légaré F, Witteman HO. Shared decision making: examining key elements and barriers to adoption into routine clinical practice. Health Aff 2013;32(2):276–84.

71. Gallagher P, Maclachlan M. Adjustment to an artificial limb: a qualitative perspective. J Health Psychol 2001;6(1):85–100.

72. Pedlow H, Cormier A, Provost M, et al. Patient perspectives on information needs for amputation secondary to vascular surgery: What, when, why, and how much? J Vasc Nurs 2014;32(3):88–98.

73. Ostler C, Ellis-Hill C, Donovan-Hall M. Expectations of rehabilitation following lower limb amputation: a qualitative study. Disabil Rehabil 2014;36(14):1169–75.

74. Murray CD. 'Don't you talk to your prosthetist?' Communicational problems in the prescription of artificial limbs. Disabil Rehabil 2013;35(6):513–21.

75. Chewning B, Bylund CL, Shah B, et al. Patient preferences for shared decisions: a systematic review. Patient Educ Couns 2012;86(1):9–18.

76. Joseph-Williams N, Elwyn G, Edwards A. Knowledge is not power for patients: a systematic review and thematic synthesis of patient-reported barriers and facilitators to shared decision making. Patient Educ Couns 2014;94(3):291–309.

77. O'Connor AM, Wennberg JE, Legare F, et al. Toward the 'tipping point': decision aids and informed patient choice. Health Aff 2007;26(3):716–25.
78. Tsulukidze M, Grande SW, Gionfriddo MR. Assessing Option Grid® practicability and feasibility for facilitating shared decision making: An exploratory study. Patient Educ Counsel 2015;98(7):871–7.
79. Scalia P, Durand MA, Berkowitz JL, et al. The impact and utility of encounter patient decision aids: Systematic review, meta-analysis and narrative synthesis. Patient Educ Counsel 2019;102(5):817–41.
80. Stacey D, Légaré F, Lewis K, et al. Decision aids for people facing health treatment or screening decisions. Cochrane Database Syst Rev 2017;4(4):Cd001431.
81. McAlpine K, Lewis KB, Trevena LJ, et al. What is the effectiveness of patient decision aids for cancer-related decisions? A systematic review subanalysis. JCO clinical cancer informatics 2018;2:1–13.
82. Yu C, Choi D, Bruno BA, et al. Impact of MyDiabetesPlan, a web-based patient decision aid on decisional conflict, diabetes distress, quality of life, and chronic illness care in patients with diabetes: cluster randomized controlled trial. J Med Internet Res 2020;22(9):e16984.
83. van Dijk LA, Vervest AM, Baas DC, et al. Decision aids can decrease decisional conflict in patients with hip or knee osteoarthritis: Randomized controlled trial. World J Orthoped 2021;12(12):1026.
84. Coronado-Vázquez V, Canet-Fajas C, Delgado-Marroquín MT, et al. Interventions to facilitate shared decision-making using decision aids with patients in Primary Health Care: A systematic review. Medicine 2020;99(32).

Health Disparities Across the Spectrum of Amputation Care: A Review of Literature

Michael Gallagher, MD, MA*, Chris Bonilla, MD

KEYWORDS

- Amputation • Rehabilitation • Health disparities • Social determinants of health

KEY POINTS

- Limb loss is a profoundly disabling event, requiring significant adaptation to accomplish mobility and activities of daily living, regardless of successful prosthesis use.
- The intersection of a variety of health disparities with the disability that occurs as a result of limb loss can worsen outcomes across the spectrum of mortality, morbidity, and day-to-day function.
- Understanding when and where disparities are likely to exist in amputation care is an initial step toward creating equitable health justice for those living with limb loss.

INTRODUCTION

Limb loss is a profoundly disabling event, presenting challenges for those who undergo amputation across a broad array of functional needs. Those living with limb loss must learn new methods for mobility and activities of daily living whether they use a prosthesis or not. In the United States, around 1.6 to 1.9 million people are living with amputation, with expectations that this number will double by around 2050.[1] The process of postoperative and prosthetic rehabilitation is costly, and as such requires significant investment relative to preventing an amputation from occurring in the first place. Additionally, despite this investment, eventual outcomes are not always desirable.

Although surgeons and rehabilitation specialists often regard amputation optimistically, with common narratives sometimes attempting to reframe the loss of a limb not as a failure of therapies, but as the next step in a journey to regaining ability from a wound, surveys of patients paint a less rosy picture, with 1 study finding three-quarters reported serious decline in social function, and only half achieving

Department of Rehabilitation Medicine, University of Washington School of Medicine, Veterans Affairs Puget Sound Health Care System, 1660 South Columbian Way, Seattle, WA 98108, USA
* Corresponding author.
E-mail address: michael.gallagher2@va.gov

Phys Med Rehabil Clin N Am 35 (2024) 851–864
https://doi.org/10.1016/j.pmr.2024.06.006
1047-9651/24/Published by Elsevier Inc.

independence with a prosthesis, among other serious impacts on physical and psychosocial well-being.[2] Certainly for successful prosthesis users, amputation may in fact present a return to some previous level of functioning if they have been markedly limited by critical limb ischemia or wounds, but data indicate that for many amputees outcomes may be less restorative, particularly in health systems where rehabilitation and prosthetist referral are limited or costly.

Barriers to functional mobility and overall independence exist across the spectrum of amputation care, including limitations in accessing rehabilitation postoperatively and for prosthesis training, cost, and access to prosthetist evaluation for fitting, and the availability of expert management for complications of amputation such as pain, wounds, and specific functional demands that may not be directly addressed by a prosthesis. As such, amputation itself presents a major challenge to community reintegration, and the intersection where amputation-related difficulties and racial, socioeconomic, regional, and sex disparities in health care meet can amplify postamputation struggles.

Disparities in the provision of medical care have been well studied across numerous disease conditions and care settings. Healthy People 2020, the United States federal initiative for public health, defines a health disparity as "a particular type of health difference that is closely linked with economic, social, or environmental disadvantage" and "adversely affect groups of people who have systematically experienced greater social or economic obstacles to health based on their racial or ethnic group, religion, socioeconomic status, gender, age, or mental health; cognitive, sensory, or physical disability; sexual orientation or gender identity; geographic location; or other characteristics historically linked to discrimination or exclusion."[3] Evidence suggests that race and ethnicity, social class/income, rural versus urban residence, gender, age, and many other contributing factors are correlated with different health outcomes across different populations, and great attention has been paid to the observation of rates at which differences occur in populations, although the literature on population-specific needs or remedies for disparities is limited. Despite a growing body of research documenting the existence of a broad intersection of health disparities and their impacts on health outcomes, disparity itself remains a tenacious challenge in care delivery. The overall picture for people with amputation means that the disparities baked into modern health care systems mete out greater impacts for certain populations. Although undergoing amputation itself is a marker for disparity, with research showing that nonwhite people are more likely to undergo primary amputation than white people, the intersections between race, sex, location, and numerous other factors can also have significant effects on the results and eventual functional outcomes of limb loss. Researchers have focused on various disparities as they occur at multiple points in the eventual road to amputation, including preventive measures such as wound care and medical management, rates of primary amputation and limb salvage, and postamputation functional outcomes, morbidity, and mortality. This article aims to provide a summary of the literature on disparities across the clinical journey that an individual patient will experience during the lead-up to and aftermath of limb loss.

PREVENTION/PREAMPUTATION

Most disparities research has focused on the various ways in which social determinants of health alter the rate or primary level of amputation, or therapies undertaken to prevent amputation. Given the degree of disability and social and functional changes after limb loss, prevention efforts are key to limiting the individual and society-wide impacts of amputation. Within the rehabilitation, podiatric, and vascular surgery literature, efforts are largely focused on secondary and tertiary prevention methods such as revascularization for peripheral arterial disease and early and expert wound care for diabetic or dysvascular wounds. Medical therapy such as statins for peripheral arterial disease and noninvasive devices like pneumatic compression devices have also been proposed as potential ways to reduce rates of progression to critical limb ischemia and amputation. Additionally, access to expert foot care is key to preventing the formation of wounds and initiating early treatment when a wound does arise, ideally preventing the progression toward chronic wounds at risk of infections like osteomyelitis or gangrene, which often lead to amputation. This care includes regular foot examinations and potentially prescription footwear and orthotics to accommodate the neuropathic foot and prevent undesired pressure that may lead to a wound.

Diabetic Foot Ulcers

Given neuropathic and dysvascular conditions lead to an estimated 80% of lower limb amputations, identifying and treating diabetic foot ulcers (DFUs) remain cornerstones of amputation prevention. However, health disparities exist in terms of the relative risks of foot ulcers among different populations and the care received for them. Primary prevention efforts for DFUs include routine foot examinations and often prescription footwear in higher-risk groups, although the primary recipients of these efforts continue to be non-Latino/a/x white populations, with Black, Latino/a/x, and indigenous groups receiving markedly less guideline-directed diabetes care overall.[4]

Particularly, longer duration of diabetes (and therefore age) are major risk factors because of the cumulative effects of hyperglycemia, although some studies have shown that younger populations tend to present with more advanced ulcers.[5] The relationship with younger adults is thought to be primarily caused by other risk factors such as smoking and more chronically elevated HbA_{1c}, which itself is an independent risk factor for DFUs.[6] Studies also consistently find Black, Latino/a/x, and other nonwhite populations are more at risk for foot wounds and tend to present at more advanced stages, which is maintained somewhat independently of socioeconomic status (ie, although poorer Black people tend to have a higher risk of DFU, the risk for a more affluent Black person does not reach parity with white populations).[7] Therefore, although lower socioeconomic status (SES) is another likely risk factor for the development of foot wounds, race and SES are closely aligned. Certain comorbidities also present a greater risk of DFUs. Particularly, chronic kidney disease, cardiovascular disease, and smoking history are independent risk factors.[6]

Disparity also exists in terms of access to secondary and tertiary prevention measures for DFUs such as wound debridement and accommodative footwear or other advanced orthoses. One interview-based study study found that Americans living in rural settings were less likely to receive multidisciplinary and specialty care such as podiatry or wound care referrals, and reported more frequent delays in referrals and accessing care.[8] A comparison of patients receiving care at a New York City triumvirate hospital system consisting of a public, private, and Veteran's Affairs (VA) hospital within a 10-block radius found that VA patients with DFUs made up a disproportionate proportion (45%) of all gangrenous wounds at presentation and had the lowest rate of healing at 17.1%, compared with 67.2% at the public hospital.[9] The study also noted that VA patients were more likely to be nonwhite and have a prior history of amputation, both independent risk factors for poor outcomes.[9] Studies also suggest that Black patients are less likely to undergo limb salvage attempts before amputation, including wound debridement, when compared with whites (11.6 vs 14.2%).[10]

Ischemic Limb

Differences in limb salvage attempts for critical limb ischemia may also contribute to variability in amputation rates among different social groups. Medical management such as statin therapy has been shown to decrease the progression of peripheral arterial disease (PAD) to critical limb ischemia. Like diabetic ulcers, wound care for venous and arterial wounds is another cornerstone of limb salvage for the dysvascular limb, as well as advanced vascular surgery interventions such as arterial bypass grafts and angioplasty with stenting.

In terms of medical management and prevention of progression to critical limb ischemia and amputation, disparities exist in statin prescribing practices. Data suggest that guideline-directed statin therapy for peripheral arterial disease reduces the progression to critical limb ischemia, can reduce rates of amputation for PAD, and may even improve the chance of limb salvage after revascularization.[11] Mentias and colleagues[12] found that women were prescribed statins at lower rates than men with PAD (48.4% vs 52.9%, $P<.001$).

A large study in Medicare patients found that on the whole, elderly Black patients were less likely to undergo wound debridement and revascularization by open and endovascular technique than white patients, and that this relationship was maintained if adjusted for regional differences for where these populations received care.[11] Several additional studies find a similar relationship, with white patients more likely to receive revascularization and Black patients more likely to undergo amputation.[13,14] A VA study examining regional and racial differences in rates of proximal amputations found that in 1 region, Black patients were more likely to undergo transfemoral amputation regardless of diabetes incidence, and in another, Latino/a/x patients were at increased risk of a transfemoral amputation regardless of diabetes incidence or prior revascularization.[15] Studies have also shown that women are less likely to undergo open revascularization for critical limb ischemia, although rates of endovascular repair appear similar.[12]

SURGICAL DECISION MAKING

Decision making when an amputation must be performed ideally considers the potential for healing the surgical incision and risks of morbidity and mortality through information obtained from vascular studies and clinical examination, as well as the functional implications of the intended level of amputation. As such, if the extent of arterial disease, the available healthy tissue for surgical coverage, and the involvement of deep structures such as bone allow, the most distal procedure possible often maximizes the functional outcome for the patient. Hence the site of primary amputation is a major consideration in surgical decision making, but evidence indicates that the decision to amputate in general and the site of incident amputation are undertaken differently in different populations. As such, not only should one expect disparities in terms of how often certain populations undergo amputations, but overall, those groups more likely to undergo amputation, and particularly those more often to undergo higher-level amputations, could be at risk for greater disability and worse functional outcomes.

Rates of Amputation and Primary Amputation

Racial disparities in the rate of amputation have been described, and growing literature indicates that there are also disparities in primary amputation (amputation as initial management for a wound or ischemic limb, without revascularization attempts). Nonwhite patients are around 20% more likely to undergo any amputation than whites, and this effect is amplified by rural place of residence.[16] Nonwhite people living in rural settings were twice as likely to undergo amputation than whites in the same settings, and had 52% higher risk of amputation versus urban nonwhite people.[16] A nationwide sample of rates of amputation by ethnicity found that Black patients made up a higher proportion of patients progressing to amputation and reiterated prior data that Black patients were less likely to undergo revascularization before amputation.[16] Mustapha and colleagues[17] demonstrated both Black and Latino/a/x patients were twice as likely to undergo amputation when compared with white patients. Black patients have also been noted to progress to amputation at faster rates. Miller and colleagues[18] showed that Black patients are 1.98 times more likely to undergo amputation within the first year of a DFU diagnosis, and that female sex is associated with a delayed amputation. Female sex is also associated with more severe ischemic limb at presentation, with higher rates of critical limb ischemia and primary amputation.[19]

Even in less common conditions such as malignant bone tumors, racial differences in choice of treatment method have been demonstrated. Lapica and colleagues[20] found in a cohort study of 5091 subjects that primary treatment with amputation for soft tissue sarcoma was 1.4 times more likely in Latino/a/x patients compared with non-Latino/a/x patients, although no differences were found with other ethnic groups. Other studies have also found disparities for Black patients; 1 study found that Black patients were about 1.1 times less likely to receive limb salvage procedures than white patients.[21] Several other studies have reported similar findings for Black and Latino/a/x populations.[22–24] Additionally, limited data find this relationship holds for Native American populations.[25] Even more alarming, a growing body of literature indicates that race is an independent risk factor for primary amputation, or amputation without prior attempts at revascularization.[26–28]

Geographic disparities have also been observed in rates of amputation, with data suggesting rural populations are 51.3% more likely to undergo amputation compared with patients in urban settings.[29] Similar to studies of racial disparities, the greater risk of amputation in rural populations has some early data to suggest it may be an independent risk for amputation also.[30]

Level of Amputation

Although any amputation can be a dramatic change for a patient, foot-level amputations present a lower overall burden of disability and eventual rehabilitative care. However, they also come with higher risk of wound failure and eventual repeat amputation, given wound healing is generally more challenging with more distal surgical incisions. The decision to pursue foot-level amputation therefore depends on the ability of the patient to heal a distal wound, as well as considering the patient's functional status and prognosticating their postoperative function, and accounting for the patient's desires and goals. Many patients will opt for a foot-level amputation despite low odds of healing because of expectations for disability and psychological distress from higher-level amputations. Additionally, because of the loss of quadriceps muscle function and a shorter residual limb lever, transfemoral amputations are typically more disabling and those undergoing transfemoral amputations are less likely to use a prosthesis.[31]

Differences in level of amputation among different racial and ethnic groups has been noted in the literature. Particularly, multiple studies in the last 3 decades have consistently shown a greater likelihood of transfemoral amputations in Black people.[32–35] Gender disparities have also been shown, with 1 retrospective chart analysis of 11,114 patients indicating that female sex was significantly associated with transfemoral amputation.[36] The same study indicated that income and insurance disparities also existed, with patients making less than $36,000 yearly and Medicare/Medicaid recipients more likely to undergo transfemoral amputation (**Table 1**).[3]

POSTAMPUTATION
Access to Care

For traumatic amputations particularly, access to care in general and ability to receive escalated care specifically can often result in better overall outcomes. For digital amputations, for example, specialized surgical care may be able to replant the amputated digit, preserving hand/finger function, or revise the amputation to allow for potential prosthesis use or functional residual digit use. Traumatic digital amputations do demonstrate regional and gender disparities. Particularly, Long and colleagues[37] showed that men were more likely to receive escalated care for revision or replantation. Additionally, higher income zip codes and those presenting to teaching trauma centers were more likely to receive escalated care, likely because of the availability of specialists. A 2008 to 2014 survey of New York State inpatient and outpatient databases found similar regional disparities in access, with replantation more likely to occur in zip codes with high-volume hospitals.[38] Similarly, Goodney and colleagues[39] found that when examining regional differences in rates of major amputation, areas with the highest rates of amputation tended to correlate with lower access to vascular care, indicating it is likely that greater vascular specialty services improve the likelihood of successful medical or procedural management of critical limb ischemia.

Postamputation rehabilitation setting plays a major role in determining outcomes. Postamputation rehabilitation should be performed at facilities equipped with an educated staff and a multidisciplinary team skilled in the unique amputee goals, such as prosthesis training. Possible facilities for rehabilitation include skilled nursing facilities (SNFs) and inpatient rehabilitation facilities (IRFs). Overall, data show a more favorable outcome following discharge from an inpatient rehabilitation facility. Patients receiving their rehabilitation at IRFs leave facilities 16 days earlier, live at home 3 months longer, have a decrease in mortality of 12%, and a decrease in readmissions.[40] In the United States, access to these facilities often depends on whether patients are insured or uninsured and where they receive their amputation; data have shown patients undergoing amputation at trauma centers are more likely to discharge to IRFs.[41]

Additionally, postamputation access to prosthetic-related care can improve functional outcomes and even mortality, with studies indicating that amputees not using prostheses have a 2.6 times (95% CI 1.16–6.25) likelihood of mortality compared with prosthesis users.[42] Differences in prosthesis access based on level of amputation are well described, with transfemoral amputees less likely to receive a prosthesis than transtibial amputees, largely because of the overall increased functional demand of transfemoral prosthesis use. As such, groups who are more likely to undergo transfemoral amputation have been shown to receive prostheses later or not at all. In the private American insurance system, women have been shown to take around 1 month longer on average to receive a prosthesis.[43] However, VA studies have indicated minimal gender differences in prosthesis receipt, perhaps due in part to access to care within socialized systems.[44]

Functional Outcomes

Those patients who undergo major amputations are faced with major challenges once they begin to reintegrate into their community and home settings. Prosthesis use in

Table 1
Overview of collated research articles and their major findings detailing health disparities in level of amputation and primary amputation

Authors, Year	Outcome Measure	Sample	Major Findings
Hurwitz et al,[15] 2021	Frequency of incident transfemoral amputation	7296	Continental region: Blacks with and without diabetes more likely to undergo transfemoral amputation (odds ratio [OR] 1.4, 95% confidence interval [CI] 1.1–1.9) Southeast: Latino/a/x at increased odds vs whites (OR > 2.9)
Minc et al,[27] 2017	Primary amputation	Meta-analysis, 8 articles included	2.52 times greater risk of primary amputation in nonwhites (95% CI 2.50–2.54)
Durazzo et al,[28] 2013	Primary amputation	774,399	Black patients more likely to undergo primary amputation (OR 1.77, 95% CI 1.72–1.84). Disparities worse in hospitals with greater revascularization capacity and wealthier zip code
Lefebvre and Metraux,[33] 2009	Level of amputation	80,845	Black race at higher risk of transfemoral amputation (OR 1.51, 95% CI 1.4–1.7), female gender at increased risk (OR 1.33, 95% CI 1.2–1.5), Medicare/Medicaid insurance at higher risk (OR 1.63, 95% CI 1.2–2.2)
Lefevbre & Chevan,[36] 2011	Frequency of incident transfemoral amputation Primary amputation	11,114	Female sex at increased risk of incident transfemoral amputation (OR 1.4, 95% CI 1.3–1.5); income less than $36,000 more at risk (OR 1.3, 95% CI 1.1–1.5). Medicare insurance more at risk (OR 1.3, 95% CI 1.3–1.6).
Holman et al,[11] 2011	Primary amputation	91,481	Black patients more likely to undergo primary amputation (23.6 vs 31.6, P<.0001) or foot-level amputation (12.9 vs 13.8%, P<.0005)
Mentias et al,[12] 2020	Primary amputation	8839	Women less likely to undergo revascularization before amputation (50% vs 53.6%, P<.001).
Minc et al,[16] 2020	Primary amputation	6795	Nonwhites more likely to undergo primary amputation (OR 1.21, 95% CI 1.05–1.39). Rural nonwhites more likely to undergo primary amputation than rural whites (OR 2.06, 95% CI 1.53–2.78) and urban nonwhites (OR 1.52, 95% CI 1.19–1.94)

particular has been shown to not only improve functional independence and ambulation, but also a significant number of psychosocial factors such as improved mood, lower rates of phantom limb pain, and reduced overall psychiatric symptoms.[45] Studies have associated prosthesis use with higher levels of employment as well, and employment status on its own may be an indicator of poorer prosthetic outcomes.[46,47]

Particularly, dysvascular amputees appear to demonstrate poor prosthetic-related function, with 1 study showing a majority (80%) of dysvascular lower limb amputees over 65 exhibiting poor functional outcomes.[47] VA studies have largely shown minimal differences in functional outcomes between male and female amputees, with 1 study showing the only difference being self-reported mobility, with women reporting slightly lower mobility than men.[44] In a study of people with lower limb amputations caused by gangrene, Black patients were significantly more likely to report being partially dependent on a caregiver a month after surgery (OR 1.373, 95% CI 1.017–1.853).[48] A study of Australian patients found that patients living in a rural setting were less likely to use a prosthesis for ambulation as well (**Table 2**).[49]

Post Amputation Mortality

Mortality rates after any major amputation remain high, with Center for Medicare and Medicaid Services data from 2000 to 2008 indicating a roughly 2-times greater risk of 1- and 3-year mortality for amputees compared with nonamputees.[50] There is also a greater mortality risk for those undergoing above-knee amputations compared with more distal amputations. A Nashville VA study of 245 lower-extremity amputees found that mortality for those who had completed high school was lower than for those who had not (62.6% vs 84.3%, $P=.001$).[51] Henry and colleagues[52] found that sociodemographic factors such as race, income, insurance status, and marital status did not appear to influence mortality rates. Mustapha and colleagues[53] found slightly higher risks of mortality after amputation in both white and Black patients relative to other races (aOR = 1.24 and 1.05 respectively), but similar mortality between geographic regions of the United States.

DISCUSSION

This article attempts to provide a comprehensive overview of existing literature on health disparities within the field of amputation rehabilitation, extending from the moment of a potentially threatening wound or ischemic limb to postamputation management and prosthesis care. Disparities across the entire clinical picture of amputation prevention and care are documented, particularly in countries like the United States with a private insurance system that can create economic barriers to access to care. Particularly, although there is an increasing recognition of the personal and societal costs of amputation and the need to prevent limb loss whenever possible, the complex interaction of an individual patient's clinical situation and his or her lived experience creates a challenge for health care workers situated in the biomedical model. Although the literature on health care inequalities has helped to identify those at higher risk for amputation and adverse postamputation outcomes in the acute phase of hospitalization and long-term outpatient settings, rates of amputation continue to increase despite growing recognition of the need for prevention, and particularly targeted prevention.

In recognition of both the overall increase in rates of amputation and the disparities in outcomes, health care systems have implemented a variety of methods to combat both issues. Within the VA system, the Prevention of Amputation in Veterans

Table 2
Overview of collated articles and major findings regarding disparities in postamputation functional outcomes

Authors, Year	Outcome Measure	Sample	Major Findings
Miller et al,[43] 2023	Time to prosthesis receipt	510	Those with diabetes/vascular disease received prosthesis early (hazard ratio [HR] 1.22, 95% CI 1.02–1.49)
			Women received prosthesis later than men (141 d vs 106 d)
Kuo et al,[44] 2023	Mobility	449	Women self-reported lower mobility than men (d = −0.26, 95% CI -0.49 to −0.02)
	Satisfaction with prosthesis services, fit, use		
Clemens et al,[47] 2023	Employment status	49	80% of lower-limb amputees not full-time employed 1 y after amputation
	Timed-up-and-go		Unemployment associated with poorer mobility and functional test scores
	2-min walk test		
	Self-reported mobility		
Spiera et al,[48] 2021	Loss of independence	5250	Black patients more likely to report dependence on a caregiver (OR 1.373, 95% CI 1.017–1.853)
de Boer et al,[49] 2022	Prosthesis use	317	Nonsignificant – urban patients more likely to use a prosthesis (OR 2.47, 95% CI 0.94–6.47)
	Mobility		

Everywhere (PAVE) initiative involves interdisciplinary committees that meet to identify patients at risk of amputation, increase collaboration for the prevention of amputation and postamputation rehabilitation, and coordinate access to preventive screenings such as foot examinations.[54] The Amputation System of Care, also a VA initiative, was created in 2008 and provides longitudinal specialty rehabilitative care to those experiencing limb loss, which increased access to amputation-related care by 34% from 2009 to 2019.[54] Several states have also passed laws requiring insurance companies to cover prosthetic-related care, although this coverage often falls short of state-of-the-art componentry.[55] Similarly, creating rehabilitation teams with specialization in amputation care and prostheses within health centers performing amputations, and increasing access to prosthetists and rehabilitation through rural centers of care or mobile care teams, can increase the number of people with amputations reached by health care workers.[56]

The existence of disparities also points to important socioeconomic considerations. Regardless of health system initiatives, the persistence of poor outcomes in specific populations often mirrors the social determinants of health – the long history of racial and ethnic bias, gender and sexuality-based discrimination, and economic structures that prioritize the ability to pay for services over society-wide parity in access and delivery of care. Although health care workers and the systems they serve can stem the effects of disparities, a major effort is required at a societal and political level to eliminate the social structures that work together to create disparities.

Many studies cited in this article are retrospective, and hence interpretation of their results is somewhat limited given the difficulties interpreting data pulled from charts and billing information. However, with existing general literature on social determinants of health and their influence on patient outcomes, it is unlikely that any bias introduced through retrospective review would change the reality of significant racial, socioeconomic, geographic, and gender disparities in the field of amputation care. Although this article helps to collate the literature around high-risk groups, addressing social determinants of health and mitigating the effects of systemic bias are necessary to mitigate the influence of health disparities on the people health care workers serve. Several studies also demonstrated the particular importance of an intersectional understanding of disparities, where multiple identified risk categories combine to influence outcomes. For example, a Black rural patient may have worse outcomes in some cases than a Black or white urban patient.

Future Directions

There is a dearth of studies on several subjects, at least within the scope of this article. Particularly, although extensive literature exists regarding disparities in providers' treatment of painful conditions in patients with different racial and ethnic backgrounds, there does not appear to be any literature specific to residual or phantom limb pain. A single article suggested a model for studying the influence of socioeconomic and demographic factors in rates of repeat amputation, but otherwise data are not available. Disparities relating to prosthesis use and functional outcomes are also similarly less studied.

CLINICS CARE POINTS

- Health care disparities in amputation rehabilitation are widespread and significant.
- Black, Native American, and Latina/o/x patients are more likely to undergo amputations, with Black patients more likely to undergo transfemoral amputations.

- Black patients are more likely to undergo amputation without prior revascularization.
- Lower socioeconomic status and female gender are also associated with higher rates of transfemoral amputation.
- Lack of access to specialized care and high-volume medical centers may result in lower likelihood of preventive care for wounds or critical limb ischemia that may lead to amputation, advanced procedures like revascularization, and replantation for traumatic digit amputations.
- Literature around disparities and postamputation outcomes, pain, and prosthesis use is limited.

DISCLOSURE

The authors report no proprietary or commercial interest in any product mentioned or concept discussed in this article.

REFERENCES

1. Molina C.S. and Faulk J.B., Lower extremity amputation, In: *StatPearls [Internet]*, 2023, StatPearls Publishing; Treasure Island (FL), Available at: https://www.ncbi.nlm.nih.gov/books/NBK546594/. (Accessed 15 November 2023).
2. Little JM, Petritsi-Jones D, Kerr C. Vascular amputees: a study in disappointment. J bioeth Inq 2022;19(1):21–4.
3. Office of Disease Prevention and Health Promotion. Disparities. Available at: https://www.healthypeople.gov/2020/about/foundation-health-measures/Disparities. [Accessed 20 November 2023].
4. Shin JI, Wang D, Fernandes G, et al. Trends in receipt of American Diabetes Association guideline-recommended care among U.S. adults with diabetes: NHANES 2005-2018. Diabetes Care 2021;44:1300–8.
5. McDermott K, Fang M, Boulton AJM, et al. Etiology, epidemiology, and disparities in the burden of diabetic foot ulcers. Diabetes Care 2023;46(1):209–21.
6. Casadei G, Filippini M, Brognara L. Glycated hemoglobin (HbA1c) as a biomarker for diabetic foot peripheral neuropathy. Diseases 2021;9(1):16.
7. Canedo JR, Miller ST, Schlundt D, et al. Racial/ethnic disparities in diabetes quality of care: the role of healthcare access and socioeconomic status. J Racial Ethn Health Disparities 2018;5(1):7–14.
8. Sutherland BL, Pecanac K, Bartels CM, et al. Expect delays: poor connections between rural and urban health systems challenge multidisciplinary care for rural Americans with diabetic foot ulcers. J Foot Ankle Res 2020;13(1):32.
9. Blumberg SN, Warren SM. Disparities in initial presentation and treatment outcomes of diabetic foot ulcers in a public, private, and Veterans Administration hospital. J Diabetes 2014;6(1):68–75.
10. Armstrong EJ, Chen DC, Westin GG, et al. Adherence to guideline-recommended therapy is associated with decreased major adverse cardiovascular events and major adverse limb events among patients with peripheral arterial disease. J Am Heart Assoc 2014;3:e000697.
11. Holman KH, Henke PK, Dimick JB, et al. Racial disparities in the use of revascularization before leg amputation in Medicare patients. J Vasc Surg 2011;54(2). 420-6, 426.e1.

12. Mentias AV-SM, Saad M, Girotra S. Sex differences in management and outcomes of critical limb ischemia in the Medicare population. Circ Cardiovasc Interv 2020;13:e009459.

13. Chew DK, Nguyen LL, Owens CD, et al. Comparative analysis of autogenous infrainguinal bypass grafts in African Americans and Caucasians: the association of race with graft function and limb salvage. J Vasc Surg 2005;42(4):695–701.

14. Nguyen LL, Hevelone N, Rogers SO, et al. Disparity in outcomes of surgical revascularization for limb salvage: race and gender are synergistic determinants of vein graft failure and limb loss. Circulation 2009;119(1):123–30.

15. Hurwitz M, Norvell DC, Czerniecki JM. Racial and ethnic amputation level disparities in veterans undergoing incident dysvascular lower extremity amputation. PM&R 2022;14(10):1198–206.

16. Minc SD, Goodney PP, Misra R, et al. The effect of rurality on the risk of primary amputation is amplified by race. J Vasc Surg 2020;72(3):1011–7.

17. Mustapha JA, Fisher BT Sr, Rizzo JA, et al. Explaining racial disparities in amputation rates for the treatment of peripheral artery disease (PAD) using decomposition methods. J Racial Ethn Health Disparities 2017;4(5):784–95.

18. Miller TA, Campbell JH, Bloom N, et al. Racial disparities in health care with timing to amputation following diabetic foot ulcer. Diabetes Care 2022;45(10):2336–41.

19. Lee MH, Li PY, Li B, et al. A systematic review and meta-analysis of sex- and gender-based differences in presentation severity and outcomes in adults undergoing major vascular surgery. J Vasc Surg 2022;76(2):581–94.e25.

20. Hughes K, Seetahal S, Oyetunji T, et al. Racial/ethnic disparities in amputation and revascularization: a nationwide inpatient sample study. Vasc Endovascular Surg 2014;48(1):34–7.

21. Downing S, Ahuja N, Oyetunji TA, et al. Disparity in limb-salvage surgery among sarcoma patients. Am J Surg 2010;199(4):549–53.

22. Collins TC, Johnson M, Henderson W, et al. Lower extremity nontraumatic amputation among veterans with peripheral arterial disease: is race an independent factor? Med Care 2002;40(1 Suppl):I106–16.

23. Abou-Zamzam AM Jr, Gomez NR, Molkara A, et al. A prospective analysis of critical limb ischemia: factors leading to major primary amputation versus revascularization. Ann Vasc Surg 2007;21:458–63.

24. Arya S, Binney Z, Khakharia A, et al. Race and socioeconomic status independently affect risk of major amputation in peripheral artery disease. J Am Heart Assoc 2018;7:e007425.

25. Rizzo JA, Chen J, Laurich C, et al. Racial disparities in PAD-related amputation rates among Native Americans and non-Hispanic whites: an HCUP analysis. J Health Care Poor Underserved 2018;29:782–800.

26. Tunis SR, Bass EB, Klag MJ, et al. Variation in utilization of procedures for treatment of peripheral arterial disease. a look at patient characteristics. Arch Intern Med 1993;153:991–8.

27. Minc SD, Fogg LF, McCarthy WJ, et al. Racial disparities in primary amputation vs revascularization for critical limb ischemia: a meta-analysis. J Am Coll Surg 2017;225:e78.

28. Durazzo TS, Frencher S, Gusberg R. Influence of race on the management of lower extremity ischemia: revascularization vs amputation. JAMA Surg 2013;148:617–23.

29. Skrepnek GH, Mills JL Sr, Armstrong DG. A diabetic emergency one million feet long: disparities and burdens of illness among diabetic foot ulcer cases within

emergency departments in the United States, 2006-2010. PLoS One 2015;10: e0134914.

30. Minc SD, Hendricks B, Misra R, et al. Geographic variation in amputation rates among patients with diabetes and/or peripheral arterial disease in the rural state of West Virginia identifies areas for improved care. J Vasc Surg 2020;71: 1708–17.e5.

31. Penn-Barwell JG. Outcomes in lower limb amputation following trauma: a systematic review and meta-analysis. Injury 2011;42(12):1474–9.

32. Lavery LA, Ashry HR, Houtum W, et al. Variation in the incidence and proportion of diabetes related amputations in minorities. Diabetes Care 1996;19:4854.

33. Lefebvre KM, Metraux S. Disparities in level of amputation: implications for improved preventative care. J Natl Med Assoc 2009;101:649–55.

34. Houtum WH, Lavery LA, Armstrong DG. Risk factors for above-knee amputations in diabetes mellitus. South Med J 1998;91:643–9.

35. de Mestral C, Hussain MA, Austin PC, et al. Regional health care services and rates of lower extremity amputation related to diabetes and peripheral artery disease: an ecological study. CMAJ Open 2020;8(4):E659–66.

36. Lefebvre KM, Chevan J. Sex disparities in level of amputation. Arch Phys Med Rehabil 2011;92(1):118–24.

37. Long C, Suarez PA, Hernandez-Boussard T, et al. Disparities in access to care following traumatic digit amputation. Hand (N Y) 2020;15(4):480–7.

38. Kurucan E, Thirukumaran C, Hammert WC. Trends in the management of traumatic upper extremity amputations. J Hand Surg Am 2020;45(11):1086.e1–11.

39. Goodney PP, Holman K, Henke PK, et al. Regional intensity of vascular care and lower extremity amputation rates. J Vasc Surg 2013;57(6):1471–9.

40. DaVanzo JE, El-Gamil A, Li JW, et al. Assessment of patient outcomes of rehabilitative care provided in inpatient rehabilitation facilities (IRFs) and after discharge. Vienna (VA): Dobson DaVanzo; 2014. Available at: https://www.amrpa.org/newsroom/DobsonDaVanzoFinalReport-PatientOutcomesofIRFvSNF-71014redated.pdf. [Accessed 31 December 2023].

41. Dillingham TR, Pezzin LE, MacKenzie EJ. Incidence, acute care length of stay, and discharge to rehabilitation of traumatic amputee patients: an epidemiologic study. Arch Phys Med Rehabil 1998;79(3):279–87.

42. Singh RK, Prasad G. Long-term mortality after lower-limb amputation. Prosthet Orthot Int 2016;40(5):545–51.

43. Miller TA, Paul R, Forthofer M, et al. Factors that influence time to prosthesis receipt after lower limb amputation: a cox proportional hazard model regression. PM&R 2023;15(4):474–81.

44. Kuo PB, Lehavot K, Thomas RM, et al. Gender differences in prosthesis-related outcomes among veterans: results of a national survey of U.S. veterans. PM&R 2023;1–11.

45. Raichle KA, Hanley MA, Molton I, et al. Prosthesis use in persons with lower- and upper-limb amputation. J Rehabil Res Dev 2008;45(7):961–72.

46. Durmus D, Safaz I, Adıgüzel E, et al. The relationship between prosthesis use, phantom pain and psychiatric symptoms in male traumatic limb amputees. Compr Psychiatry 2015;59:45–53.

47. Clemens SM, Kershaw KN, McDonald CL, et al. Disparities in functional recovery after dysvascular lower limb amputation are associated with employment status and self-efficacy. Disabil Rehabil 2023;45(14):2280–7.

48. Spiera Z, Ilonzo N, Kaplan H, et al. Loss of independence as a metric for racial disparities in lower extremity amputation for diabetes: a national surgery quality

improvement program (NSQIP) analysis. J Diabetes Complications 2022;36(1): 108105.

49. de Boer M, Shiraev T, Waller J, et al. Patient and geographical disparities in functional outcomes after major lower limb amputation in Australia. Ann Vasc Surg 2022;85:125–32.

50. Jones WS, Patel MR, Dai D, et al. High mortality risks after major lower extremity amputation in Medicare patients with peripheral artery disease. Am Heart J 2013; 165(5):809–15.

51. Henry AJ, Hevelone ND, Hawkins AT, et al. Factors predicting resource utilization and survival after major amputation. J Vasc Surg 2013;57(3):784–90.

52. Corey MR, St Julien J, Miller C, et al. Patient education level affects functionality and long-term mortality after major lower extremity amputation. Am J Surg 2012; 204(5):626–30.

53. Mustapha JA, Katzen BT, Neville RF, et al. Determinants of long-term outcomes and costs in the management of critical limb ischemia: a population-based cohort study. J Am Heart Assoc 2018;7(16):e009724.

54. Webster J, Scholten J, Young P, et al. Ten-year outcomes of a systems-based approach to longitudinal amputation care in the US Department of Veteran Affairs. Fed Pract 2020;37(8):360–7.

55. Fish D. The development of coverage policy for lower extremity prosthetics: the influence of the payer on prosthetic prescription. J Prosthet Orthot 2006;18(6): 125–9.

56. Ham R, Regan JM, Roberts VC. Evaluation of introducing the team approach to the care of the amputee: the Dulwich study. Prosthet Orthot Int 1987;11(1):25–30.

Reintegration Following Amputation

A Biopsychosocial Approach

Nicolette Carnahan, PhD, Lindsey Holbrook, PhD, Eric Brunk, DO,
Jennifer Viola, DO, Marlís González-Fernández, MD, PhD*

KEYWORDS

- Amputation • Biopsychosocial approach • Limb loss
- Social, Psychological, and physical adjustment to limb loss • Driving after limb loss
- Community reintegration after limb loss
- Depression, anxiety, and PTSD associated with limb loss

KEY POINTS

- Biopsychosocial factors interact to influence reintegration after limb loss.
- Reintegration and associated barriers may differ for upper versus lower extremity amputees.
- Mental health screening and early intervention are critical to successful reintegration into the community.

INTRODUCTION

Historically, amputation literature has placed focus on physical aspects of adjustment to amputation and reintegration. Important shifts in research have refocused attention toward a biopsychosocial model that incorporates the interaction among physical, social, and psychological well-being.[1,2] It has become increasingly apparent that the overlap between these factors is imperative to successful reintegration postamputation. However, there are multiple domain-specific barriers (eg, social and psychological adjustment, activity restriction, satisfaction with prostheses, and pain experience) identified across the amputation literature that impact reintegration as a whole. Further, reintegration postamputation and barriers experienced by patients may differ between lower versus upper extremity amputation. This study (1) provides an overview of reintegration postamputation from a psychological, social, and biological perspective that incorporates barriers to reintegration and factors to promote resilience and

Department of Physical Medicine and Rehabilitation, Johns Hopkins University School of Medicine, 600 North Wolfe Street, Suite 160, Baltimore, MD 21287, USA
* Corresponding author.
E-mail address: Marlis@jhmi.edu

Phys Med Rehabil Clin N Am 35 (2024) 865–877
https://doi.org/10.1016/j.pmr.2024.06.007
1047-9651/24/© 2024 Elsevier Inc. All rights reserved, including those for text and data mining, AI training, and similar technologies.

positive adjustment across domains (**Fig. 1**) and (2) discusses screening, prevention, and treatments to effectively prevent reintegration challenges, identify difficulties early, and treat patients who have persistent or severe problems.

PSYCHOLOGICAL ADJUSTMENT

Amputation is a major life event, and it is common for patients to experience psychological distress following amputation. However, it is worth emphasizing that psychological distress is not universally experienced. Even when distress is experienced, there is a significant range in symptomology and most people do not develop a major psychiatric disorder.[3] While the psychological effects of amputation are unique to the individual, the most common affective complaints may include depression, anxiety, and posttraumatic stress symptoms.[1] Body image issues, stigmatization, changes in self-identity, and social functioning also commonly arise.[1] Further, it is important to note that research has found greater risks of psychological distress in traumatic amputations than planned or scheduled amputations (ie, vascular, infectious, or tumor pathology) due to the unexpected nature of the injury and a lack of preparedness for such loss.[4,5]

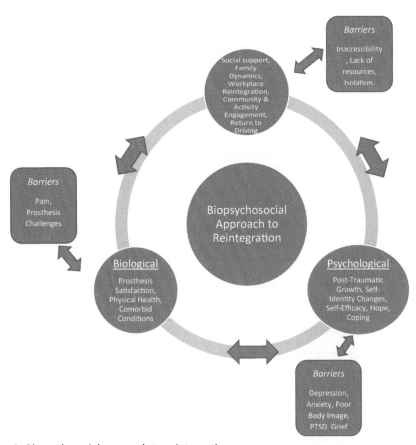

Fig. 1. Biopsychosocial approach to reintegration.

POSITIVE OUTCOMES

Much of the mental health research on patients with amputation have focused on psychopathology and negative psychological outcomes. However, it is important and relevant to highlight the greater proportion of patients who experience posttraumatic growth (PTG) and adjust effectively.[6] PTG is defined as a positive psychological change following a difficult experience, and there is a small literature base that has examined this concept and factors that predict PTG in the amputation population.[7] Some reports have found that up to 77% of patients described a positive outcome postamputation, with factors such as social support, humor, and active coping contributing to positive outcomes.[6,8] In addition, positive cognitive processing within the first 9 week postamputation was found to lead to a greater likelihood of PTG at 12 months postamputation.[9] Higher levels of self-efficacy have also been highlighted as related to adapting to a new normal and maintaining a positive attitude postamputation.[10] Given the large number of patients who adjust well and reintegrate effectively, more literature is needed to better identify factors that lead to positive outcomes.

DEPRESSION, GRIEF, AND RELATED SYMPTOMS

Some literature purports that 21% to 35% of patients may experience depressive symptoms following amputation, which is markedly increased from the general population (10%–15%).[4] Etiology of the depressive experience is likely multifactorial and may include social isolation/withdrawal, a decreased sense of control, guilt, grief, helplessness, changes in self-esteem and body image, and somatic symptoms (eg, pain and phantom sensations).[11] For those with planned amputations, the preoperative period may contain "anticipatory grief" and associated stage-based reactions:[12]

- Denial (eg, refusal to engage in discussion surrounding procedure)
- Anger (eg, conflicts with medical team and feelings of being "tricked" into procedure)
- Bargaining (eg, attempts to stall surgery)
- Depression (eg, feelings of helplessness and overwhelm)
- Acceptance (eg, which may not be reached until the rehabilitation process)

In the postoperative period, there may be significant postamputation grief, in which the individual grieves "the loss of their limb, body integrity, and the [person] they used to be."[13] Further, some may experience guilt and a sense of responsibility for their actions or inactions that preceded their amputation, such as blaming oneself for their accident or health conditions/status.[13] The presence of pain or fear of anticipatory pain may also negatively impact quality of life and subsequently increase depressive symptoms. Individuals may experience pain at the site of injury, phantom pain, or pain associated with a prosthesis.[14] Individuals who experienced continued pain postamputation demonstrate lower levels of acceptance of injury compared to counterparts who experienced lesser levels of pain postamputation. As pain experience is reported to be highest in the immediate postoperative stage, lasting hours to days, timely and appropriate pain management is a crucial component in optimizing patient reactions to amputation.[4]

An additional factor that decreases quality of life and is related to depression is negative body image, which is a common phenomenon after amputation.[15] In addition, Senra and colleagues found that beyond body image, individuals with amputation also experience changes with the self, overall requiring the individual to embrace a new self-identity.[16]

Depression rates are highest within the first 2 years of amputation, and it has been found that time since amputation is an important factor to consider in assessing depression.[3] Compared to other hospitalized populations, rates of depression are found to be higher in amputation patients.[14] Depression may negatively affect the rehabilitation process due to lack of engagement, decreased perception of self-abilities, fatigue, and so forth. Given the acute onset of depressive symptoms postamputation, it is particularly important to address these symptoms to improve rehabilitative trajectories, as delays in intervention may serve to prolong the patients with amputation return to engagement with social, occupational, and recreational activities discussed throughout this article.[12]

ANXIETY AND TRAUMA SYMPTOMS

Studies show that rates of anxiety are also significantly higher in the first 2 years postamputation than in the general population.[11,17] Symptoms of anxiety are especially observed in the early phase of adjustment, as individuals may experience "panic attacks, worry, fear, avoidance behavior, irritability, trouble sleeping, difficulty concentrating, and muscle tension."[3] There is also concern for preoperative anxiety, in which patients may begin to anticipate pain and adjustment difficulties, with some literature suggesting an association between preoperative anxiety state and postoperative acute pain, including phantom limb pain.[12,18] In a series of postamputation interviews, Rosca and colleagues found that patients reported numerous negative thoughts leading to rumination and insomnia including negative projections about the future, fear, existential uncertainty, lack of control, and further anticipations of loss.[11] Some may also experience anxiety due to concerns/fear of a change in ability status in preparation for return to work or in reorganizing family roles (eg, provider and caretaker).[4]

Particularly concerning for increased anxiety reactions are traumatic amputations, in which literature suggests up to 60% of patients may experience significant anxiety within the first 6 months postamputation.[4,19] Following traumatic amputations, it is especially indicated to assess for acute stress disorder or post-traumatic stress (dependent on length of time since injury), as the unexpected nature of the trauma may lead to a higher prevalence of the disorders.[3,20] One study found that 39% of patients with traumatic upper extremity amputation endured posttraumatic stress that amounted to pathologic grief and suggested increased incidence of posttraumatic stress in upper versus lower traumatic amputations.[5] However, planned amputations are not impervious to symptoms of post-traumatic stress and may be observed in approximately 5% of patients.[4] In a cohort of nontraumatic patients with amputation, Pedras and colleagues found posttraumatic stress was associated with worse general and social adjustment and adjustment to limitations.[21] These authors also found that social support mediated the relationship between posttraumatic stress symptoms and adjustment to limitations; however, as posttraumatic stress symptoms may include interpersonal difficulties and social detachment, it is particularly important to assess for and address these concerns in traumatic and nontraumatic amputations.[21]

SCREENING

The literature on screening for psychological adjustment postamputation has largely focused on assessing body image concerns, self-esteem, depression, anxiety, and quality of life, specifically for lower limb amputation.[2] However, more recently, there have been efforts to assess and examine predictors of positive adjustment such as resilience, hope, and social support.[8,22] In addition, there have been a few recent studies examining measures of psychosocial adjustment for upper limb amputation.[23]

There are a handful of amputation-specific screening tools for psychosocial adjustment that have been widely used and studied. The Amputation-Related Body Image Scale and the Amputee Body Image Scale measure body image concerns for patients with amputation and have been associated with other measures of psychosocial well-being as well as significant predictors of psychosocial adjustment.[2] The Trinity Amputation and Prosthetic Experience Scale is a widely used measure assessing psychosocial adjustment in multiple important domains (eg, social adjustment, activity restriction, satisfaction with prostheses, and pain experience).[2] However, this measure has been criticized for a lack of applicability for patients with amputation who do not use prostheses. Thus, Renik and colleagues[23] modified the survey and generated new items for those who do not use prostheses, increasing generalizability for the 20% to 40% of the upper limb amputation population that do not use a prosthesis. In addition to the amputation-specific screening tools, anxiety and depression are commonly assessed in this population using the Hospital Anxiety and Depression Scale, the General Health Questionnaire, and the Center for Epidemiologic Studies-Depression Scale, among other self-report measures.[2] Specifically, these 3 tools consistently demonstrate convergent validity with other self-report measures in the population with lower extremity amputation.[2]

Measuring predictors of positive adjustment to amputation has garnered growing attention in the literature. There have been numerous studies to examine the role of perceived social support, typically measured by the Multidimensional Scale of Perceived Social Support, as a significant mediator between amputation and negative mental health outcomes; with higher levels leading to significantly better adjustment.[8,24] Additionally, hope at the beginning of rehabilitation, measured by the Hope Scale, and effectively adjusting goals postamputation, measured by the Goal Adjustment Scale, have been shown to lead to positive adjustment following a lower limb amputation.[8,25] Finally, self-esteem, measured by the Rosenberg Self Esteem Scale, is commonly assessed and has been found to be a significant predictor of positive adjustment.[26,27] The literature suggests that screening for various mental health symptoms, as outlined earlier, as well as assessing for predictors of positive adjustment, may provide insight into interventions and preventative strategies for providers and patients to improve positive adjustment and reintegration.

PREVENTION AND INTERVENTION

Distress immediately following amputation is common but may resolve overtime as individuals adjust and reintegrate into their lives.[3] Factors that may aid in the prevention of prolonged and severe distress include instilling hope in the beginning of the rehabilitation process,[8] having a strong social support system, and readjusting important goals postamputation.[28] Additionally, a recent qualitative study by Ostler and colleagues[29] found that patients with amputation identified important domains for readjustment and emotional well-being as the ability to participate in valued activities, comfortable and easy prostheses, effectively managing pain, and accepting their new normal. A final important distress prevention factor highlighted in the literature is interdisciplinary teamwork and patient-centered care to promote self-efficacy and empower patients.[3] There is minimal research on trauma-informed care for this population that is particularly relevant due to the higher prevalence of trauma symptoms for patients with amputation compared to the general population.[3,20]

Despite prevention efforts, a portion of patients will experience prolonged and/or severe distress that may require intervention. With regular mental health and psychosocial adjustment screening as outlined earlier, amputation patients with adjustment difficulties may be readily identified and treated. Options for treatment that have been highlighted in the literature include peer support, individual psychotherapy, medications, and learning self-management skills for coping.[3] Prevention efforts, regular mental health screening, and early intervention will help a greater proportion of patients reintegrate effectively into their lives in the community and reengage in valued activities such as driving.

SOCIAL AND COMMUNITY REINTEGRATION

Social factors that are essential to reintegration postamputation include the family unit, redefinition of roles, community integration, romantic relationships, reentering the workforce, and adapting to sports and recreation. The majority of limb loss is in the lower extremities and the literature reflects this. With the intersectionality of common risk factors, some generalizations can be made for adults with limb loss. For example, in industrialized countries, the etiology of limb loss is largely due to vascular disease seen in older male adults with comorbid conditions.[30–34] This sample tends to report more positive experiences since their chronic pain was resolved and they often experience relief.[10,35] In emergent countries, the etiology is often traumatic and occurs in younger male individuals where rehabilitative resources and accessible environments may be limited.[36] Thus, these patients may be at a higher risk to experience more challenging psychological adjustments as outlined earlier. Younger patients with transtibial amputations that are further out from their limb loss are more likely to report higher quality of life, return to work, and community participation. In fact, most patients have positive adjustments in long term.[33,34,37–40]

There are several modifiable factors that predict positive community adjustment and return to work. These include improving physical activity, improving function of the extremity, lack of phantom limb pain, psychological adjustment, high self-efficacy, and prosthetic use. Conversely, factors that can indicate negative community adjustment are inadequately controlled pain, depression, inaccessible environments, and poor body image. These areas can become significant barriers and they are important to address to encourage successful community reintegration.[10,35,37,41–44] Reintegration is multifactorial and promoting positive predictors while identifying and addressing barriers early and effectively can lead to better outcomes.

As discussed previously in relation to mental health, strong social support both preamputation and postamputation is important for successful community reintegration. Additionally, connecting with the limb loss community through peer support networks can also help facilitate positive adjustment.[10,41,44,45] Some individuals with limb loss rely on family and friends as caregivers, which may impact social dynamics. Many individuals endorse fear of "burdening" their support system.[10,30,44] Yet, 78% of people who experienced limb loss reported high social support and satisfaction in life in another study,[31] emphasizing the significance of resilience and PTG as previously discussed. According to one cross-sectional study on caregiver burden when taking care of someone with an amputation, 15.1% of caregivers experienced high burden, 23.3% had mild-to-moderate burden, and 61.6% had no or little burden. Those who experienced the highest burden were those who cared for people with transfemoral amputations.[46] The patients with amputation who expressed conflicts with their support system endorsed greater levels of depression, highlighting the significant interaction between social and psychological factors in reintegration postamputation.[31] Caregiver burden should be openly addressed as there tends to be a disconnect between perceived burden by the individual and experienced burden reported by caregivers.

A majority of caregivers are spouses, yet there is very limited research on romantic relationships, dating, and sex after amputation. More research is needed to understand and provide holistic patient-centered treatment and education while dispelling internal and external stigmatizing attitudes (eg, feeling judged by strangers and inferior to their partners, traditional beauty standards, and self-esteem).[45,47] While sexual functioning and satisfaction vary greatly among patients with amputation, one literature review found that all participants reported a negative impact and/or concerns about their limb loss on their sexual functioning.[48] Negative contributing factors were single status, male gender, phantom or residual limb pain, older age, and more proximal amputation sites.[45,47]

Another major factor in navigating and reintegrating into the community, from a physical perspective, is the prosthesis itself. Research shows that better comfort of the prosthesis is associated with longer duration of use, greater ambulation, and increased engagement in family, community, recreational activities, and work.[30,33,37–41,43] Therefore, having a positive relationship with the rehabilitation team, including the prosthetist, will directly impact reintegration. Selecting a prosthesis and writing the prosthesis prescription must be a patient-centered and goal-directed approach accounting for patient's preferences of prosthesis appearance and desire to participate in certain work, driving, or leisure activities.

Globally, individuals with limb loss fear stigma. Many cultures consider amputation to be a taboo topic either related to death, or self-inflicted or spiritual punishment, and those with limb loss in those cultures may prefer to hide their injury.[10,35,45,47] Therefore, many patients with amputation grapple with body image especially in public areas around strangers and elect to make cosmetic adjustments (eg, shoes and clothing). Some cultures view cosmetic prostheses as a symbol of hope, reintegration, empowerment, and improved functional independence.[10,42,47]

RETURN TO DRIVING

The ability to drive represents freedom and independence to individuals with mobility restrictions such as amputations.[49] The feeling of dependence upon others has been identified as a significant barrier to reintegration following amputation as the patient with amputation commonly does not want to burden caregivers.[50] This may be mitigated for the patients with amputation with reliable access to public transportation. Generally speaking, the ability to drive improves self-esteem and allows for greater autonomy, employment, and recreation.[51]

The Bureau of Transportation Statistics reported that over 90% of people aged 18 to 64 years without disabilities drove a vehicle; though only 60% of respondents with disabilities drove. They also showed that regardless of driving status, respondents with disabilities took fewer trips for social and recreational purposes than those without disabilities but had a similar number of trips for the purposes of errands and attending medical appointments. The reason for this discrepancy is unclear. Current literature on the social and leisure engagement of people with disabilities emphasizes the significant physical and psychological impact of increased engagement, namely increased sense of meaning, belonging, and autonomy, among others.[52] As noted earlier, a large barrier to this engagement is the ability to drive, and more importantly, drive for recreational purposes. There are multiple components and barriers when considering returning to driving postamputation that will be outlined later.

Following an amputation, there are several trends identified throughout the literature in relation to returning to driving. Male individuals are more likely to return to driving compared to female individuals, and patients with upper extremity amputation are more likely to drive compared to patients with lower extremity amputation.[49,53] There are no significant differences in either upper or lower extremity amputations comparing driving rates after left-sided versus right-sided amputations. After lower extremity amputations, those with amputations distal to the knee were more likely to drive compared to amputations proximal to the knee and comparison of upper limb amputations showed no significant differences between proximal and distal to the elbow amputations.[54]

Basic Requirements of Driving

Regardless of the type of amputation, there are some basic requirements all drivers must be able to perform. The act of driving may be broken down into a hierarchy of the strategic tier, the maneuvering tier, and the operational control tier. The strategic tier entails designing a route to safely get to the destination. The maneuvering tier requires a driver to actively negotiate typical driving situations. The operational tier is the most basic tier and encompasses the driver's need to perform essential mechanical tasks such as operating the pedals and turning the steering wheel.[55] The operational control tier is the area most heavily impacted by an amputation as the individual has to learn to perform these essential tasks in a new way. Additionally, as manual and automatic transmission vehicles require different demands from upper, lower, right, and left extremities, the location of amputation is important when considering return to driving due to specific operational barriers.

Lower Extremity Amputation

The reported rate to return to driving after lower extremity amputation ranges between 40% and 80%, with wide ranges likely attributed to broad and international study populations.[49,54] Overall, vehicles with automatic transmissions are best suited for unilateral lower extremity amputations regardless of laterality, as the person with amputation may operate the gas and brake pedals with 1 foot.

It is generally accepted that left lower extremity amputations do not hinder the ability to drive an automatic transmission vehicle. Right lower extremity amputations with an appropriately fitted prosthesis have several options including (1) operate the pedals exclusively with the right prosthesis, (2) use the left foot to operate the pedals in the standard configuration, or (3) modify the car by adding a left-sided accelerator and operating the pedals with the left foot. Meikle and colleagues[56] investigated these 3 configurations in patients with right transtibial amputations wearing a prosthetic device and found that there was no significant difference in response times between them. This study was done in a laboratory, but it does suggest that there is reasonable potential for a right transtibial amputation with a prosthesis to operate an automatic vehicle without modification. Despite these findings, we do not recommend patients to operate vehicle pedals with a prosthesis due to the lack of proprioception. We further do not recommend using a "2 feet technique" to operate the pedals, where 1 foot operates the accelerator and 1 foot the brake, regardless of the laterality of the amputation. In addition, our clinical recommendation for right lower extremity amputations is to operate the pedals with the left foot in standard configuration or to use the left foot with the addition of a left-footed accelerator.

No significant difference was identified in return to driving rates when comparing transfemoral and transtibial amputations of the right side. Regardless of amputation level, most patients with right lower extremity amputation simply drove with their left foot with standard pedal configuration.[49]

Upper Extremity Amputation

Similar to lower extremity amputations, those with upper extremity amputations are best served with an automatic transmission vehicle, as this eliminates the need to operate the gear. In unilateral arm amputations, regardless of the level of the amputation, a spinner knob attached to the steering wheel is the most recommended assistive device.[51] As technology continues to improve, some of these spinner knobs also have integrated vehicle controls that allow the driver to always keep their hand on the steering wheel. These types of spinner knobs are more frequently recommended to those with a transhumeral amputation or higher.[51]

Multiple Limb Amputations

For those with multiple limb amputations, a combination of devices may be required. Occupational therapists can make recommendations for vehicle modifications, provide training with the adaptations, and can optimize the ergonomics of driving. In these more complex scenarios, the patient with amputation is best served by undergoing a formal evaluation by a qualified Driver Rehabilitation Professional (DRP). The Association for Driver Rehabilitation Specialists is the credentialing authority for DRPs in the United States and Canada. Each state in the United States maintains a list of DRPs who can perform an evaluation, make recommendations, and provide training on driving adaptation devices. The cost of an assessment varies depending on location and typically is not covered by medical insurance.

In the United States, each state's licensing authority has their own requirements and processes related to clearing a patient with amputation to drive. It is also worth noting that the Americans with Disabilities Act prohibit insurance companies from charging a higher premium to a disabled driver based solely on their disability. These considerations are essential when discussing reintegration as driving has a significant impact on the ability of the individual to reintegrate back into the community and participate in social and recreational activities.

EXERCISE

Exercise leads to benefits mentally, physically, and, at times, socially. The patients with amputation who participate in physical activities report higher self-esteem and quality of life and increased perceptions of social support, physical functioning, and acceptance of their disability. Between 10% and 60% of individuals with lower limb amputation participate in sports, with preferred activities to be fishing, swimming, golf, walking, and cycling.[32,34] For more competitive sports, specialized prostheses and individualized training programs are preferred.[32] Limb loss may put individuals at increased risk for sport-related injuries; however, many believe that the psychosocial benefits outweigh the risks.[34] Age, gender, etiology of amputation, site of amputation, comorbid conditions, and prosthetic characteristics all affect return to sports.[30,41] Barriers to participating in recreational activities include access to suitable prostheses, prosthetic cost, and inaccessible facilities.[37]

RETURNING TO WORK

Returning to work is multifactorial; however, the largest contributing factor is mobility, which depends on one's prosthesis and access to rehabilitative services.[36,43] A study of Bengali patients with amputation reported up to 60% of individuals did not return to work, resulting in lost wages, poor treatment access, high medical costs, and ultimately high rates of impoverishment (up to 80%).[36] Taken together, poor return to work may lead to adverse outcomes such as financial strain, decreased access to care, and deleterious psychological effects such as depression, grief, and a loss of/change in identity (ie, provider). However, the majority of people with limb loss worldwide (60%–70%) do return to work. Positive return to work factors, which overlap with the previously mentioned community integration factors, are younger age, longer period of time since the amputation, higher education level, amputation site, use of and satisfaction with a prosthesis, and work self-efficacy.[33,37,39,40] Return to work may require workplace accommodations or transition to a less physically demanding role that is also apparent among service members.[33,39,40]

SUMMARY

In summary, when considering reintegration postamputation from a biopsychosocial perspective, it is important to understand and recognize the significant interaction between each respective domain. While most patients with amputation report positive psychological adjustment, those who experience more significant mental health symptoms may have greater reintegration difficulty in other areas. For instance, an amputation can impact a person's ability to drive which may make it harder to participate in recreation. With less recreation, they may begin to feel isolated and depressed that can impact intimate relationships, and so forth. Pain and access to comfortable prostheses can create significant barriers to reintegration in the community and can lead to difficulties with psychological adjustment. Therefore, it is imperative to complete early and frequent mental health screenings for patients with amputation, implement early intervention, assess the biopsychosocial barriers to reintegration outlined earlier, and to address these barriers early and efficiently.

CLINICS CARE POINTS

- Regular and early mental health screening is imperative to identify patients with amputation at risk for developing more severe symptoms that may hinder reintegration and require intervention.

- Location of amputation is important to consider when assessing and considering barriers to reintegration from a biopsychosocial perspective.

- Interdisciplinary teams should consider the psychological, social, and biological aspects of patients with amputation and their life for optimal reintegration.

DISCLOSURE

The authors declare that they have no relevant or material financial interests that relate to the research described in this article.

REFERENCES

1. Hamill R, Carson S, Dorahy M. Experiences of psychosocial adjustment within 18 months of amputation: an interpretative phenomenological analysis. Disabil Rehabil 2009;32(9):729–40.

2. Wolfe DL, Hebert JS, Miller WC, et al. Psychological adjustment to lower limb amputation: an evaluation of outcome measurement tools. Psychoprosthetics 2019;67–90.

3. Wegener ST, Hofkamp SE and Ehde DM, Interventions for psychological issues in amputation: a team approach, In: Psychoprosthetics, 2008, Springer London; London, 91–10.

4. Jo SH, Kang SH, Seo WS, et al. Psychiatric understanding and treatment of patients with amputations. Yeungnam Univ J Med 2021;38(3):194–201.

5. Pomares G, Coudane H, Dap F, et al. Psychological effects of traumatic upper-limb amputations. J Orthop Traumatol: Surgery & Research 2020;106(2): 297–300.

6. Dunn DS. Well-being following amputation: salutary effects of positive meaning, optimism, and control. Rehabil Psychol 1996;41(4):285–302.

7. Stutts LA, Stanaland AW. Posttraumatic growth in individuals with amputations. Disabil Health J 2016;9(1):167–71.

8. Unwin J, Kacperek L, Clarke C. A prospective study of positive adjustment to lower limb amputation. Clin Rehabil 2009;23(11):1044–50.

9. Phelps LF, Williams RM, Raichle KA, et al. The importance of cognitive processing to adjustment in the 1st year following amputation. Rehabil Psychol 2008; 53(1):28–38.

10. Yip K, Yip Y, Tsui W. Thoughts and experiences regarding leg amputation among patients with diabetic foot ulcers: a phenomenological study. Int Wound J 2023; 20(6):2159–68.

11. Roşca AC, Baciu CC, Burtăverde V, et al. Psychological consequences in patients with amputation of a limb. an interpretative-phenomenological analysis. Front Psychol 2021;12:537493.

12. Bhuvaneswar CG, Epstein LA, Stern TA. Reactions to amputation: recognition and treatment. Prim Care Companion J Clin Psychiatry 2007;9(4):303–8.

13. Belon HP, Vigoda DF. Emotional adaptation to limb loss. Phys Med Rehabil Clin N Am 2014;25(1):53–74.

14. Calabrese L, Maffoni M, Torlaschi V, et al. What is hidden behind amputation? quanti-qualitative systematic review on psychological adjustment and quality of life in lower limb amputees for non-traumatic reasons. Healthcare 2023;11(11): 1661.

15. Holzer LA, Sevelda F, Fraberger G, et al. Body image and self-esteem in lower-limb amputees. PLoS One 2014;9(3):e92943.

16. Senra H, Oliveira RA, Leal I, et al. Beyond the body image: a qualitative study on how adults experience lower limb amputation. Clin Rehabil 2012;26(2):180–91.

17. Waqar S, Noor R, Khan MMH. Depression, anxiety & psychological adjustment among amputees. Int J Rehabil Res 2015;4:14–8.

18. Raichle KA, Hanley MA, Molton I, et al. Prosthesis use in persons with lower- and upper-limb amputation. J Rehabil Res Dev 2008;45(7):961–72.

19. Mckechnie PS, John A. Anxiety and depression following traumatic limb amputation: a systematic review. Injury 2014;45(12):1859–66.

20. Copuroglu C, Ozcan M, Yilmaz B, et al. Acute stress disorder and post-traumatic stress disorder following traumatic amputation. Acta Orthop Belg 2010; 76(1):90–3.

21. Pedras S, Carvalho R, Pereira MG. A predictive model of anxiety and depression symptoms after a lower limb amputation. Disabil Health J 2018;11(1):79–85.

22. Miller MJ, Mealer ML, Cook PF, et al. Psychometric assessment of the connor-davidson resilience scale for people with lower-limb amputation. Phys Ther 2021;101(4):pzab002.
23. Resnik L, Ni P, Borgia ML, et al. A psychosocial adjustment measure for persons with upper limb amputation. Can Prosthet Orthot J 2022;5(1):37873.
24. Pedras S, Vilhena E, Carvalho R, et al. Quality of life following a lower limb amputation in diabetic patients: a longitudinal and multicenter study. Psychiatry 2020; 83(1):47–57.
25. Mireille NN, Nadège FOJE N. Social resilience and self-esteem among amputees: a case study of amputees with positive self-esteem. J Med Clin Res Rev 2019; 3(3). https://doi.org/10.33425/2639-944x.1088.
26. Kizilkurt OK. Quality of life after lower extremity amputation due to diabetic foot ulcer: the role of prosthesis-related factors, body image, self-esteem, and coping styles. Düşünen Adam J Psychiatry Neurol Sci 2020. https://doi.org/10.14744/dajpns.2020.00070.
27. Pedras S, Vilhena E, Carvalho R, et al. Psychosocial adjustment to a lower limb amputation ten months after surgery. Rehabil Psychol 2018;63(3):418–30.
28. Coffey L, Gallagher P, Desmond D. A prospective study of the importance of life goal characteristics and goal adjustment capacities in longer term psychosocial adjustment to lower limb amputation. Clin Rehabil 2013;28(2):196–205.
29. Ostler C, Donovan-Hall M, Dickinson A, et al. Exploring meaningful outcome domains of recovery following lower limb amputation and prosthetic rehabilitation: the patient's perspective. Disabil Rehabil 2023;45(23):3937–50.
30. Urva M, Donnelley CA, Challa ST, et al. Transfemoral amputation and prosthesis provision in Tanzania: patient and provider perspectives. Afr J Disabil 2023;12: 1084.
31. Brier MJ, Williams RM, Turner AP, et al. Quality of relationships with caregivers, depression, and life satisfaction after dysvascular lower extremity amputation. Arch Phys Med Rehabil 2018;99(3):452–8.
32. Matthews DJ, Sukeik M, Haddad F. Return to sport following amputation. J Sports Med Phys Fitness 2014;54(4):481–6.
33. Schoppen T, Boonstra A, Groothoff JW, et al. Factors related to successful job reintegration of people with a lower limb amputation. Arch Phys Med Rehabil 2001;82(10):1425–31.
34. Bragaru M, Dekker R, Geertzen JHB, et al. Amputees and sports: a systematic review. Sports Med 2011;41(9):721–40.
35. Abouammoh N, Aldebeyan W, Abuzaid R. Experiences and needs of patients with lower limb amputation in Saudi Arabia: a qualitative study. East Mediterr Health J 2020;27(4):407–13.
36. Sayeed MSI, Oakman J, Dillon MP, et al. Disability, economic and work-role status of individuals with unilateral lower-limb amputation and their families in Bangladesh, post-amputation, and pre-rehabilitation: a cross-sectional study. Work 2022;73(4):1405–19.
37. Sions JM, Seth M, Pohlig RT, et al. Key modifiable factors in community participation among adults with lower limb amputation. Am J Phys Med Rehabil 2023; 102(9):803–9.
38. Damiani C, Pournajaf S, Goffredo M, et al. Community ambulation in people with lower limb amputation. Medicine 2021;100(3):e24364.
39. Darter BJ, Hawley CE, Armstrong AJ, et al. Factors influencing functional outcomes and return-to-work after amputation: a review of the literature. J Occup Rehabil 2018;28(4):656–65.

40. Journeay WS, Pauley T, Kowgier M, et al. Return to work after occupational and non-occupational lower extremity amputation. Occup Med 2018;68(7):438–43.
41. Hutchison A, D'Cruz K, Keeves J, et al. Barriers and facilitators to community reintegration in adults following traumatic upper limb amputation: an exploratory study. Disabil Rehabil 2024;46(16):3691–701.
42. Bernhoff K, Björck M, Larsson J, et al. Patient experiences of life years after severe civilian lower extremity trauma with vascular injury. Eur J Vasc Endovasc Surg 2016;52(5):690–5.
43. Clemens SM, Kershaw KN, McDonald CL, et al. Disparities in functional recovery after dysvascular lower limb amputation are associated with employment status and self-efficacy. Disabil Rehabil 2023;45(14):2280–7.
44. Keeves J, Hutchison A, D'Cruz K, et al. Social and community participation following traumatic lower limb amputation: an exploratory qualitative study. Disabil Rehabil 2023;45(26):4404–12.
45. Ward Khan Y, O'Keeffe F, Nolan M, et al. "Not a whole woman": an interpretative phenomenological analysis of the lived experience of women's body image and sexuality following amputation. Disabil Rehabil 2021;43(2):251–61.
46. Alessa M, Alkhalaf HA, Alwabari SS, et al. The psychosocial impact of lower limb amputation on patients and caregivers. Cureus 2022;14(11). https://doi.org/10.7759/cureus.3124.
47. Mathias Z, Harcourt D. Dating and intimate relationships of women with below-knee amputation: an exploratory study. Disabil Rehabil 2013;36(5):395–402.
48. Geertzen JHB, Van Es CG, Dijkstra PU. Sexuality and amputation: a systematic literature review. Disabil Rehabil 2009;31(7):522–7.
49. Boulias C, Meikle B, Pauley T, et al. Return to driving after lower-extremity amputation. Arch Phys Med Rehabil 2006;87(9):1183–8.
50. Liu F, Williams RM, Liu HE, et al. The lived experience of persons with lower extremity amputation. J Clin Nurs 2010;19(15–16):2152–61.
51. Burger H, Marincek C. Driving ability following upper limb amputation. Prosthet Orthot Int 2013;37(5):391–5.
52. Labbé D, Miller WC, Ng R. Participating more, participating better: Health benefits of adaptive leisure for people with disabilities. Disabil Health J 2018. https://doi.org/10.1016/j.dhjo.2018.11.007.
53. Engkasan JP, Ehsan FM, Chung TY. Ability to return to driving after major lower limb amputation. J Rehabil Med 2012;44(1):19–23.
54. Fernández A, López MJ, Navarro R. Performance of persons with juvenile-onset amputation in driving motor vehicles. Arch Phys Med Rehabil 2000;81(3):288–91.
55. Heikkilä VM, Kallanranta T. Evaluation of the driving ability in disabled persons: a practitioners' view. Disabil Rehabil 2005;27(17):1029–36.
56. Meikle B, Devlin M, Pauley T. Driving pedal reaction times after right transtibial amputations. Arch Phys Med Rehabil 2006;87(3):390–4.

Innovations in Amputation Rehabilitation and Prosthetic Design

Mary E. Matsumoto, MD[a,b,*], Juan Cave II, MSPO, CPO[a],
John Shaffer, BS, CPO[a]

KEYWORDS

- Amputation rehabilitation • Prosthesis • Artificial limb • Osseointegration
- Targeted muscle reinnervation • Sensory restoration

KEY POINTS

- New socket designs and interfaces seek to improve common challenges with traditional socket design, which include discomfort, skin problems, residual limb volume fluctuations, and sweating.
- Osseointegration is a surgical procedure that allows for direct attachment of the prosthesis to the skeleton via a percutaneous, bone-anchored implant, eliminating the need for a socket altogether.
- Increasingly sophisticated prosthetic componentry is now available with microprocessor and hydraulic control, powered joints, and crossover feet. There are benefits and drawbacks to each type of componentry. Selection should be based on the patient's condition, goals, and environment.
- Despite advances in prosthetic design and componentry, prosthetic users are still limited by lack of intuitive prosthetic control and sensory feedback from their prosthesis. Muscle and sensory reinnervation procedures such as targeted muscle reinnervation are of great interest in their ability to provide these. Some have been shown to have the additional benefit of improving postamputation pain.

INTRODUCTION

The history of human advancements in amputation rehabilitation and prosthetic design goes back millennia to fossils from ancient Egypt that have been found with cosmetic additions to replace missing toes.[1] The oldest known prosthetic limb, the "Capula leg," discovered by archeologists in 300 B.C., was made of wood and bronze.[1]

---

[a] Department of Physical Medicine and Rehabilitation, Minneapolis VA Health Care System, 1 Veterans Drive, Minneapolis, MN 55417, USA; [b] Department of Rehabilitation Medicine, University of Minnesota, Minneapolis, MN, USA
* Corresponding author. Department of Physical Medicine and Rehabilitation, Minneapolis VA Health Care System, 1 Veterans Drive, Mail Stop 117, Minneapolis, MN 55417.
E-mail address: Mary.Matsumoto@va.gov

Phys Med Rehabil Clin N Am 35 (2024) 879–896
https://doi.org/10.1016/j.pmr.2024.06.008
1047-9651/24/Published by Elsevier Inc.

Although this history goes back to ancient times, innovation has accelerated in modern times. In the last several decades, there were groundbreaking advancements such as the ischial containment socket in the 1970s, gel liners in the 1980s, energy-storing carbon fiber feet, and microprocessor componentry in the 1990s.

Today, advances in materials, technology, and surgical techniques seek to address challenges and limitations of artificial limbs. New techniques in casting and new socket design focus on making prosthetic care more accessible and less time-intensive, as well as making sockets more comfortable and adjustable. Prosthetic componentry continues to grow more technologically sophisticated, seeking to mimic the functions of the missing joints. Finally, surgical procedures are expanding the horizons of prosthetic rehabilitation: for the first time, osseointegration offers an alternative to the traditional socket and motor and sensory reinnervation offer the potential for more intuitive motor control and sensory restoration.

As in past times, all of these innovations seek to address challenges with prosthetic use and improve the experience, function, and quality of life of the user. It is the challenge of clinicians to understand the multitude of different prosthetic and surgical options available after amputation and provide the most appropriate and up-to-date rehabilitation and prosthetic management to help their patients achieve the best possible outcome after amputation.

SURGICAL INNOVATIONS
Osseointegration

Osseointegration is a surgical technique that involves direct anchorage of an implant in bone by the formation of bony tissue around the implant. This technique was pioneered by Per-Ingvar Branemark in the 1950s, who developed a commercially pure titanium implant, which was well tolerated within living bone and relatively resistant to infection. Since the 1990s, percutaneous osseointegrated implants have been used for the attachment of a prosthesis directly to the skeleton.[2]

By allowing for the attachment of a prosthesis directly to the skeleton, the need for socket, interface, and suspension of a traditional socket is eliminated. In some cases, challenges with the use of a traditional socket are the limiting or prohibitive factor in terms of prosthetic use. Common challenges include

- Sweating or dermatologic issues,
- Residual limb volume fluctuations,
- Inadequate suspension particularly in the case of short residual limbs,
- Difficulty donning and doffing the socket, and
- Socket discomfort especially when sitting.[3]

A study of persons with lower extremity amputations reported that half had socket problems and 22% to 41% had skin problems.[4] Additionally, eliminating the socket could reduce the need for prosthetic follow-up care in terms of socket replacements and adjustments.

In addition to eliminating socket-related complications, osseointegration has additional potential benefits such as increased sitting comfort, increased ease of donning and doffing the prosthesis, improved hip range of motion (ROM) and walking ability, reduced energy expenditure, and increased sensory feedback, termed "osseoperception."[5]

Patient selection
Patient selection is very important for the success of the procedure. Although inclusion and exclusion criteria vary slightly depending on implant type and institution, inclusion criteria generally include

- Skeletally mature adult
- Challenges using a traditional socket prosthesis
- Bony anatomy of the residual limb can accommodate the implant (ie, bone length, endosteal diameter, and cortical thickness)
- Able to follow the rehabilitation protocol

The risks of the procedure include infection; implant loosening and failure; and skeletal fracture. Because of these risks, populations with a higher risk of infection, impaired healing, and fracture are not eligible for this procedure. Contraindications include[5]

- Diabetes
- Peripheral vascular disease
- Immunocompromise
- Active or dormant infection
- Smoking
- Osteoporosis
- Atypical bony anatomy
- Skin disease of the amputated limb

Moreover, there are lifetime precautions against:

- High-impact activities such as running and jumping
- Activities that would put excessive torque on the implant
- Swimming in community pools, ponds, and lakes

In general, the ideal candidate is someone in good health who is or has the potential to be an active prosthetic user but is limited by complications from their socket. They must also be able to commit the necessary time to the surgical and rehabilitation protocols.

Implant systems

Osseointegrated prostheses for the rehabilitation of amputees. The osseointegrated prostheses for the rehabilitation of amputees (OPRA; Integrum) was first performed in Europe in the 1990s using the osseointegration implant developed by Branemark. It is currently the only implant system to have Food and Drug Administration (FDA) premarket approval, having been approved for use at the transfemoral level in December, 2020.[5]

The OPRA system is implanted in a 2 stage surgery.[5] Componentry consists of a fixture, a threaded intramedullary implant, an abutment, and an abutment screw (**Fig. 1**). The implant is composed of commercially pure titanium.

Integral leg prosthesis. The integral leg prosthesis (ILP; OrthoDynamics) was developed in Germany in the late 1990s.[5] It is currently used in the Netherlands and Australia. It has been used at the transfemoral, transtibial, and transhumeral levels. It has not been approved for use in the United States.

Like OPRA, the ILP is implanted in a 2 stage surgery. Unlike OPRA that uses a screw-style implant, the ILP uses a press-fit intermedullary implant composed of cobalt-chrome-molybdenum and transcutaneous dual cone adapter to which the prosthesis attaches.[5]

Osseointegrated prosthetic limb. The osseointegrated prosthetic limb (OPL; OrthoDynamics) was introduced in Australia in 2011.[6] It is also used in the Netherlands. Similar to the ILP, it is used at the transfemoral, transtibial, and transhumeral levels and is not approved for use in the United States.[5]

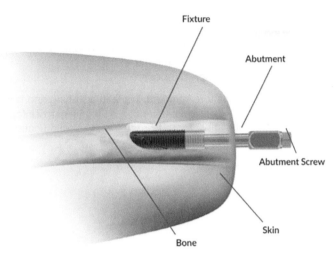

Fig. 1. Fixture and abutment components of the OPRA implant system placed in the femur bone of the residual limb. (With permission from Integrum.)

The OPL can also be implanted in a 2 stage surgery, although more recently, a single-stage procedure has been developed.[6] The componentry is similar to the ILP with press-fit intermedullary implant and transcutaneous dual cone adapter. The OPL implant is composed of titanium alloy (Ti6A14V) with a plasma-sprayed surface coating to promote osseointegration.[5]

Percutaneous osseointegrated prosthesis. The percutaneous osseointegrated prosthesis (POP; DJO Global) was developed at the University of Utah for use at the transfemoral level. An FDA-approved early feasibility study was completed.[7]

The POP is implanted in a 2 stage surgery. The componentry consists of a press-fit intermedullary implant composed of titanium alloy (Ti6A14 V) with the distal implant and collar having an additional porous titanium coating, as well as a percutaneous post and a prosthetic device adapter.[7]

Surgical procedure
Prior to surgery, radiologic imaging is obtained to assess bone length, endosteal diameter, and cortical thickness to make sure the implant is compatible with bony anatomy.

In most cases, the osseointegration procedure involves a 2 stage surgery. In the first stage, the intermedullary implant is inserted into the residual bone. In the second stage, the percutaneous component is attached, and the soft tissue is closed around it. For OPRA, there is a period of 3 to 6 months between the first and second stages to allow the bone to grow into the fixture to anchor it in the femur, whereas for the ILP, OPL, and POP systems, the interval between first and second surgeries is 4 to 8 weeks.[5,6]

Rehabilitation protocol
The rehabilitation protocol for OPRA begins 6 weeks after the second surgery. A short training prosthesis is used for progressive weight-bearing, starting at 20 kg, and increasing by 10 kg every week. At 3 to 6 months postoperatively, full weight-bearing is achieved, and a full-length prosthesis is provided. The loading program may take up to a year after the second surgery. If there is pain near the implant, the loading program is postponed until the pain resolves.[2]

For the press-fit devices, rehabilitation begins soon after the second surgery and progresses more quickly. For the ILP, partial weight-bearing begins immediately after the second surgery with progression to full weight-bearing at 4 to 6 weeks. In the case of the OPL, limited weight-bearing is allowed on day 3 and most progress to unaided walking in 4 to 5 months.[6] After POP implantation, rehabilitation begins on the first day after surgery with partial weight-bearing following a 10 day rehabilitation protocol prior to discharge from the hospital. In the pilot study, most participants achieved independent ambulation at 5 weeks postoperatively.[7]

Prosthetic management

In terms of prosthetic componentry, most systems recommend the use of an additional fail-safe component to prevent excessive torque from being transmitted to the implant. In the case of the OPRA system, the Axor II safety device is coupled between the distal end abutment and the prosthesis.[8] Osseointegration is compatible with all commercially available prosthetic componentry except for powered componentry.

Outcomes

Complications. Superficial skin infections are the most common complication with rates most often reported in the 20% to 55% range.[5] Deep infections were generally less common (2%–5.9%) though one study reported a higher rate of 21.6% and septic failure was rare (0%–3.3%). Aseptic failure and femoral fracture were also less common (0%–10% for both). Additionally, with advances in implant design, surgical technique, and rehabilitation protocols, lower rates of complications have been observed.[6]

Function and quality of life. Studies of all systems consistently report improvements in prosthetic usage, mobility, physical function, and quality of life after osseointegration.[5,6] After osseointegration, patients reported using their prosthesis more compared to their traditional prosthesis as well as being more mobile with it. They also reported less problems with their prosthesis and better prosthesis-related quality of life.

In terms of quantitative measurements, a study showed improvements on the 6 min walk test and Timed Up-and-Go test after osseointegration and showed increased walking distance and speed with less oxygen requirements.[9]

Other benefits noted were improved sitting comfort, less time needed to manage the prosthesis, "osseoperception," and incorporation of the prosthesis into body image.[6]

Motor and Sensory Reinnervation

Another new frontier in amputation rehabilitation is motor and sensory reinnervation to provide more intuitive motor control and sensory feedback from the prosthesis. These procedures have initially been used in upper extremity amputations where existing prosthetic options poorly replicated the sensory feedback and degrees of freedom of motion of the arm and hand leading to poor acceptance, even with the advent of myoelectric prostheses.[10]

A 2013 survey reported that patients with amputation wanted enhanced, intuitive motor control and the ability to feel with their prosthesis.[11] The goal of motor and sensory reinnervation is to restore these abilities. Other benefits of sensory restoration include not having to rely solely on visual input and being able to modulate motor control based on sensory input.

Furthermore, many of these procedures have been found to improve postamputation neuroma pain in both the residual limb and the phantom limb.[12–15] This may occur through inhibiting neuroma formation and reversing maladaptive cortical reorganization.

Targeted muscle reinnervation

Targeted muscle reinnervation (TMR) is a surgical procedure that was developed by Kuiken at Northwestern to provide improved prosthetic control of upper extremity myoelectric prostheses. He first reported its use in a human subject with a shoulder disarticulation amputation in 2004.[16] It was initially not considered in lower extremity amputations because of infrequent use of myoelectric prostheses.

Surgical procedure. In this procedure, amputated nerve endings are either coapted to recipient motor nerves or implanted directly into the muscle. The targeted muscles are no longer biomechanically functional after amputation, and once reinnervated by the amputated nerve, their contraction can be recorded by surface electrodes to provide control signals for a myoelectric prosthesis[17] (**Fig. 2**). Postoperatively, it takes 3 to 6 months for electromyogram (EMG) signals from transplanted nerves to become robust.

At the transhumeral level, median, ulnar, and radial nerves can be transferred into the short head of the biceps, the brachialis and the lateral head of the triceps to provide signals for closing the hand, wrist motion, and opening the hand, respectively. At the shoulder disarticulation level, the musculocutaneous, median, radial, and ulnar nerves can be transferred into the pectoralis major, pectoralis minor, and latissimus dorsi.[2]

Contraindications to the surgery include

- Brachial plexopathy,
- Lack of muscle targets,
- Poor quality of local soft tissue, and
- Inability to tolerate the surgical procedure that typically lasts 2.5 to 5 hours.[2]

Prosthetic control. In TMR, implantation of the severed nerves into the muscles of the residual limb provides additional myosites, which allows for simultaneous prosthetic control of different joints. For example, instead of having to switch between using 2 myosites (biceps and triceps) to control 4 actions (elbow flexion and extension, hand opening and closing), there could be 4 myosites (2 in biceps, 2 in triceps) to control each action.

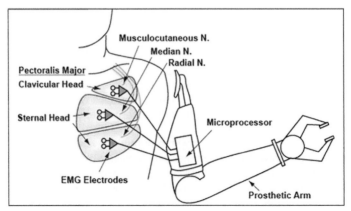

Fig. 2. TMR in person with shoulder disarticulation. EMG, electromyogram; N, nerve. (*From* Shirley Ryan Ability Lab; with permission.)

It also provides more intuitive prosthetic control with the amputated nerves controlling physiologically appropriate functions in the prosthesis. An example of this would be implanting the severed median nerve into the short head of the biceps after a transhumeral amputation. Once reinnervation occurs, when the subject thinks of closing their hand, the short head of the biceps will contract, creating an electromyographic signal. The myoelectric prosthesis can be programmed so that this signal causes the prosthetic hand to close. In short, when the subject thinks of closing their hand, their prosthetic hand will close.

In a series of 3 patients with transhumeral amputations undergoing TMR with amputated median and radial nerves being transplanted into the median heads of the biceps and motor nerve of the brachialis respectively, 2 of the 3 had successful nerve transfers resulting in 4 myosites instead of 2. Following surgery, both were fit with a modified prosthesis with 4 myosites and were able to simultaneously operate the elbow and hand. Moreover, both showed improvement on functional outcome measures, and both preferred this prosthesis.[17]

Pain control. Studies suggest that TMR improves residual limb pain and phantom limb pain in upper and lower extremity amputations.[12,13]

Sensory restoration and targeted sensory restoration. After undergoing TMR, some patients have had sensation in the missing hand and arm restored to the skin over the reinnervated muscles, implying cutaneous reinnervation was occurring as well.[18] The referred sensations were intermixed with native skin sensation and did not precisely correlate with the sensory map of the transferred nerve. The surgical technique has been further refined with the goal of reliably recreating the sensory map of the hand on the skin of the residual limb.[19] If this can be accomplished, the next step is creating an interface that can transmit sensation from the prosthetic hand onto this sensory map on the residual limb.

Targeted nerve implantation
In targeted nerve implantation (TNI), a severed nerve ending is implanted into a secondary motor point of a muscle of the residual limb. Similar to TMR, TNI involves transfer of an amputated nerve to a surgically denervated muscle to encourage orderly reinnervation. However, unlike TMR, the goal of TNI is not to create defined EMG signals for prosthetic control, but to prevent or improve postamputation pain. Because of this, more distal nerve transfer is possible, and denervation of proximal muscles can be avoided.

Both TNI and TMR can be done primarily at the time of amputation or secondarily afterward. A study of primary and secondary TNI showed that both improved neuroma pain.[14]

Regenerative peripheral nerve interfaces
Regenerative peripheral nerve interfaces (RPNIs) involve implanting severed peripheral nerves into free, devascularized muscle grafts. This differs from TMR and TNI, which have living muscle targets for nerve transplantation. The benefit is that muscle can be harvested from a distant donor site if it is not available due to scar tissue or soft tissue damage. Reinnervation of the graft occurs as early as 1 month postoperatively.[20]

Potential benefits of RPNI include improvement in postamputation pain, prosthetic control, and sensory restoration. To date, its use for postamputation pain is the most well studied with multiple studies showing improvement in neuroma and phantom limb pain with RPNI.[15,21]

In terms of prosthetic control, there is a case study of 2 participants with upper extremity amputations implanted with RPNIs that produced EMG signals which they could use to control a virtual prosthesis.[22]

With regard to sensory restoration, Vu reported a study of 2 patients who underwent RPNI with the median and ulnar nerves. Stimulation of these implanted nerves by an electrode placed on the muscle graft surface produced sensation in the phantom hand in the respective nerve sensory distribution.[23]

Sensory restoration through neural interfaces

Another method of restoring sensation currently under investigation is through implanted neural interfaces in which electrodes are implanted in nerves of the residual limb. Implantation can be epineural, interneural, or intraneural. Signals captured by sensors on the prosthesis are transmitted to the implanted electrodes, which stimulate the peripheral nerve using a current proportional to the original input, restoring the sensation from the missing limb. Investigation is ongoing into the long-term stability of this interface and its potential impact on the health of the nerve due to scarring.[20]

PROSTHETIC INNOVATIONS
Casting Techniques

Traditional socket fabrication requires the prosthetist to cast the patient's residual limb with either fiberglass or plaster bandage. During casting, the clinician must expose anatomy such as fibular head or distal tibia to ensure that they are not impinged upon in the final socket. Once the cast is obtained, modifications are performed to apply pressure to the tolerant areas and to relieve pressure over the intolerant areas. From this model, a clear diagnostic socket is fabricated prior to the final carbon fiber socket. This workflow is very laborious and time-consuming for both patient and clinician. To expedite this process, orthotic and prosthetic manufacturers have developed novel techniques to decrease the fabrication time. These new techniques are known as direct-to-socket or compression-based casting.

Currently, there are 2 different direct-to-socket options on the market. The primary goal of this design is to provide a well-fitting carbon fiber socket as quickly as possible without use of a diagnostic socket. The Ossur Direct Socket System utilizes carbon fiber weave, where acrylic resin is pushed evenly over the patient's limb.[24] Next, a rubber bladder is slid over the patient's limb, where it is pumped up to the desired amount of pressure, which is determined by the patient's residual limb soft tissue type (soft, medium, or firm). The pressure is evenly spread over the limb so that no areas of direct pressure are noticeable. Once cured, the socket is removed and finished for the patient to take home. A study of 38 transfemoral prosthetic users fit with the Direct Socket saw a 29.8% increase in prosthetic satisfaction and a 14.8% increase in satisfaction with their service.[25]

The Ottobock Amparo direct-to-socket design uses a prefabricated carbon fiber mold, which is selected based on the measurement of the patient's residual limb.[26] The carbon mold is preheated for 10 minutes in a heating hood, during which time it becomes malleable. It is placed on the limb and manually manipulated on the patient as it cools. Air is drawn from the mold to produce a well-fitting socket. Once completely cooled, the socket is removed and smoothed for the patient to take home.

These novel casting techniques allow patients to mobilize quicker than they would with traditional techniques. Due to portability and ease of fabrication, these techniques can be used outside of the clinic, which expands the reach of a prosthetist. Mobility of prosthetic care provides the opportunity to improve access and improve outcomes.[26,27]

Another novel casting technique is water casting with the Symphonie Aqua System, which has been commercially available for a few years, primarily in Europe, but with growing popularity in the United States (**Fig. 3**). This technique is conceptually similar to the aforementioned systems, in that it provides total surface pressure evenly distributed across the residual limb. Unlike those systems, this technique requires a cast of the limb while the patient is weight-bearing. The patient's limb is wrapped with plaster bandage and placed in a cylindrical chamber, where the walls are lined with rubber bladders which are subsequently filled with water. The amount of pressure applied to the limb is based on the patients' weight and residual limb tissue type. These variables are applied to a mobile application (Symphonie VC App) that produces the desired, constant pressure for the limb.[28,29] During the casting process, the patient is required to stand for the entire time while the plaster dries, which is approximately 5 minutes.

The cast produced from this technique can go straight to a diagnostic or definitive socket without any plaster modification. Research has shown that this technique is equally as comfortable as traditional methods and takes about the same amount of time from start to finish.[30,31] It is important to note that the requirement to stand during casting can be challenging for patients with lower mobility.

New casting and fabrication techniques are frequently introduced to the field of prosthetics and orthotics. It is the job of the clinician to determine which technique works best for their patients given their specific needs. The downside of these novel techniques is that there is a learning curve that could lead to poor initial results.

Socket Design

During the modern era of prosthetics (post-WWI), socket designs have gone through a variety of changes.[1] Advancements have not only been made due to advances in

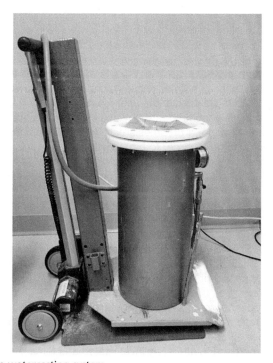

Fig. 3. Symphonie watercasting system.

materials, but also because of an increased emphasis on patient comfort while wearing their device. Transtibial socket designs have by in large stayed the same over the years, utilizing a patella tendon bearing bar to aid in offloading the distal end of the limb. The most common variation is capturing the patella and the medial tibial flare while ignoring the patella tendon, which will spare the patella tendon from damage due to prolonged excessive pressure.

In contrast, transfemoral sockets have gone through various iterations over the years. Beginning in the 1950s, the quadrilateral socket or quad socket was the gold standard due to ease of fitting. In this design, the patient's ischium sits on top of the posterior wall to aid in offloading the distal end of the limb. Currently, the quad-socket design is rarely used due to socket-based gait deviations.

From the late 1970s and early 1980s on, the most prevalent socket design has been ischial containment, where the socket encapsulates the ischium. By controlling the ischium, the socket is less likely to rotate during ambulation, while also offloading the distal end. A downside of this design is that it can cause discomfort while sitting.

To improve socket comfort and increase hip ROM, sub-ischial socket designs are increasing in popularity.[32] The benefit of this socket design is that increased ROM not only improves sitting comfort but also makes it easier for the user to toilet or maneuver into and out of a car.[32-34] Sub-ischial sockets utilize passive suction suspension and circumferential pressure around the limb to prevent individualized pressure points.[32-34] However, due to the decrease in pelvic control with this design, increased muscular strength and pelvic stability are necessary to control the prosthesis. Because of this, it tends to be more appropriate for higher level ambulators due to their strength.

Adjustable sockets

Prosthetic sockets are often identified as the most problematic component of a prosthesis, despite being custom molded and fabricated. The volume of the residual limb can change from day to day and within the same day due to many factors. In addition, long-term residual limb changes such as muscle atrophy mean that the fit of rigid sockets will inevitably alter overtime, necessitating socket replacements.[35] Within the socket of a lower limb prosthesis, the user often experiences a decrease in limb volume that traditionally is accommodated by use of socks or pads. Without accommodations for volume change, a prosthesis can become uncomfortable and cause skin problems, which can be a barrier to prosthetic use.

To address the challenge of limb volume change and socket fit in lower limb prostheses, many adjustable socket designs have become available (**Fig. 4**). Designs available to users range from custom fit, prefabricated adjustable sockets with buckles and straps to adjustable dials and spectra cables integrated into 3 dimensional printed or traditionally laminated sockets. Prefabricated adjustable sockets allow quick, early prosthetic fitting after amputation and can more easily address rapid limb volume and shape change. They may be of particular benefit in low resource settings.[36] Custom adjustable designs, such as the Martin Bionics Socket-less Socket, allow users to fine-tune the socket fit, may offer improved ROM, and have received positive feedback from users.

While there are positive reports with the use of adjustable sockets, many lack appropriate safety features to limit over or under tightening, which may present a risk of tissue damage or inadequate suspension. In addition, the relationships between design and comfort or function are rarely investigated and remain a significant gap in the literature.[36]

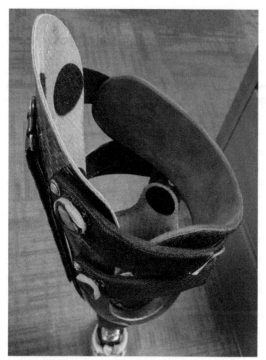

Fig. 4. Adjustable transfemoral socket with Boa system.

Liners

Prosthetic liners are designed to be an interface between the residual limb and the socket, which protects the limb from skin irritation and provides some shock absorption during ambulation. Liner materials such as silicone and thermoplastic elastomer gel have predominately stayed the same for the last 10+ years. A common complaint among prosthetic wearers is overheating and sweating of their residual limb, which can lead to skin irritation or loss of suspension. To combat this, the Alpha SmartTemp Gel Liner by WillowWood was developed, featuring heat absorption technology. Research participants in a study by Wernke demonstrated that perspiration and temperature were significantly reduced pre-exercise and post-exercise by those who used this liner.[37]

Suspension Systems

Traditional prosthetic distal locking suspension systems are pin lock and lanyard. A newer suspension mechanism, Maglock 2.0, uses a strong magnet on the distal end of the socket that is attracted to the base of the liner which is infused with metal.[38,39] This is a great option for patients who struggle with lining their pin into the lock or those who do not have the dexterity for a hand-driven system such as a lanyard. This design is more forgiving, still locking in place when up to 10° off center.[38]

Prosthetic Componentry

Hydraulic ankles

Traditional dynamic response feet use mechanical elements, such as carbon fiber, to store and release energy during walking. This energy return helps in propelling the user forward, contributing to a more efficient and less fatiguing gait. These feet can incorporate additional elements that absorb shock, rotation, and allow multiaxial motion. Unfortunately, they typically fail to replicate the full ROM of the anatomic ankle joint, instead providing a fixed foot/ankle position that can only be affected by compression or deflection of the material.

Prosthetic feet with hydraulic ankle motion use fluid to control the movement and resistance of a mechanical ankle joint through gait. The amount of resistance the fluid provides, along with the desired end ROM, can be adjusted to suit the needs of the user.

Studies have shown that hydraulic ankles

- Mimic natural ankle joint motion[40]
- Adapt to changes in terrain[40] and slopes
- Provide shock absorption[40]
- Reduce forces on the residual limb contributing to increased comfort[41]
- Increase toe clearance in swing phase
- Enhance stability[42]
- Reduce the risk of falls[42]
- Ease transition from sit to stand

Though studies have shown several positive outcomes, it has also been shown that lower functioning participants walked with lower prosthetic energy efficiency with a hydraulic ankle than with a flexible keel foot.[42]

Powered componentry

As technology advances, so does prosthetic componentry. Microprocessor-regulated prosthetic componentry is predominately employed in prosthetic feet and knees. The microprocessor and gyroscope work together to determine which phase of gait the user is in. Subsequently, the microprocessor regulates the flow of hydraulic fluid controlling the level of resistance provided.[43] Microprocessors are traditionally reserved for unlimited community ambulators due to the amount of muscular strength and control required to fully benefit from them.

Most microprocessor components are passive and have no propulsion; however, powered propulsion is also rising to prominence. Powered technology has always lived on the fringes of the prosthetic field due to its cost, battery life, and weight. By facilitating navigation of stairs more effectively and helping to decrease energy expenditure over level ground, powered devices decrease fatigue compared to passive prosthetic devices.[44,45] Furthermore, studies have also found that there is a significant increase in walking speed and decrease in knee and back pain.[46,47]

Microprocessor-controlled ankles

Microprocessor-controlled ankles offer the same benefits of hydraulic ankles with the addition of electronic force and position sensors that continuously monitor movement. Some offer powered ankle position and propulsion. Evidence shows that microprocessor-controlled ankles reduce energy expenditure of users, improve swing clearance, and reduce risk of falls compared to hydraulic ankles and dynamic response feet.[44,45,47]

A consideration when selecting these components is their durability and need to be charged daily for proper function. High-activity users may find that the products require excessive maintenance and may not provide adequate energy return.

Crossover feet

One prosthetic foot is not optimal for all activities, especially when comparing walking to running. In response to this, manufacturers have developed activity-specific feet. The problem with using specialized prosthetic feet is that they require a user to have multiple prosthetic devices, use quick disconnect devices to alternate feet, or adjust prosthetic alignment without the assistance of a prosthetist. This can be challenging for a person with lower limb loss.

Crossover dynamic response feet have been developed to meet most of the daily needs of active users with 1 prosthesis. The Ossur Cheetah Xplore was the first to combine the dynamics of a running blade with the stance dynamics of a walking foot by adding a carbon heel (**Fig. 5**). It must be bonded directly to the socket without adjustable components. The Fillauer AllPro was designed to provide the dynamics of the Cheetah Xplore with the simplicity of attachment to a socket with endoskeletal components.

There is limited but promising research that shows benefits of crossover feet over energy-storing feet. Crossover feet offer increased prosthetic ankle ROM and energy return and are preferred by users for a variety of higher level activities, such as running and playing sports.[48] In a pilot study, participants exhibited, on average, better mobility at comfortable and fast speeds, improved endurance, reduced perceived exertion, increased speed, faster cadence, and longer sound side steps while wearing a crossover foot compared to an energy-storing foot.[49]

Gait Analysis

Equally important as a well-fitting prosthesis with the appropriate componentry is the alignment of the prosthesis. Prosthetic alignment provides the patient with increased

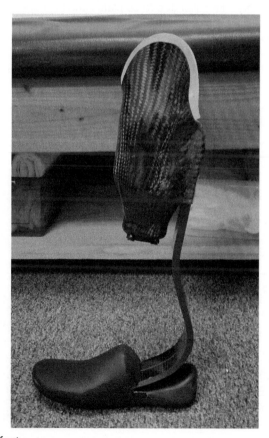

Fig. 5. Crossover foot.

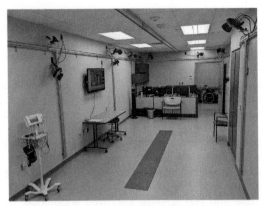

Fig. 6. Motion analysis laboratory at Minneapolis Veterans Affairs Health Care System.

stability and safety while ambulating. This is performed by aligning the foot, pylon, and socket to provide a smooth and energy-efficient gait. Traditionally, prosthetists evaluate gait with their trained eye and adjust alignment based on their observations and patient feedback. A novel way to perform gait analysis is by utilizing a motion analysis laboratory. A laboratory with calibrated force plates and high-speed cameras can be used to perform real-time assessments (**Fig. 6**). By recording the patient walking, the patient does not have to walk as much and the clinician can utilize the ground reaction forces from force plates to check alignment more accurately (**Fig. 7**).[50] Kinematic reports can also be generated to quantify the patient's gait by providing step length, step

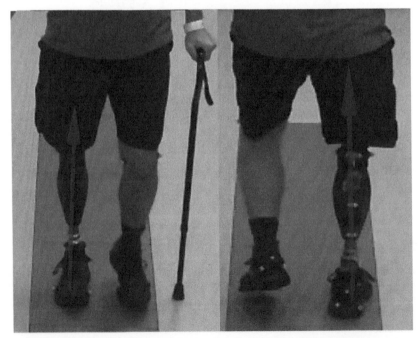

Fig. 7. Gait analysis performed using motion capture system and force plates.

time, and step width, which is not easily obtained. Performing prosthetic alignment in a motion laboratory not only aids in educating clinicians and patients about gait but assists with critical clinical thinking.[50] This technology is not available widely due to cost and training but is a viable option in larger hospital systems that have a motion analysis laboratory.

SUMMARY

Amputation rehabilitation and prosthetic design have been continually evolving over the course of history.

Modern innovations include

- New casting techniques to facilitate early prosthetic fitting
- New socket designs to increase comfort and adjustability
- Powered prosthetic technology
- Osseointegration
- Motor and sensory reinnervation

These innovations seek to address challenges with prosthetic use and to improve the experience, function, and quality of life of the user. There are pros and cons compared to existing options. The best options for a specific patient are determined by their condition, goals, and environment.

CLINICS CARE POINTS

- When determining prosthetic prescription, socket design, and componentry selection are key factors that ultimately affect prosthetic acceptance.

- Comfort of a prosthetic device sometimes outweighs functionality.

- There are benefits and drawbacks to new socket designs and advanced componentry. Selection should be based on the patient's condition, goals, and environment.

- Patient selection is crucial with regard to osseointegration because the outcome depends on a wide range of patient factors from the medical to the psychosocial. For the appropriate patient, it can be hugely beneficial in improving their prosthetic mobility and quality of life.

- TMR can be considered for prosthetic control in proximal upper extremity amputations. TMR or TNI can be considered to improve postamputation neuroma pain in upper or lower extremity amputations.

DISCLOSURE

The contents of this article and opinions expressed do not represent the views of the Department of Veterans Affairs or United States Government. The authors have no relevant financial relationships.

REFERENCES

1. Prosthetics Through the ages, *NIH Medlin Mag*, 18 (2), 2023, 20–22. Available at: https://magazine.medlineplus.gov/pdf/Prosthetics_Through_Ages.pdf_.final_.042823.pdf.
2. Krajbich JI, Pinzur MS, Potter BK, et al. Atlas of amputations and limb deficiencies: surgical, prosthetic, and rehabilitation principles. Rosemont, IL: Lippincott Williams & Wilkins; 2023.

3. Hagberg K, Brånemark R, Gunterberg B, et al. Osseointegrated trans-femoral amputation prostheses: Prospective results of general and condition-specific quality of life in 18 patients at 2-year follow-up. Prosthet Orthot Int 2008;32(1): 29–41.

4. Hoaglund FT, Jergesen HE, Wilson L, et al. Evaluation of problems and needs of veteran lower-limb amputees in the San Francisco Bay Area during the period 1977-1980. J Rehabil RD 1983;20(1):57–71.

5. Zaid MB, O'Donnell RJ, Potter BK, et al. Orthopaedic osseointegration: state of the art. J Am Acad Orthop Surg 2019;27(22):e977–85.

6. Hebert JS, Rehani M, Stiegelmar R. Osseointegration for lower-limb amputation: a systematic review of clinical outcomes. JBJS Rev 2017;5(10):e10.

7. Sinclair S, Beck JP, Webster J, et al. The First FDA approved early feasibility study of a novel percutaneous bone anchored prosthesis for transfemoral amputees: a prospective 1-year follow-up cohort study. Arch Phys Med Rehabil 2022; 103(11):2092–104.

8. Li Y, Felländer-Tsai L. The bone anchored prostheses for amputees – Historical development, current status, and future aspects. Biomaterials 2021;273:120836.

9. Van De Meent H, Hopman MT, Frölke JP. Walking ability and quality of life in subjects with transfemoral amputation: a comparison of osseointegration with socket prostheses. Arch Phys Med Rehabil 2013;94(11):2174–8.

10. Biddiss EA, Chau TT. Upper limb prosthesis use and abandonment: A survey of the last 25 years. Prosthet Orthot Int 2007;31(3):236–57.

11. Judy J. DARPA RE-NET Government Oversight Program Review. Arlington, VA: Defense Advanced Research Projects Agency; 2013.

12. Dumanian GA, Potter BK, Mioton LM, et al. Targeted muscle reinnervation treats neuroma and phantom pain in major limb amputees: a randomized clinical trial. Ann Surg 2019;270(2):238–46.

13. Souza JM, Cheesborough JE, Ko JH, et al. Targeted muscle reinnervation: a novel approach to postamputation neuroma pain. Clin Orthop 2014;472(10):2984–90.

14. Pet MA, Ko JH, Friedly JL, et al. Does targeted nerve implantation reduce neuroma pain in amputees? Clin Orthop 2014;472(10):2991–3001.

15. Kubiak CA, Kemp SWP, Cederna PS, et al. Prophylactic regenerative peripheral nerve interfaces to prevent postamputation pain. Plast Reconstr Surg 2019; 144(3):421e–30e.

16. Hijjawi JB, Kuiken TA, Lipschutz RD, et al. Improved myoelectric prosthesis control accomplished using multiple nerve transfers. Plast Reconstr Surg 2006; 118(7):1573–8.

17. O'Shaughnessy KD, Dumanian GA, Lipschutz RD, et al. Targeted reinnervation to improve prosthesis control in transhumeral amputees: a report of three cases. J Bone Jt Surg 2008;90(2):393–400.

18. Hebert JS, Elzinga K, Chan KM, et al. Updates in targeted sensory reinnervation for upper limb amputation. Curr Surg Rep 2014;2(3):45.

19. Hebert JS, Olson JL, Morhart MJ, et al. Novel targeted sensory reinnervation technique to restore functional hand sensation after transhumeral amputation. IEEE Trans Neural Syst Rehabil Eng 2014;22(4):765–73.

20. Nghiem BT, Sando IC, Gillespie RB, et al. Providing a sense of touch to prosthetic hands. Plast Reconstr Surg 2015;135(6):1652–63.

21. Woo SL, Kung TA, Brown DL, et al. Regenerative peripheral nerve interfaces for the treatment of postamputation neuroma pain: a pilot study. Plast Reconstr Surg - Glob Open 2016;4(12):e1038.

22. Lawera N, Vu P, Irwin Z, et al. Abstract 22: real-time dextrous fine motor control of an advanced prosthetic arm using regenerative peripheral nerve signals. Plast Reconstr Surg - Glob Open 2019;7(4S):16–7.

23. Vu PP, Lu CW, Vaskov AK, et al. Restoration of proprioceptive and cutaneous sensation using regenerative peripheral nerve interfaces in humans with upper limb amputations. Plast Reconstr Surg 2022;149(6):1149e–54e.

24. Walker J, Marable WR, Smith C, et al. Clinical outcome of transfemoral direct socket interface (PART 2). Can Prosthet Orthot J 2021;4(1).

25. Marable WR, Smith C, Bþ Sigurjónsson, et al. Transfemoral socket fabrication method using direct casting: outcomes regarding patient satisfaction with device and services. Can Prosthet Orthot J 2020;3(2):34672.

26. Barbareschi G, Teerlink W, Njuguna JG, et al. Evaluating the use of a thermoplastic socket in Kenya: A pilot study. Prosthet Orthot Int 2022;46(5):532–7.

27. Coughlin SS, Clary C, Johnson JA, et al. Continuing challenges in rural health in the United States. J Environ Health Sci 2019;5(2):90–2.

28. Cutti A, Osti G, Migliore G, et al. Clinical effectiveness of a novel hydrostatic casting method for transfemoral amputees: results from the first 64 patients. O&P News 2018.

29. Denune J., Comparative observational study – blind test hydrostatic casting vs. other residual limb impression methods. Symphonie Aqua Line, Available at: https://www.cypressadaptive.com/_files/ugd/31187c_a466bc5915474eb1b63eb581a 3c63525.pdf?index=true. (Accessed 18 December 2023).

30. Cutti AG, Fatone S. Technique to assess shape captured by two casting approaches. Guadalajara, Mexico: Presented at: International Society for prosthetics and orthotics World Congress; 2023.

31. Fatone S, Cutti AG. Effect of casting approach on initial comfort: interim results of clinical trial. Guadalajara, Mexico: Presented at: Effect of Casting Approach on Initial Comfort: Interim Results of Clinical Trial; 2023.

32. Fatone S, Caldwell R, Angelico J, et al. Comparison of Ischial Containment and Subischial Sockets on Comfort, Function, Quality of Life, and Satisfaction With Device in Persons With Unilateral Transfemoral Amputation: a Randomized Crossover Trial. Arch Phys Med Rehabil 2021;102(11):2063–73.e2.

33. Fatone S, Stine R, Caldwell R, et al. Comparison of Ischial Containment and Subischial Sockets Effect on Gait Biomechanics in People With Transfemoral Amputation: a Randomized Crossover Trial. Arch Phys Med Rehabil 2022;103(8): 1515–23.

34. Fatone S, Caldwell R, Major M, et al. Sub-Ischial Prosthetic Sockets Improve Hip Range of Motion and Performance for Individuals with Transfemoral Amputations. 2015. Available at: https://www.semanticscholar.org/paper/Sub-Ischial-Prosthetic-Sockets-Improve-Hip-Range-of-Fatone-Caldwell/730af1c1d7cf91e8ef66a40f7f3af 369939c845f. [Accessed 18 December 2023].

35. Sanders JE, Fatone S. Residual limb volume change: Systematic review of measurement and management. J Rehabil Res Dev 2011;48(8):949.

36. Baldock M, Pickard N, Prince M, et al. Adjustable prosthetic sockets: a systematic review of industrial and research design characteristics and their justifications. J NeuroEng Rehabil 2023;20(1):147.

37. Wernke MM, Schroeder RM, Kelley CT, et al. SmartTemp prosthetic liner significantly reduces residual limb temperature and perspiration. JPO J Prosthetics Orthot 2015;27(4):134–9.

38. MAGLOCK 2.0 & MAGLOCK 2.0 PLUS | Akder Medikal. 2020. Available at: https://www.akdermedikal.com/product/maglock-2-0-maglock-2-0-plus/. [Accessed 18 December 2023].

39. Magnetic Suspension with MAGLOCK 2.0 - OPEDGE.COM. Available at: https://progress.oandp.com/ShowcaseProducts/NEWS_2017-03-01_05/NEWS_2017-03-01_05. [Accessed 19 December 2023].

40. Ernst M, Altenburg B, Schmalz T, et al. Benefits of a microprocessor-controlled prosthetic foot for ascending and descending slopes. J NeuroEng Rehabil 2022; 19(1):9.

41. Portnoy S, Kristal A, Gefen A, et al. Outdoor dynamic subject-specific evaluation of internal stresses in the residual limb: Hydraulic energy-stored prosthetic foot compared to conventional energy-stored prosthetic feet. Gait Posture 2012; 35(1):121–5.

42. Chang SR, Miller CH, Kaluf B. Effects of hydraulic ankle-foot prostheses on gait in individuals with transtibial limb loss: a scoping review. JPO J Prosthetics Orthot 2021;33(2):101–9.

43. Kaluf B, Cox C, Shoemaker E. Hydraulic- and microprocessor-controlled ankle-foot prostheses for limited community ambulators with unilateral transtibial amputation: pilot study. JPO J Prosthetics Orthot 2021;33(4):294–303.

44. Au SK, Weber J, Herr H. Powered ankle–foot prosthesis improves walking metabolic economy. IEEE Trans Robot 2009;25(1):51–66.

45. Russell Esposito E, Aldridge Whitehead JM, Wilken JM. Step-to-step transition work during level and inclined walking using passive and powered ankle–foot prostheses. Prosthet Orthot Int 2016;40(3):311–9.

46. Cacciola CE, Kannenberg A, Hibler KD, et al. Impact of a powered prosthetic ankle-foot component on musculoskeletal pain in individuals with transtibial amputation: a real-world cross-sectional study with concurrent and recalled pain and functional ratings. JPO J Prosthetics Orthot 2022. https://doi.org/10.1097/JPO.0000000000000442.

47. Ferris AE, Aldridge JM, Rábago CA, et al. Evaluation of a powered ankle-foot prosthetic system during walking. Arch Phys Med Rehabil 2012;93(11):1911–8.

48. Slater C, Hafner BJ, Morgan SJ. Effects of high-profile crossover feet on gait biomechanics in 2 individuals with Syme amputation. Prosthet Orthot Int 2023. https://doi.org/10.1097/PXR.0000000000000295.

49. Hafner BJ, Halsne EG, Morgan SJ, et al. Functional outcomes in people with transtibial amputation using crossover and energy-storing prosthetic feet: a pilot study. JPO J Prosthetics Orthot 2018;30(2):90–100.

50. Talaty M, Esquenazi A. Determination of dynamic prosthetic alignment using forceline visualization. JPO J Prosthetics Orthot 2013;25(1):15–21.

Approaches to Prosthetic Limb Restoration in Resource-Limited Settings/ Countries: 3 Dimensional Printing

Stephanie Rand, DO[a],*, Tushara Surapaneni, MD[b],
Matthew N.M. Bartels, MD, MPH[a], Andrew Gitkind, MD[a]

KEYWORDS

- Amputees • Prosthetics • Developing countries • Resource-limited health care
- 3 dimensional printing

KEY POINTS

- The World Health Organization estimates that while 10% of the worldwide population has a disability, 80% of these individuals live in developing countries with limited access to health care and rehabilitation services, and only 5% to 15% of the world population has access to the assistive products that they need.
- Three dimensional (3D) printing can be used for "point of care manufacturing," a system of producing items when the need arises.
- 3D-printed prostheses can be designed specifically for use in resource-poor settings, including developing countries, to minimize the cost of consumable parts while optimizing durability in harsh environmental conditions.

INTRODUCTION

Much of the burden of living with a disability is concentrated among those populations least financially able to bear the burden. The World Health Organization (WHO) estimates that while 10% of the worldwide population has a disability, 80% of these individuals live in developing countries with limited access to health care and rehabilitation services.[1–3] According to the 2017 WHO standards for prosthetics and orthotics, only 5% to 15% of the world population has access to the assistive products that they need. This is caused, in part, by the significant cost associated with manufacturing and repairing traditional prosthetic and orthotic devices.[4] Leveraging decreasing

[a] Department of Rehabilitation Medicine, Montefiore Medical Center, Albert Einstein College of Medicine, 111 East 210th Street, Bronx, NY 10467, USA; [b] Department of Emergency Medicine, Eden Medical Center, 20103 Lake Chabot Road, Castro Valley, CA 94546, USA
* Corresponding author.
E-mail address: srand@montefiore.org

Phys Med Rehabil Clin N Am 35 (2024) 897–904
https://doi.org/10.1016/j.pmr.2024.06.009
pmr.theclinics.com

costs and increasing availability of high-tech solutions such as 3 dimensional (3D) printing and scanning provides an opportunity to introduce advanced medical technologies in resource-limited environments[5] consistent with the WHO model of community-based rehabilitation model.[3]

The advantages of 3D printing are heralded in academia, in popular media, and by leaders of technology, business, engineering, politics, and medicine. Compared to traditional manufacturing, 3D printing allows for creative freedom, point-of-care production, patient-matching, and limited waste.[6] In some circles, 3D printing has become so popular that many postulate that it will usher in the end of assembly lines producing spare parts.[7] As the price of 3D printing decreases, individual access to this technology increases. In a world that is more digitally connected than ever, there are several digital repositories of open-source designs that are free to download. These online resources allow hobbyists to industry experts the opportunity to share, adapt, and troubleshoot designs.

The ability to create complex shapes and rapidly test prototypes with 3D prints lends itself to many applications in medicine.[8] Common medical applications of 3D printing are diverse; these include printed clinical and surgical tools, medical equipment and devices (including but not limited to prostheses/orthoses), and anatomic models for education or surgical planning.[9] Despite increasing opportunities to explore medical applications of 3D printing in developing countries, there is less literature on these applications.[10] We will explore the use of this increasingly common technology as a viable solution to meet the unique needs of low-resource settings. In addition, the authors will recount our introduction of 3D printing to an underserved community in a rehabilitation hospital in Kingston, Jamaica, and our ongoing collaboration with their medical teams.

Challenges Faced by Resource-Limited Health Care Settings

In this article, "resource-limited" or "low-resource" is used to describe a health care setting with low funds, limited supply of medical devices, technology, medicines, difficulty maintaining or replacing equipment, inconsistent infrastructure (Internet connectivity, electricity, and temperature and humidity controls), human resource shortages, and/or other challenges. Although expensive equipment is often donated to developing countries, this can end up being inefficient and wasteful for a variety of reasons. Frequently, there is a lack of spare parts for older medical equipment that is donated to hospitals in low-resource settings, rendering up to 75% of these devices unusable. In addition, because many low-resource facilities are located in areas with harsh climates, certain equipment cannot withstand the environmental challenges. Technology that is designed specifically for use in resource-poor settings minimizes the cost of consumable parts while optimizing durability in harsh environmental conditions. Recognizing the unique limitations of low-resource health care settings, several nongovernmental organizations, private companies, and academic institutions are working to create sustainable, low-cost medical equipment and diagnostic tests.[11]

Barriers to disseminating newly designed technology include design, production, and distribution.

Design
All new devices must meet the standard of care.

Production
To scale production for use in another country, researchers either contract formally with a manufacturer or use informal (local) manufacturing channels.

Distribution

Regardless of whether the device is sold or donated, financing to support the project is required, including but not limited to shipping fees and import taxes. Financial support may be secured through international donations, direct sales, or via local distributors.

Distribution of such novel medical devices in a developing country typically uses 1 of 3 channels: the public or government sector, private or corporate sector, and/or the nongovernmental organization (NGO) sector. If done through government channels, stringent bureaucratic regulations on procurement, testing, and safety can cause delays of months to years until novel technology is accessible to the public. Conversely, private health care companies with greater resources and funds can sooner offer novel technologies at the expense of higher fees. Because many patients cannot afford private sector fees, NGOs and faith-based organizations provide a large bulk of health services in developing countries. Researchers often partner with NGOs to gain governmental connections, thereby gaining more efficiency and flexibility than the public sector can provide.[12]

3D Printing: Background and Overview

The initial research on 3D printing for medical applications fell under 1 of 4 categories: (1) printing of organ/body part models for medical education or perioperative planning; (2) printing customized nonbioactive implants, most commonly used in dentistry and orthopedics; (3) creating bioactive "scaffolds" upon which cells can adhere and proliferate; and (4) printing bioactive tissues and organs.[13] As the integration of this technology evolves, more attention has been paid to the use of 3D printing for bracing, as well as prosthetic sockets and limbs (**Fig. 1**).[14–16]

Materials

3D printers fashion prints from a computer-aided design (CAD) drawing. The CAD drawing is digitally "sliced" into hundreds of individual layers. There are a variety of different 3D printers, and each type is best suited for different applications. Methods of 3D printing include material extrusion, material jetting, binding jetting, power bed fusion, directed energy deposition, sheet lamination, and vat photopolymerization. Depending on the type of machine, prints can be fashioned from plastics, metals, ceramics, or bioactive materials.

The majority of our 3D-printing efforts utilizes extrusion-based printing, also known as fused deposition modeling (FDM). In FDM, a nozzle heats and deposits semimelted filament onto the build plate one layer at a time. Each layer cools and hardens in seconds just as another layer is deposited over it, until the print is complete. Such printers can produce complex, accurate shapes within hours. Another benefit to extrusion-based printers is that they are less expensive compared to other printer types such as powder-based, droplet-based, and vat photopolymerization printers.[8,17] Printers that utilize FDM can handle polymer materials such as polylactic acid (PLA), acrylonitrile butadiene styrene, polyethylene, or polypropylene. Polymers vary in hardness and melting point, but, in general, they are among the most affordable, lightweight, and adaptable options for medical devices such as prosthetic limbs.[7]

3D printing is a prime example of "point of care manufacturing," a system of producing items when the need arises. In traditional manufacturing, the design, production, and shipment of a product are decentralized. The design–build–test cycle of product development is all done on-location, and so 3D printing closes the distance between supply and demand. Prototype iterations can be rapidly tested, redesigned, and reprinted at one facility. Greater complexity and customization are both achievable at no extra cost. Fulfilling the demand for a product locally decreases the reliance

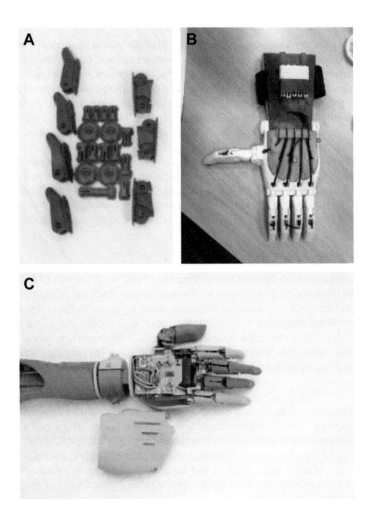

Fig. 1. (*A*) 3D-printed prosthetic fingers, unassembled, with rafts still attached. (*B*) 3D-printed body-power prosthetic hand. (*C*) 3D-printed myoelectric transradial prosthesis.

on complex international supply chains, which saves both time and money.[18] Moreover, when using 3D printing as a supply option, consumables such as dental crowns, finger splints, or surgical instruments can be printed on an as-needed basis and replenished easily, quickly, and affordably so long as printing filament is available. Beyond the cost-effectiveness of low-volume production, 3D printing also saves space. Traditional bulk production methods entail keeping an inventory of equipment, which requires storage. Perishable items that require climate-controlled rooms pose an even greater challenge. On-demand 3D printing of medical devices, consumables, or small parts involves less inventory upkeep, thereby decreasing the burden on facilities where space is a premium. When medical devices are personalized to the anatomy of the patient, waste is minimized.

Despite its many advantages, 3D printing is not without its limitations. The cost of a commercially available printer can be prohibitive in many parts of the world. Another barrier is the technical expertise required to design prints using CAD software.

Although the field is growing, there may still be a scarcity of experts in developing countries who can design, manufacture, and troubleshoot 3D prints on-site. One study investigating the use of 3D printing in Brazil found that initial community excitement about 3D printers was quickly tempered after the steep learning curve of using CAD for design was realized.[14] Although large repositories of open-source designs are available for free online, for local manufacturers to customize objects, they will need someone experienced with CAD. Another challenge is printing large objects. Many printers, particularly those that are low to midrange in price, can only print smaller sized objects. Larger prints need to be digitally "sliced" into different components and then joined together. For child-sized 3D-printed prosthetics, this is less of an issue. However, the same prosthetic design scaled for an adult patient would require longer print time and multiple separate prints to be joined together. When larger sized products are made by joining multiple small size prints, there is an increased likelihood of product failure in the future.

3D printing in a box: a program to establish 3D printing at Sir John Golding Rehabilitation Centre in Kingston, Jamaica.

Jamaica is a country with a population of almost 2.95 million.[19] According to the most recent data from the World Bank,[20] Jamaica's health care expenditure per capita was US$327.49 in 2019. This number is striking when compared to the US$10,921.01 per capita spent by the United States in 2010. The average health care expenditure of all countries in the "Caribbean small states" region was US$621.24 per capita in 2018. Notably, Jamaica's health care expenditure per capita was the third lowest in the region. Although Jamaica is an "upper-middle income country" by World Bank measures, there is a clear incongruence between Jamaica's wealth and the proportion allocated to health care.

Through a variety of partnerships, the Department of Physical Medicine and Rehabilitation at Montefiore Medical Center (MMC) in the Bronx, NY, piloted a 3D printing program at Sir John Golding Rehabilitation Centre in Kingston, Jamaica. The program aims to empower rehabilitation colleagues working in a resource-limited setting to produce cost-effective medical devices. Beginning in 2016, attending faculty, fellows, residents, and interdisciplinary staff from the Department of Rehabilitation Medicine at Montefiore traveled semiannually to the Sir John Golding Rehabilitation Center (Golding) until the onset of the coronavirus disease 2019 pandemic in early 2020, restarting in July 2023. This facility serves thousands of Jamaicans annually while relying on limited resources. At Golding, our providers worked in both inpatient and outpatient settings to participate in patient care and assess needs and opportunities to implement 3D printing. During rounds at Golding, Montefiore staff identified candidates for 3D-printed splints, prosthetic fingers, and other small medical devices. One frequently identified area of need was in the field of prosthetic limbs. Many patients have partial or complete amputations, particularly of the upper extremity. While the hospital does have access to a traditional local prosthetics and orthotics laboratory, this facility is overburdened by excessive demand and limited insurance coverage for devices. In addition, materials to create traditional splints and braces are often difficult to source. Recognizing the time and cost-saving value of 3D printing, Golding staff were enthusiastic about adopting the technology.

In April 2018, faculty from MMC brought a computer with CAD software and a Universal Serial Bus (USB) thumb drive with ready-to-print files to Jamaica. A Montefiore research fellow trained a small group of locally engaged staff from Golding how to design 3D models using the software. Three months later, MMC Department of Rehabilitation Medicine donated and personally transported a MakerBot (MakerBot Industries LLC, NY) Replicator fifth-generation printer, and spools of compatible filament to Golding. The

MakerBot utilizes FDM for its prints, as discussed previously. Almost immediately after its arrival at the hospital, the printer was set up for use. Within 4 hours of being unpacked, the first 3D print was successfully created by Golding rehabilitation staff on-site.

Future Goals

For hospitals in resource-limited countries to be self-sufficient in 3D printing, there must exist equipment maintenance to fulfill the needs of their patient population. The costliest expense is a replacement extruder head as it wears down. The MakerBot Smart Extruder+ is currently priced at approximately $200. The cost of PLA filament ranges from $25–$50 per kilogram, depending on the company. If the filament is bought in the United States, shipping fees are another important consideration. Institutions can consider charging a fee to recipients of 3D prints to help cover expenses.

Limitations

A study of outcomes of 3D-printed upper extremity prostheses for children in Nepal showed that while all 76 children participating could lift small objects, including bottles of water, with e-NABLE community 3D-printed prosthetic hands, only 61.8% were completely satisfied. Although only a few participants could lift heavier objects with the devices, the main source of dissatisfaction revolved around durability of the device.[21]

SUMMARY

3D printing can produce cost-effective medical devices in resource-limited settings while minimizing waste and storage requirements. By manufacturing medical devices and consumables on-site, the logistical and environmental burden associated with worldwide shipment of parts is minimized. As the price of printers and materials continues to become more affordable, the power to design and execute novel medical devices is increasingly democratized. Although there are limitations to the current technology, 3D printing can be a viable solution for many health care settings. Transnational collaboration like the MMC and Sir John Golding Rehabilitation Centre project can serve as a model for developed countries to make 3D printing possible in low-resource settings worldwide.

CLINICS CARE POINTS

> - As healthcare inequities have been increasing internationally, we can and should leverage technological advances to maximize access in resource-limited areas.
> - Costs advantages of 3D printing highlighted in this article are noted after one-time start up costs, generally ranging from $5,000–$10,000. Much of this cost was offset and/or donated by private companies and donors. Pursuing such collaborations allows for strengthened opportunities in resource-limited health systems both locally and internationally.
> - Tutorials for learning 3D printing and CAD software are available open-source for clinicians interested in learning, but are not required as many opportunities exist for collaborative efforts.

ACKNOWLEDGMENTS

No grants were received for this research.Special thanks to Makerbot, The Everest Foundation and Albert Einstein College of Medicine for their support of our 3D prinitng and international medical work.

DISCLOSURE

None.

REFERENCES

1. Elde A, Øderud T, Disability & International Development. Towards inclusive global health. 1st edition. New York: Springer Science+Business Media; 2009. p. 149–60. Chapter 10. Assistive Technology in Low-Income Countries.
2. Borg J, Lindström A, Larsson S. Assistive technology in developing countries: a review from the perspective of the Convention on the Rights of Persons with Disabilities. Prosthet Orthot Int 2011;35(1):20–9.
3. World Health Organization. World report on disability. 1st edition. Geneva: WHO Press; 2009.
4. World Health Organization. WHO standards for prosthetics and orthotics. France: WHO Press; 2017.
5.. Silva K, Rand S, Cancel D, et al. Three-dimensional (3-D) printing: a cost-effective solution for improving global accessibility to rostheses. PM&R 2015;7(12): 1312–4.
6. US Food and Drug Administration. Discussion paper: 3d printing medical devices at the point of care. 2022. Available at: https://www.fda.gov/media/154729/download. [Accessed 18 February 2022].
7. Garrett B. 3D printing new economic paradigms and strategic shifts. Global Policy 2014;5(1):70–5.
8. Shahrubudin N, Lee T, Ramlan R. An Overview on 3D Printing Technology: Technological, Materials, and Applications. Procedia Manuf 2019;35:1286–96.
9. Liaw C-Y, Guvendiren M. Current and emerging applications of 3D printing in medicine. Biofabrication 2017;9(2):024102.
10. Dotz AD. A pilot of 3D printing of medical devices in Haiti. In: Hostettler S, Hazboun E, Bolay J-C, editors. Technologies for development. New York City: Springer International Publishing; 2015. p. 33–44.
11. Richards-Kortum R, Oden M. Devices for low-resource health care. Science 2013;342(6162):1055–7.
12. Malkin R, von Oldenburg Beer K. Diffusion of novel healthcare technologies to resource poor settings. Ann Biomed Eng 2013;41(9):1841–50.
13. Yan Q, Dong H, Su J, et al. A review of 3D printing technology for medical applications. Engineering 2018;4(5):729–42.
14. Choo YJ, Boudier-Revéret M, Chang MC. 3D printing technology applied to orthosis manufacturing: narrative review. Ann Palliat Med 2020;9(6):4262–70. Epub 2020 Sep 24. PMID: 33040564.
15. Olsen J, Day S, Dupan S, et al. 3D-Printing and Upper-Limb Prosthetic Sockets: Promises and Pitfalls. IEEE Trans Neural Syst Rehabil Eng 2021;29:527–35. Epub 2021 Mar 3. PMID: 33587701.
16. Ngan CGY, Kapsa RMI, Choong PFM. Strategies for neural control of prosthetic limbs: from electrode interfacing to 3D printing. Materials (Basel) 2019;12(12): 1927. PMID: 31207952; PMCID: PMC6631966.
17. Ibrahim AM, Jose RR, Rabie AN, et al. Three-dimensional printing in developing countries. Plastic and Reconstructive Surgery Global Open 2015;3(7).
18. Chan HN, Tan MJA, Wu H. Point-of-care testing: applications of 3D printing. Lab Chip 2017;17(16):2713–39.
19. The World Bank. Jamaica. 2022. Available at: https://data.worldbank.org/country/jamaica?view=chart. [Accessed 14 March 2022].

20. The World Bank. Current health expenditure per capita (current US$). 2022. Available at: https://data.worldbank.org/indicator/SH.XPD.CHEX.PC.CD. [Accessed 14 March 2022].
21. Shrestha S, Gautam S. Outcome of Three Dimensional Printed Functional Prostheses for Children with Upper Limb Deficiency in Nepal. Kathmandu Univ Med J (KUMJ) 2023;21(81):52–7. PMID: 37800426.

UNITED STATES POSTAL SERVICE®

Statement of Ownership, Management, and Circulation
(All Periodicals Publications Except Requester Publications)

1. Publication Title	2. Publication Number	3. Filing Date
PHYSICAL MEDICINE AND REHABILITATION CLINICS OF NORTH AMERICA	009 – 243	9/18/2024

4. Issue Frequency	5. Number of Issues Published Annually	6. Annual Subscription Price
FEB, MAY, AUG, NOV	4	$352.00

7. Complete Mailing Address of Known Office of Publication (Not printer) (Street, city, county, state, and ZIP+4®)

ELSEVIER INC.
230 Park Avenue, Suite 800
New York, NY 10169

Contact Person: Malathi Samayan
Telephone (Include area code): 91-44-4299-4507

8. Complete Mailing Address of Headquarters or General Business Office of Publisher (Not printer)

ELSEVIER INC.
230 Park Avenue, Suite 800
New York, NY 10169

9. Full Names and Complete Mailing Addresses of Publisher, Editor, and Managing Editor (Do not leave blank)

Publisher (Name and complete mailing address)

Dolores Meloni, ELSEVIER INC.
1600 JOHN F KENNEDY BLVD. SUITE 1600
PHILADELPHIA, PA 19103-2899

Editor (Name and complete mailing address)

MEGAN ASHDOWN, ELSEVIER INC.
1600 JOHN F KENNEDY BLVD. SUITE 1600
PHILADELPHIA, PA 19103-2899

Managing Editor (Name and complete mailing address)

PATRICK MANLEY, ELSEVIER INC.
1600 JOHN F KENNEDY BLVD. SUITE 1600
PHILADELPHIA, PA 19103-2899

10. Owner (Do not leave blank. If the publication is owned by a corporation, give the name and address of the corporation immediately followed by the names and addresses of all stockholders owning or holding 1 percent or more of the total amount of stock. If not owned by a corporation, give the names and addresses of the individual owners. If owned by a partnership or other unincorporated firm, give its name and address as well as those of each individual owner. If the publication is published by a nonprofit organization, give its name and address.)

Full Name	Complete Mailing Address
WHOLLY OWNED SUBSIDIARY OF REED/ELSEVIER, US HOLDINGS	1600 JOHN F KENNEDY BLVD. SUITE 1600 PHILADELPHIA, PA 19103-2899

11. Known Bondholders, Mortgagees, and Other Security Holders Owning or Holding 1 Percent or More of Total Amount of Bonds, Mortgages, or Other Securities. If none, check box. ► ☐ None

Full Name	Complete Mailing Address
N/A	

12. Tax Status (For completion by nonprofit organizations authorized to mail at nonprofit rates) (Check one)
The purpose, function, and nonprofit status of this organization and the exempt status for federal income tax purposes:
☒ Has Not Changed During Preceding 12 Months
☐ Has Changed During Preceding 12 Months (Publisher must submit explanation of change with this statement)

PS Form 3526, July 2014 [Page 1 of 4 (see instructions page 4)]   PSN: 7530-01-000-9931   PRIVACY NOTICE: See our privacy policy on www.usps.com.

---

13. Publication Title		14. Issue Date for Circulation Data Below
PHYSICAL MEDICINE AND REHABILITATION CLINICS OF NORTH AMERICA		AUGUST 2024

15. Extent and Nature of Circulation			Average No. Copies Each Issue During Preceding 12 Months	No. Copies of Single Issue Published Nearest to Filing Date
a. Total Number of Copies (Net press run)			122	119
b. Paid Circulation (By Mail and Outside the Mail)	(1)	Mailed Outside-County Paid Subscriptions Stated on PS Form 3541 (Include paid distribution above nominal rate, advertiser's proof copies, and exchange copies)	73	69
	(2)	Mailed In-County Paid Subscriptions Stated on PS Form 3541 (Include paid distribution above nominal rate, advertiser's proof copies, and exchange copies)	0	0
	(3)	Paid Distribution Outside the Mails Including Sales Through Dealers and Carriers, Street Vendors, Counter Sales, and Other Paid Distribution Outside USPS®	32	30
	(4)	Paid Distribution by Other Classes of Mail Through the USPS (e.g., First-Class Mail®)	14	17
c. Total Paid Distribution (Sum of 15b (1), (2), (3), and (4))			119	116
d. Free or Nominal Rate Distribution (By Mail and Outside the Mail)	(1)	Free or Nominal Rate Outside-County Copies included on PS Form 3541	3	3
	(2)	Free or Nominal Rate In-County Copies Included on PS Form 3541	0	0
	(3)	Free or Nominal Rate Copies Mailed at Other Classes Through the USPS (e.g., First-Class Mail)	0	0
	(4)	Free or Nominal Rate Distribution Outside the Mail (Carriers or other means)	0	0
e. Total Free or Nominal Rate Distribution (Sum of 15d (1), (2), (3) and (4))			3	3
f. Total Distribution (Sum of 15c and 15e)			122	119
g. Copies not Distributed (See Instructions to Publishers #4 (page #3))			0	0
h. Total (Sum of 15f and g)			122	119
i. Percent Paid (15c divided by 15f times 100)			97.74%	97.48%

* If you are claiming electronic copies, go to line 16 on page 3. If you are not claiming electronic copies, skip to line 17 on page 3.

PS Form 3526, July 2014 (Page 2 of 4)

16. Electronic Copy Circulation		Average No. Copies Each Issue During Preceding 12 Months	No. Copies of Single Issue Published Nearest to Filing Date
a. Paid Electronic Copies	►		
b. Total Paid Print Copies (Line 15c) + Paid Electronic Copies (Line 16a)	►		
c. Total Print Distribution (Line 15f) + Paid Electronic Copies (Line 16a)	►		
d. Percent Paid (Both Print & Electronic Copies) (16b divided by 16c × 100)	►		

☒ I certify that 50% of all my distributed copies (electronic and print) are paid above a nominal price.

17. Publication of Statement of Ownership
☒ If the publication is a general publication, publication of this statement is required. Will be printed in the NOVEMBER 2024 issue of this publication.   ☐ Publication not required.

18. Signature and Title of Editor, Publisher, Business Manager, or Owner

Malathi Samayan   *Malathi Samayan*   Date 9/18/2024

Malathi Samayan - Distribution Controller

I certify that all information furnished on this form is true and complete. I understand that anyone who furnishes false or misleading information on this form or who omits material or information requested on the form may be subject to criminal sanctions (including fines and imprisonment) and/or civil sanctions (including civil penalties).

PS Form 3526, July 2014 (Page 3 of 4)   PRIVACY NOTICE: See our privacy policy on www.usps.com.

Moving?

Make sure your subscription moves with you!

To notify us of your new address, find your **Clinics Account Number** (located on your mailing label above your name), and contact customer service at:

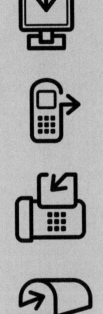

Email: journalscustomerservice-usa@elsevier.com

800-654-2452 (subscribers in the U.S. & Canada)
314-447-8871 (subscribers outside of the U.S. & Canada)

Fax number: 314-447-8029

Elsevier Health Sciences Division
Subscription Customer Service
3251 Riverport Lane
Maryland Heights, MO 63043

Printed and bound by CPI Group (UK) Ltd, Croydon, CR0 4YY

12/05/2025

01869433-0001